CANCER

THE
WAYWARD
CELL

PERSPECTIVES IN MEDICINE

Leo van der Reis, M.D., General Editor

The
Wayward
Cell

CANCER

Its
Origins,
Nature, and
Treatment
by
Victor
Richards,
M.D.

Second edition

UNIVERSITY OF CALIFORNIA PRESS
BERKELEY, LOS ANGELES, AND LONDON

University of California Press
Berkeley and Los Angeles
University of California Press, Ltd.
London, England
© 1978 by The Regents of the University of California
First edition published 1972

ISBN 0-520-03596-8
Library of Congress Catalog Card No. 77-88138
Printed in the United States of America
Designed by W. H. Snyder

EDITOR'S FOREWORD

During the last decade, general public interest in medicine has greatly increased. Today there is a real need for reliable and intelligible information about developments in the science and art of medicine. A wide gap exists between technical scientific papers in the journals and popular—and sometimes erroneous or misleading—accounts written for a mass audience.

This new series of books is intended for serious readers who wish to learn more about current medicine but who cannot and should not be expected to read textbooks or scientific journals intended for physicians and medical students. Our intention is to present the fundamentals of each subject in terminology that is understandable to the educated reader who is not trained in medicine. We hope, also, that the volumes will be useful to students in the biological sciences and to those whose work brings them into contact with medical issues: social workers, jurists, pharmacists, psychologists, and others. Perhaps, too, the practicing physician will find help in formulating answers to the questions of his patients, since a better understanding of diseases and of bodily functions can dispel fears and superstitions that sometimes delay or hamper treatment. If some of these purposes are served, the books will justify the effort expended by the authors.

Each book offers a concise, comprehensive, and illustrated essay on a major disease, or a body system and its fundamentally related parts, or a specialized area of research, or an aspect of our society that affects the public health. Historical and sociological factors have been included where appropriate.

LEO VAN DER REIS, M.D., *General Editor*

CONTENTS

PART FOUR—*Psycho-Social Problems*
           by DENISE SCOTT

PREFACE

The aim of this book is to present in clear and concise terms the main currents of biological knowledge which are essential to an understanding of the nature and treatment of cancer. I have attempted to combine scientific and humanistic approaches, thereby tempering the cold facts of science with personal concern for the patient and for the reader.

Dramatic advances in science during the past decade have revolutionized our understanding of the gene, the mechanisms of inheritance, and the processes of cellular growth and function. Clarification of the basic principles of cells has demonstrated a simple, comprehensible logic, which can be appreciated by all. With it the scientist hopes to solve the mysteries of cell differentiation, immunity, neurofunction, and malignant transformation. With it society hopes for intervention, prevention, and intelligent control of many of the more formidable diseases, chief of which is cancer. Real comprehension of any field of science involves the understanding of inherent limitations and hazards. In the field of cancer, the limitations and hazards dispel optimism for a quick, glamorous, and single cure, but our present understanding of normal and abnormal human biology offers promise in enlarging the scope and productivity of lives compromised by abnormal cell mechanisms.

My approach to the understanding of cancer is an outgrowth of two major groups of experience: first, observations of patients afflicted by cancer and members of their families, and second, explorations of the nature of cancer with many research scientists, medical practitioners and students, and through interchanges with lay audiences, who have usually been strongly motivated to learn more about the disease. I have observed many patients with cancer and have followed their treatment through all phases of the disease with every conceivable type of therapy available in our major medical centers. The perplexing questions that enter the minds of cancer patients and their families, the happiness of cures, the temporary joys of remissions, and the bitter agonies of failure have all been encountered. Numerous classes and lectures to general medical audiences and to community groups have permitted a systematic study of the questions about cancer that puzzle layman and scientist alike. These conferences have offered invaluable lessons in ways to elucidate and simplify basic scientific concepts. The questions to be answered have required a synthesis of knowledge from diverse disciplines, all of which bear on the nature of cancer. The book strives to answer, insofar as possible, the questions most often asked about cancer. It is divided into four major parts: (1) the biology of the cell, including a discussion of normal and abnormal growth; (2) the history, ecology, and environmental origins of cancer, emphasizing early diagnosis and prevention; (3) current methods of treatment of cancer; and (4) the psychological and social problems relevant to this perplexing disorder. Throughout, innovative attempts to translate advances in cancer research to application in human cancer have been analyzed, with particular emphasis on prevention, control, and treatment.

The basic nature and origins of cancer are complex—research so far has shown that more than 110 viruses and 1,000 chemicals are capable of producing cancer in animals. The vagaries, manifestations, and courses of the disease and its prognosis are countless. But, in the past 25 years revolutionary advances in genetics, virology, biochemical studies of protein synthesis, membrane function, and immunology have brought about a set of organizing principles governing normal and abnormal cell growth and the transfer of hereditable information. Central to the understanding of cancer is the fundamental biology of the cell.

Part One traces the origins and present state of knowledge of the molecular events in the cell which have been so magnificently elucidated since 1950. No quick or glamorous cure for cancer has emerged from this brilliant work, but the foundations on which eventual solutions will be built have been immeasurably broadened.

Part Two reviews the history of cancer and discusses environmental agents which can initiate cancer. Geographical variations in cancer incidence and types of cancer suggest preventable environmental and social factors. Cancer prevention offers greater possibilities for the control of cancer and the saving of human lives than any other measure at the present time. Next to prevention the early diagnosis and treatment of cancer, prior to its spread by invasion of the blood or lymphatic systems, seem to have the most important influence on the results of therapy. The effectiveness of Papanicolau testing in improving the prognosis of cervical cancer in women is ample testimony to the value of early diagnosis and treatment. Cancer screening, including chemical and immunological tests for early detection, seems promising and the social implications of this approach are fascinating to contemplate but still unevaluated because of requisite social changes in health evaluation on a mass scale. The need for genetic counseling and public education is also emphasized.

The treatment of cancer is covered in Part Three. The surgical treatment of cancer is analyzed, with cancer of the breast being used to typify this method of therapy. Irradiation therapy in its conventional form is exemplified by the treatment of cancer of the cervix, but additional instances are given in the application of irradiation to lymphomas and Hodgkin's disease. Discussion of the chemotherapy of cancer relates drug therapy to the molecular basis of the origin of cancer. With all forms of such treatment the patient is exposed to physical and emotional hardship, but is occasionally blessed by a complete cure. Throughout Part Three, areas of current and future research are appraised, and concern is evidenced for the total value of life with emphasis on the distinction between mere existence and a positive mode of living to accompany the treatment.

The interrelationship of psychological and social problems with cancer is discussed in Part Four. Individual responsibility in the prevention, treatment, and research of cancer must be shaped into programs for social action, so that the shared purposes of science and society can be blended into a meaningful whole. The imponderables of smoking, living with cancer, secrecy about cancer, family attitudes toward the afflicted, and dying with cancer are honestly confronted. The principal orientation is a strong belief in the resilience of the human spirit. Gloom and despair, both individually and socially, can be relieved by intellectual appraisal of psycho-social problems. Hope, warmth, and understanding on an individual level can banish despair, and on a social level can lead to dignified constructive action.

During the past 20 years my personal research in cancer has been supported by many generous individuals and organizations, among them the American Cancer Society, the Damon Runyon Fund, and the United States Public Health Service through its National Cancer Institute. The United Commercial Travelers Benevolent Foundation, Inc. gave me great freedom in the utilization of their funds, and I am particularly grateful to them for defraying secretarial and artistic costs incident to the completion of this manuscript. The opportunity for research stimulated the intellectual curiosity to synthesize into a comprehensible whole the achievements of many scientific disciplines bearing on cancer. I hope the book transmits to the reader the intellectual excitement that comes from contact with and understanding of these impressive human achievements, despite the drastic condensation that has been necessary.

I am grateful to several old friends for reading the manuscript and for offering helpful comments, particularly to Henry Kaplan, Professor of Radiobiology at Stanford University, David Linder, Associate Professor of Pathology at the University of Oregon, and J. Englebert Dunphy, Professor of Surgery at the University of California Medical Center, San Francisco. I express my sincere appreciation to Denise Scott for her contribution on psycho-social problems relevant to cancer (Part Four). She also rendered invaluable aid in simplifying the expression of difficult scientific material and in encouraging an easy, readable style. Hajime Okubo has embellished the book with his drawings, conveying complex scientific material with admirable simplicity and precision. I also wish to thank members of the staff of the University of California Press, particularly William McClung and Joel Walters, for their help in seeing the book through the publishing process.

My wife and children have not only given me the free time to complete this work, but have sustained in countless ways the intellectual effort and ingredients essential to its construction. Why they permitted the work to continue and encouraged my devotion to it is far more than I can understand. Such support defies adequate comprehension and precludes appropriate thanks.

VICTOR RICHARDS, M.D.

PROLOGUE

One morning I walked into the fifth-floor solarium of the old and antiquated hospital in which I had been working for a number of years. Here, sitting upright in bed, with legs crossed under her, was a beautiful young girl, fresh and vivacious, looking out over the city of San Francisco, resplendent in the sunshine and breathtaking in its beauty.

"What are you thinking about, Gertrude?" I asked. She answered with a flood of profound and disturbing questions. "Doctor, where does life come from? Can one inherit cancer? What is the nature of cancer and can anyone like me ever get well of it? How much longer will I live? What will death be like when it comes?"

I looked at this young woman sitting proudly erect in bed, her long hair flowing over her lovely shoulders. She had been my patient for approximately a year and we were now reaching the time when we could speak freely about the crucial questions that plagued her.

Gertrude's mother had died when she was young, her father had remarried when she was fifteen, and although both her father and her stepmother had been good to her she had sought independence early in life. She had come to San Francisco to go to school, to find the happiness and beauty she was looking for in life through a study of the arts. Two years ago she had fallen in love with one of her classmates, who was interested in art and philosophy. He was a gifted artist and had persuaded her to become a Zen Buddhist. Against the wishes of her family they were married. She had worked for a year to support her husband, had then become pregnant, and soon afterwards had noticed a change in her right breast. She could feel a hard lump in the enlarged breast.

Her obstetrician thought that the change in her breast was consistent with the course of her pregnancy, but, as she kept complaining about her condition and wondering about a possible tumor, he took some X-rays of both breasts. These proved to be extremely difficult to interpret; the radiologist's conclusion was that the condition of the right breast was probably due to pregnancy and he was unable to detect any tumor in either breast.

However, Gertrude became more and more concerned about the localized lump. This was understandable since her mother had died of cancer of the breast at an early age. Gertrude decided to seek additional consultation, and I had been called into the case for the first time approximately nine months before. She was then in the sixth month of her pregnancy. From a clinical standpoint the nature of the hardness in her right breast was indeterminate and I suggested that a biopsy be performed. At this juncture I told her that if the tumor proved to be malignant I would recommend the classical operation for cancer of the breast, the so-called *radical mastectomy*. This consists of the total removal of the breast and the pectoral muscles from the chest wall, together with the axillary lymph nodes (lymph nodes under the arm) to which a cancer of this area would have an initial tendency to spread. She accepted this with the basic questions and concerns—namely, what would be done about her pregnancy, and would she be able to nurse the baby if she were allowed to bear it.

To these questions there are no unequivocal answers. I told her that many doctors would advise her to terminate her pregnancy, but that in my opinion there was very little evidence to support such a view. In fact, several clinical studies were available which indicated that the outcome of cancer in pregnant women was not different from that in nonpregnant women. On the question of nursing the child I told her that there was evidence that in experimental animals mammary cancer was transmitted to the young through the breast milk. But I emphasized that mammary cancer in the mouse was caused by a virus, a microscopic particle visible only under the intense magnification of the electron microscope, and that cancer of the breast in a human was not known to be due to a virus or to be transmitted through the breast milk. I asked her how she felt about her pregnancy. She quickly replied: "Doctor, I can think of no experience more wonderful than having a child and I would certainly want to nurse it."

I told her that in a young woman there was a 10 to 20 percent chance of the cancer appearing in the other breast. I also added that in a young person there was evidence that cancer of the breast was susceptible to ovarian hormones circulating through the body and that some doctors felt that the ovaries should be removed, thereby making her sterile but hopefully retarding the growth and recurrence of the malignancy. I added that if her ovaries were removed the adrenal glands would tend to take over the ovarian function, and that if she got a good response from the operation the removal of the adrenal glands should be considered at a later date.

She asked me how conclusive the evidence was in favor of the removal of the other breast and of the ovaries. I informed her that the clinical and biological evidence was liable to a wide range of error, that the benefit from such an intervention was not proved, but was assumed on the basis of indirect evidence only, and I asked her how she felt about retaining her other breast and her ovarian function. Her prompt answer was that she wished to keep the other breast and to remain a normal woman, looking forward to having more children.

We decided to go ahead with the biopsy. The tumor was malignant. The classical radical mastectomy was performed. Nothing was done about the pregnancy.

These events had taken place about nine months before. Some time after the operation Gertrude had given birth to a baby whom she nursed with great pleasure and satisfaction. Shortly after delivery we had taken some mammograms of the left breast to make sure that no tumor had been left undiscerned; these had been interpreted by the radiologist as normal.

Since then Gertrude had had six months of complete happiness, living normally, contentedly, and indeed passionately with her husband, nursing her child. I had seen her at regular intervals. At the end of these six months I had discovered small swellings under her left arm which were obviously in her lymph nodes. She herself was not aware of these. My colleagues and I had now to consider whether the swellings were due to *metastasis*, that is, a spread from the original cancer in the right breast, or whether she had a latent cancer in the left breast which had escaped our attention during the period that she was lactating. Because of the lactation process the left breast felt firm and hard, but no localized lump was noticeable. Therefore it was not possible to diagnose a tumor clinically. The mammograms were repeated and again the reading was equivocal.

We had therefore, some months previously, taken out some of the lymph nodes in the left axilla, and they were shown to contain cancer cells identical to those which had been present in the right breast. This finding still left unanswered the question as to whether this was a spread from the original cancer in the right breast or whether there had been a latent cancer in the left breast.

I discussed the situation with Gertrude and her husband and presented them with the dilemma. X-rays of her chest and bones were taken and showed no evidence of cancer spread beyond the axilla. Gertrude was not anxious to have her remaining breast removed, and inquired about other therapy. The possibility of using chemotherapy (treatment with drugs) was discussed. I told her that the cancer was probably present in other parts of her body even though we could not find it, and that it would be wise to try drug therapy. She agreed. But after three months, as so often happens in drug therapy, she felt sick; she had lost her youthful zest for life. There was no regression in the size of the lymph nodes, and indeed there was a diffuse extension in the hardness of the left breast.

We then talked at length about the fact that cancer was still present in her left breast and in her axilla. New X-rays were taken of her chest and bones; no evident cancer was detectable. She asked the obvious question: "Doctor, how do you know that the cancer is still not limited to the left breast and the axilla and that you can't cure me by removing the breast and cleaning out the axilla?"

This simple logic, coming from one who had borne cancer with such fortitude, struck a responsive chord in my heart and I hoped, against all the reasoned counsels of my experience, that Gertrude was right. Her query had occasioned her re-entry into the hospital, her contemplative mood, and my visit prior to the operation. Her barrage of questions at this time kindled an urge to respond with all the knowledge I possessed.

Thus began an attempt to portray what was known and what was still unknown about the origins, nature, mutations, and responses of those wayward cells that have evaded human inhibition and control and that have caused unparalleled suffering and destruction of life. To Gertrude and to patients like her who must bear with all the courage at their command the ravages of this dread disease, to relatives and friends, and indeed to all others who wish to understand cancer, I offer this account.

THE BIOLOGY OF CANCER

1
THE EVOLUTION
OF LIFE

*"It is often said that all the
conditions for the first production of
a living organism are now present which could
ever have been present. But if (and oh! what a big if!)
we could conceive in some warm little pond with all
sorts of ammonia and phosphoric salts, light,
heat, electricity, etc., present, that a protein
compound was chemically formed ready to undergo
still more complex changes, at the present
day such matter would be instantly devoured
or absorbed, which would not have been
the case before living creatures
were formed."*
CHARLES DARWIN (1871)

Cancer cells are very much alive. They have a lust for life and for their own reproduction, but they are a form of life that is totally selfish, unconcerned with the well-being of the organism within which they dwell. They divide and reproduce themselves without any order- ly or specific purpose, invading neighboring tissues and organs. In their need for "vital space" they may reach to distant parts of the bodies they inhabit, traveling through the blood and lymph streams. They show a total contempt for the right of other cells to accomplish their task without interference; if they are not stopped in their destructive course their uncontrolled proliferation will ultimately result in the death of the carrier organism. Life and nonlife are thus seen to be united in the entity of the cancer cell.

Because of the nature of cancer, any consideration of the disease confronts us rather quickly with certain fundamental questions. What is life? How does it originate? Did it originate as a single cataclysmic event in time or is it the result of a prolonged chemical and biological evolution? What is the nature of life? Can we assign life to an individual cell or is it a property of larger groupings of matter? We know, for example, that the late Dr. Alexis Carrel kept some cells from an embryo chicken heart alive for 40 years, yet we may like to think that only an entire organism should be called alive. We would consider this to be true beyond question with regard to human beings, who have the capacity not only for physical existence and freedom of movement, but for mental and spiritual life.

In very simple terms, life is the ability to utilize energy and to reproduce itself, to change and to pass changes to progeny. In nature such an ability has existed for billions of years: it existed much before the appearance of animal and human species; it originated with the coming into existence of large molecules called *nucleic acids*. These form the material our genes are made of, and they are contained in the nuclei of our cells. How did these "living" elements, the nucleic acids, appear on the surface of the earth? How did nonliving elements (incapable of reproducing themselves) such as hydrogen, oxygen, carbon, nitrogen, and phosphorus ever combine into living molecules capable of reproducing themselves?

To understand the origin of life would require a long and many-branched exploration back into time. Scientists have made at least part of this exploration comprehensible for us in chemical and biological terms. Science has given us simple, quantitative definitions of various aspects of life which we can use to enlarge our understanding of all living things, whether these living things are normal or abnormal, benevolent or destructive of life itself.

Without question, however, any quantitative scientific definition of life is far too simple and most of us will reject it as incomplete, for the essence of life, the basic quality which each human being knows to belong to his own life, is felt but cannot be defined. The diversity of life startles us. When we watch a healthy animal, a growing child, an active adult, a man in his declining years whose capacities have turned to the contemplative, a sick person who struggles for health, and also think of a bird singing, a flower blooming, a tree bursting with colorful blossoms, we realize that in all these forms of life there is a common essence which eludes definitions. Like truth, beauty, or happiness, the concept of life refuses to be imprisoned in formulas. It cannot be reduced to simple, rigid concepts; these destroy its meaning rather than clarify its nature. The simple distinctions between quality and quantity in life are most eloquently evident to the cancer patient who is faced with the difference between the enjoyment of a full life and mere existence. When he must submit to medical procedures which alter the quality of life, when he must ultimately contemplate the possibility of his death, he knows acutely then that life is not survival but something infinitely more which must be recaptured if he is to feel whole again.

Nevertheless the patient, indeed all of us, must make a beginning in understanding cancer by utilizing those definitions of life provided by the advancing tools and techniques of science. Scientifically life can be defined in terms of the elements, forms, constructions, interactions, and communications between identifiable parts. Although one need only see a person alive at one moment and dead at the next to realize that life is indefinable in terms of elements alone, all living things must do two things:

1. Transfer and transform energy.
2. Communicate and transfer information so that reproduction and replication can take place.

The simplest forms of life we know are the *virus*, which is composed of an inner core of nucleic acid and an outer coat of protein; the *bacterium*, which is a single cell, alive and ubiquitous in the universe; and the plant or animal cell which is the unit of life for all organisms in both the plant and animal kingdom. The cell in the plant kingdom operates on a *chlorophyll* or *anaerobic* system; the cell in the animal kingdom on an *aerobic*, or respiratory system. Chlorophyll, the green pigment of plants, captures the energy of sunlight and transforms carbon dioxide into sugars; this takes place in the absence of oxygen and for that reason is referred to as anaerobic. The process does, however, return oxygen to the atmosphere; in turn oxygen is utilized by animals and human beings in respiration. The animal system, the aerobic system, is utterly dependent on oxygen and is especially designed to obtain maximal energy from carbohydrates and other foods, and to return carbon dioxide to the atmosphere. The mutual relationship of these two systems is essential for the continuation of plant and animal life (fig. 1–1).

CHEMICAL AND BIOLOGICAL EVOLUTION

Our earth is 4.5 to 5 billion years old. When it was still young, 1.7 to 3.5 billion years ago, the first unicellular organisms appeared on the earth's surface. Chemical evolution, that is, the development of single-celled organisms from the primitive atoms through a long chain of transformations, has taken approximately 2 billion years. One of these unicellular organisms contains 10^{10} molecules, or 10 billion molecules! But man himself is made of 10^{10} cells, or, in terms of molecules, of 10^{20} molecules: 1 followed by 20 zeros! It is not surprising, then, that biological evolution, the evolution from single-celled organisms to a multicellular organism such as man, took another 2 billion years.

A crucial question in considering the evolution of cells and their interrelation is the matter of how they are able to "communicate." How do we know that cells have a way to "speak" to one another? How in fact do cells "know" when to grow, when to stop, and when to divide? Within the last ten to twenty years we have begun to understand the problems of communication between molecules, the essence of cell growth and differentiation, and the nature of information transfer between living cells. The answer to these puzzles resides within the cell itself. For example, if several normal cells are placed on a glass surface the cells stop moving and growing when and only

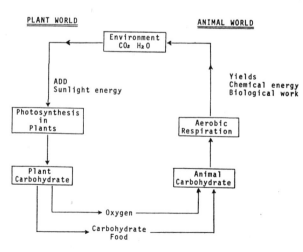

FIGURE 1–1. *Stylized representation of the "carbon cycle," the interaction between photosynthetic and nonphotosynthetic cells in the breakdown of carbohydrates using different forms of energy.*

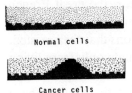

FIGURE 1–2. *Schematic diagram of the growth of normal cells and of cancer cells on a glass surface. Normal cells (left) grow in a single layer displaying contact inhibition. Cancer cells, however, grow in a heaped-up multilayer.*

when they touch each other; it is presumed that in this contact exists a "language," a mechanism inhibiting further growth, a so-called *contact inhibition*. If cancer cells, however, are placed on a glass surface, they do not stop moving and dividing when they touch each other (fig. 1–2). This indicates that in cancer there must be some disturbance in the natural communication between cells. That there is communication between normal cells has been established by inserting a microelectrode into one cell and another microelectrode into an adjacent cell; an electric current passes. An ion flux (movement of electrically charged atoms) is involved in intercellular communication. If the same procedure is repeated with cancer cells, one discovers that there is a high resistance to such a movement; the ion flux necessary for cells to communicate is absent, thus the cancer cells are unable to "speak" to one another, to tell one another to stop proliferating (Lowenstein and Kanno, 1966; Lowenstein *et al.*, 1967).

There are a number of things about cells that scientists have not yet elucidated. Still completely unexplained are such obvious questions (to a biologist if not to everyone) as the essential communication between the nucleus, or center of the cell, and its surrounding cytoplasm, the nature of the cell membranes, the origins of changes and mutations within cells, the actions of extracellular factors on cell functions, and the origin within cells of "organizers" for structuring their functions and their form.

The idea that living organisms have arisen on the surface of the earth as a natural outgrowth of chemical transformation of basic molecular elements is relatively recent. Charles Darwin, in his classic paper, "On the Tendency of Species to Form Varieties; and on the Perpetuation of Varieties and Species by Natural Means of Selection," first read in 1858, postulated the processes of mutation, of natural selection, and of survival of the fittest. He was able to explain the evolution and perpetuation of varieties of species by natural selection once they were alive. In 1863 Louis Pasteur, the great French scientist, performed experiments indicating to him that life could not originate on the surface of the earth from conditions that then existed, and he unequivocally stated that life could originate only from living things.

Neither Pasteur nor Darwin (who sensed that there might be a chemical evolution which antedated the biological evolution he so brilliantly clarified), however, had the tools or the techniques for the study of chemical evolution. They could not have discovered how lifeless, inert chemicals ever united with one another to form living substances capable of reproducing themselves. For it is only recently that the concept of chemical evolution could be given serious consideration because of the availability of magnificent analytical instruments. Appropriate instrumentation, combined with a flood of knowledge in chemistry, physics, and biology, and a richer understanding of energy metabolism, has enabled three new theoretical approaches to the study of chemical evolution. These are: (1) the study of patterns of energy metabolism, both in the presence of oxygen (aerobic) and in its absence (anaerobic); (2) the analysis of the earliest discovered fossils by refined chemical instrumentation such as mass spectrometry and other techniques; and (3) the simulation of the synthesis of life by reproducing in the laboratory the chemical pathways essential for the construction of compounds, substances, and systems which we accept as living. Each of these three new theoretical approaches will be briefly discussed below.

EVOLUTION OF ENERGY METABOLISM

All living things require energy to perform work. All energy is either potential, that is, stored; or kinetic, actually being used. Potential energy can be likened to a boulder at the top of a hill, which must be pushed to roll down the slope; as soon as the push is given the energy becomes kinetic, or energy of movement. Among many types of energy and of particular importance to living organisms are chemical, electrical, and radiant energy. The work performed by such organisms may be mechanical, electrical, or osmotic, osmosis being the passage of one fluid into another through a membrane, as when food gets into our blood through the wall of the intestines.

The unit of life, the site of life's prodigious energy, is the single cell. Cells, and all living things, are endowed with complex, efficient, and almost miraculous devices for transforming energy. The curious and central point is that life in animals and in man requires oxygen for the utilization of energy and the performance of work. In other words, life in man and animals, as we know it, requires an aerobic environment. But the primitive atmosphere of the world of several billion years ago must of necessity have been anaerobic, devoid of free oxygen. If oxygen had been present the molecules composing living organisms would simply have undergone combustion and would have disappeared. Life would not have been sustained.

What little oxygen there was in the primitive atmosphere was bound to hydrogen in the form of water molecules. Hydrogen was the main reducing gas of the atmosphere and the most abundant; it was light and slowly disappeared from the surface of the earth, but its concentration was sufficiently great for it to combine with carbon, nitrogen, and oxygen, forming simple gases such as ammonia, carbon dioxide, and water vapor. It is postulated that, later, these simple gases reacted slowly but continuously with one another to form small organic molecules, that is, complex molecules containing carbon. Called the basic element of life, carbon has the ability to combine with other atoms in a great number of ways. Such chemical activations took place under the influence of the sun, whose ultraviolet rays were powerful reactors and also under the influence of electrical discharges in the atmosphere, which had the power of "sticking" atoms together.

If we try to picture this primitive earth, its atmosphere, and its slow transformation, we see a sphere surrounded by a vapor atmosphere and a coat of gases; the vapor condensed into water and oceans were formed; the gases and newly formed molecules on the surface of the earth dropped into the waters of the sea. When the ultraviolet rays of the sun penetrated the depths of the oceans, strange things began to happen to the chemicals in these waters; the hydrogen and oxygen of water split, the carbon and hydrogen of methane split, and the nitrogen and hydrogen of ammonia split. These elements then recombined with other elements into very large molecules which could make copies of themselves; in this manner chemical evolution began and life eventually appeared in our universe.

The essential elements of life—carbon, nitrogen, hydrogen, and oxygen—had the special property of becoming extremely stable after gaining and sharing electrons, and they regularly formed double and triple bonds in doing so. Two other elements, phosphorus and sulfur, also played a large part in organic evolution since they, too, had the special ability of forming high-energy bonds by accepting and donating electrons.

The result of the splitting of water molecules into oxygen and hydrogen in the primeval atmosphere was the dispersion of hydrogen into space and the formation of ozone (O^3), which spread densely over the surface of the earth, screened the ultraviolet rays of the sun, and permitted the gentler *actinic rays* to nourish the newly formed plant kingdom. Living organisms formerly hidden in the depths of the oceans rose to the surface and algae appeared on their shores. Carbon dioxide made its appearance, and with oxygen also present, a flow of energy between the plant and animal kingdoms was eventually made possible, since the plants "breathe in" carbon dioxide and emit oxygen and the reverse is true for the organisms of the animal kingdom.

It took millennia for such "simple" changes to occur in nature; it is estimated to be about 400 million years ago that the newly formed organisms attached to themselves a complex molecule, the green chlorophyll, which is so essential to the life of the plant world. The succeeding stage was undoubtedly an anaerobic process akin to fermentation, which provided a chemical source of energy by converting sugars into alcohol, carbon dioxide, and high-energy phosphate compounds.

Probably the next type of anaerobic metabolism was the hexose monophosphate cycle which has only been elucidated recently. This process develops hydrogen and carbon dioxide. The hydrogen thus synthesized was most necessary in the universe in remote times since the primitive hydrogen had disappeared from the earth at the time life is known to have originated.

The subsequent process and probably the most important one to evolve was the process of *photophosphorylation*. It was during this stage of chemical evolution that special pigments such as chlorophyll and metalloporphyrins developed, and then were acted upon by sunlight to produce high-energy phosphate. Soon, *photosynthesis,* which is the metabolic system of present-day plants, emerged, largely integrating the previous evolutionary steps. In photosynthesis the energy of sunlight is transduced to synthesize glucose, through high-energy phosphates. Photosynthesis captures the radiant energy of sunlight in the green cells of plant life and transforms it into chemical energy, producing carbohydrates and oxygen. This production of oxygen from carbon dioxide and water paved the way for the animal kingdom to utilize oxygen in the process of respiration.

The next evolutionary stage in the flow of energy leading to higher forms of life was the development of respiration, in which the chemical energy of carbohydrates and other foodstuff molecules is transformed into a more useful kind of energy yielding large amounts of high-energy phosphates and returning carbon dioxide to the atmosphere for reutilization by green plants. The oxygen-using cells comprise the bulk of living cells, although it should be remembered that some living cells do not require oxygen.

It may sound strange to say that oxygen is not necessary to have oxidation reactions, but if one keeps in mind that an oxidation reaction is a reaction in which the atom of oxygen attracts electrons from another atom, it is logical to consider that a reaction in which an element other than oxygen behaves in the same manner may be called oxidation. The process by which foodstuff molecules undergo oxidation in the absence of oxygen is fermentation. In all cells, however, it is the process of oxidation which is the main source of energy. In both aerobic and anaerobic cells the energy yielded from foodstuffs during oxidation is conserved, not as heat, but as chemical energy. We know now that the specific compound in which chemical energy is preserved is *adenosine triphosphate* (ATP); it serves as the carrier of energy, whether derived from aerobic or anaerobic processes.

In animal cells the chemical energy of ATP is used to perform the chemical, mechanical, or osmotic work of the cell. In providing the chemical energy, ATP is converted into its discharged form, *adenosine diphosphate* (ADP). This energy carrier system is charged during the oxidation of foodstuffs and discharged during the performance of work in a continuous dynamic cycle, just as carbon dioxide is converted by photosynthesis into carbohydrates and oxygen, and the oxygen is reutilized in respiration of cells for the liberation of chemical energy.

During the long span of chemical evolution there was a natural selection of the chemical processes which were most essential to the development of photosynthesis and aerobic respiration. Chemicals changed to facilitate essential reactions and those elements survived which were best suited for energy metabolism. George Wald (1964) has expressed this scientific truth in almost poetic terms: "We living things are a late outgrowth of the metabolism of our galaxy. The carbon that enters so importantly in our composition was cooked in the remote past in a dying star. From it, at lower temperatures, nitrogen and oxygen were formed. These, our indispensable elements, were spewed into space in the exhalation of red giants and such solar catastrophes as supernovae, there to be mixed with hydrogen and form eventually the substances of the sun and planets and ourselves. The waters of ancient seas set the pattern of irons in our blood, the ancient atmosphere molded our metabolism."

ANALYSIS OF FOSSILS

The prehistoric past and the present are linked together most notably by fossil remains. In recent years fossil analysis has yielded astounding information concerning the origins of life. This is largely related to the development of brilliant analytical tools which have facilitated the examination of fossils at the molecular level. Such tools include the mass spectrometer, a unique instrument which permits the ionization of compounds into their fundamental elements and the subsequent precise measurement of these elements according to their weight or mass; gas chromatographs, which make possible accurate and rapid identification of gases according to their molecular weight; and, finally, the electron microscope, which permits the intense magnification of materials so that an infinitesimal amount can actually be viewed for identification and verification of its structure.

With the aid of such special tools, Melvin Calvin and his associates have searched the geological records of the past. The Green River shale of western North America of 60 million years ago has revealed hydrocarbons that are quite typical of biological organisms.

Living things, therefore, are presumed to have been present on the earth at that time. Also found were other types of hydrocarbons which are linked to the production of chlorophyll. These were discovered in the Green River shale, in the None Such shale of northern Michigan (1,000 million years old), more recently in the Soudan shale of Minnesota (2,700 million years old), and in South African shales (2,200 million years old).

As a result of his investigations, Calvin (1967) has written: "The possibility exists that many of the organic compounds now believed to be the proximate substrate for organic evolution might have been present in the original cosmic dust that gave rise to the earth itself. . . . We are searching for still older rocks, rocks which have ages beyond 3,000 million years ago, and which contain carbon. The amounts of carbon we need are of course getting smaller as our analytical tools are becoming more sophisticated, and I believe that we will be able to determine the nature of the carbon-containing molecules present in even the oldest rocks."

LABORATORY SYNTHESIS OF COMPOUNDS ESSENTIAL TO LIFE

Scientists agree that the fundamental atoms in the primitive earth were those of hydrogen, carbon, nitrogen, and oxygen, the latter, as mentioned above, not in the form of free oxygen, but bound to hydrogen in the form of water molecules. The basic question then is: "Is it possible, by introducing energy in such an aggregation of molecules, to achieve the synthesis of compounds now known to be essential to life, namely, proteins, sugars, nucleic acids, and fats?" (See fig. 1–3.)

Recently Calvin and other chemists interested in the synthesis of vital compounds from basic atoms have given an answer to this question. They have taken primitive organic molecules, such as water, carbon monoxide, carbon dioxide, methane, hydrogen, and ammonia (the original gases existing in the atmosphere of the earth) and have energized these molecules with ultraviolet light, irradiation, or electrical discharge, thus reproducing the conditions which must have been present on primeval earth. They have found that they could break and recombine these primitive molecules. After a series of reactions, they finally obtained the common materials essential to life,

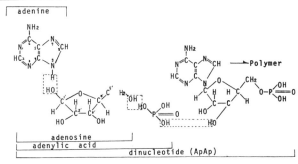

PROTEINS

$$\underset{R_1}{H_2N-CH-\overset{\overset{O}{\|}}{C}-\underset{}{[OH+H]}-\overset{H}{N}-\underset{R_2}{CH-CO_2H}} \longrightarrow \underset{\underset{\underline{\text{dipeptide}}}{\overset{R_1 \qquad R_2}{}}}{H_2N-CH-\overset{\overset{O}{\|}}{C}-NH-CH-CO_2H} \longrightarrow Polymer$$

amino   carboxyl

POLYSACCHARIDES

→Disaccharide→Polymer

NUCLEIC ACIDS (3 STAGES) RNA SHOWN - DNA LACKS OH ON 2 POSITION

adenine

NH₂

→Polymer

adenosine

adenylic acid

dinucleotide (ApAp)

FIGURE 1–3. *Chemical structure of generalized models of proteins, polysaccharides, and nucleic acids.*

namely, the amino acids, sugars, the hydroxy acids, and the dicarboxylic acids.

Of special significance in these primitive reactions (during the first breaking and recombining of the initial molecules) is the synthesis of hydrocyanic acid (HCN) for it has recently been shown that HCN plays a role in the formation of *adenine*. Adenine is an essential building block of nucleic acids and proteins, both of which are essential for life, are used for performance of specific functions by cells, and enter into the transcription of genetic information from cell to cell.

The steps in the long process of chemical evolution were undoubtedly facilitated by the intervention of chemical agents called *catalysts*. A catalyst is a substance which does not initiate but which helps bring about a chemical reaction. If compound A, for example, can be converted into either compound B, C, or D, and if a catalyst favorable for its conversion to D is present, compound A will invariably be transformed into compound D. The action of an important catalyst is illustrated by the chemical combining pattern of iron. Iron is instrumental in the conversion of hydrogen peroxide to water and free oxygen, but this reaction ordinarily takes place very slowly. If, however, the iron atom is surrounded by a catalyst, *heme*, the capacity of the iron to react is enhanced a thousandfold. If heme is further surrounded by protein, a complex enzyme, *catalase*, results. Catalase stimulates the conversion of hydrogen peroxide to water and free oxygen several times more readily than does heme alone. When these conditions are present in a suitable environment the catalytic power residing in the iron atom is enhanced by more than a millionfold.

To this juncture several aspects of the generation of living material have been described. They can be grouped into two general phases: first, the conversion of simple compounds into more complex ones in a random fashion; second, the autoselection of certain compounds favorable to life from these precursors through association with catalysts. These compounds are capable of storing and converting energy. Let us turn now to the origin of chemical compounds capable not only of storage and conversion of energy but also of transmission of inheritable information from one cell to another.

TRANSFER OF INFORMATION IN LIVING TISSUES

The most complicated and intricate chemical components of animal structures are the proteins and nucleic acids. Despite their complexity, these substances can now be synthesized in the laboratory. A protein results from the synthesis and fusion of amino acids. From this action a chain of polymers is obtained, which ultimately becomes the protein itself. Nucleic acids are formed in a similar way (and so are sugars and lipids).

Although nucleic acids are complex molecules they are the simplest manifestation of life, since they have been found to be the first compounds in the hierarchy of molecules capable of reproducing themselves and of transmitting their characteristics to their progeny. In that sense, they are extremely important to chemists, biologists, and geneticists and to others interested in the study of the origins of life.

Proteins and nucleic acids show a definite tendency to intrinsic order. The proteins coil into a helical form which has been given the name of *alpha helix*. Nucleic acids, or more precisely, *nucleotides*, the many lesser divisions of these complex molecules, come together in an intricate and beautiful figure in space. They form themselves into the shape of a *double helix*, which may be described as two ribbons coiling around a common center, or two spiral staircases winding parallel to each other (fig. 1–4). The coils of the double ribbons are composed of phosphates and sugars, and "hanging" from these two strands are four different bases: *adenine, guanine, cytosine,* and *thymine.* Any of these four bases can hang from either strand and they are held together across the strand by hydrogen bonds. Curiously enough, the amount of adenine in the double-stranded helix is always equal to the amount of thymine, and the amount of guanine is always equal to the amount of cytosine—a fact of some importance in the unique qualities of nucleic acids (their reproduction and information transfer). Thymine invariably pairs with adenine and guanine invariably pairs with cytosine. The amino acids, which are the building blocks of proteins, have very much the same structure except that they form single helixes.

One type of nucleic acid, containing deoxyribose sugar, is called

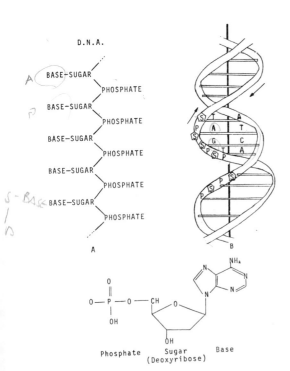

FIGURE 1–4. *Two representations of the structure of deoxyribonucleic acid (DNA). (A) Schematic listing of the chemical compounds in a single chain of DNA; (B) Diagram of the double helix. The two ribbons symbolize the sugar-phosphate chains; the horizontal bars, the pairs of bases holding the chains together.*

deoxyribonucleic acid (DNA). DNA is to be found in the nuclei of our cells and it is the material of which our genes are composed. Another type of nucleic acid, containing ribose sugar (and the base uracil instead of the base thymine) is named *ribonucleic acid* (RNA). RNA is found in the cytoplasm of the cell. The DNA of the cell nucleus is the repository of all the information necessary for the formation of protein and for the reproduction of the cell. The genetic message of the nucleus can be carried from the nucleus to the cytoplasm on a strand of RNA termed the messenger RNA. This substance wraps itself around the *ribosomes* in the cytoplasm and gives them the information necessary for identical genetic replication.

It has been said that the four bases of DNA, namely, adenine, guanine, thymine, and cytosine, or to use their initials, A, G, T, C, form the language of life; all that can be passed on about life in the recesses of our cells would therefore require only the code A-G-T-C. The sequence of any three of the four letters determines the specificity of a given amino acid, that is, what its role and duty are. The same is true of any information essential to the life and reproduction of the cell. DNA is the knower, yielding messenger RNA, the carrier. The protein synthesis actually takes place in the ribosomes. So the cell harbors within itself the knowledge of and the capacity for its own reproduction.

Once in a great while (perhaps once in a million times) a different grouping occurs than in a normal chain of DNA. Cytosine might, let us say, pair with thymine, or a segment of the DNA chain may be substituted or deleted, thereby altering the composition of the DNA. A new DNA is born, a mutation has occurred. These mutations are of great interest to the cancer researcher, for the cancer cell is a changed cell, which does not behave like a normal cell and may thus be the outcome of a mutation. Cancer may be the result of a direct mutation within the *genome* (or entire genetic information) of the cellular DNA. But the cell may also be influenced by carcinogenic agents from without. The origin of malignancy, of cancer, and its variabilities is wrapped up in these genomal and extragenomal changes in the normal cell.

PAST AND FUTURE EVOLUTIONS

Life slowly emerged on our earth through chemical and biological evolutions that have spanned 2 to 3 billion years. To go from hydrogen to man, or as Calvin has put it, from "atom to Adam," has involved enormous periods of time. If life, as it is now accepted, has evolved from the favorable conjunction of molecules, temperature, and environment, similar events might be expected to have occurred on other planets. The possibility of extraterrestrial life thus becomes of interest in further elucidation of life on earth.

Since the moon has no atmosphere, our kind of life cannot exist on its surface. But the low temperature of the moon does not preclude its being a cold storage repository for fragments of biological material it may have captured in its travels through space. Mars and Venus may offer more suitable environments for some sort of life than does the moon. Sampling devices have been created to obtain specimens, and tools have been perfected to analyze particles from the surface of these two planets.

Undoubtedly man will continue to explore the planets and beyond to achieve a more thorough understanding of the nature of life on earth. As Wald has said: "Surely this is a great part of our dignity as men that we can know and that through us matter can know itself; at the beginning were protons and electrons; out of the womb of time and the vastness of space we can begin to understand that, organized as in us, the carbon, the nitrogen, the oxygen, the hydrogen, the sixteen to twenty-one elements, the water, sunlight—all, having become us, can begin to understand what they are, and how they came to be."

On the cellular level, too, we are approaching new paths. We can now envision means of selectively transforming and transducing the genes, thereby hoping to control which gene may be transcribed and which deleted. Inherent in this approach is the control of hereditary diseases, of cancer, and perhaps of disease in general. The possible alteration of intelligence and emotions is linked to similar biological undertakings and understanding.

Calvin (1964) offers the following thoughts: "We have the power to intensify certain human traits, delete others, and perhaps even develop new ones. An important corollary of this is the approaching ability to control man's mind by chemical means, bringing with it the major problems of how and by whom this power should be exercised.

"Today the world is as awesome to contemplate as it must have been at its beginning, for today man is here and he has a little knowledge! With each thread of new truth there is, the possibility to weigh the consequences of its application becomes more critical. The rate of evolution can change tremendously man's new knowledge and the responsibility to control the rate and direction of change must depend on wisdom. As it has to this day time will record our success—or failure."

Man's long and laborious chemical and biological evolution may yield eventually to a psycho-social evolution, yet such a process will undoubtedly come into being very slowly, owing to the immense psychological and social complexities which are befalling mankind in modern times. Psychologically and socially man possesses an instinctive resistance to change and innovation. Psychologically man finds comfort in the perpetuation of the past and socially he fears a future that threatens established privileges, accepted ideas, and even the concept of self.

2
THE LIVING CELL

*"All cells are born
from a cell."*
RUDOLF VIRCHOW

All the activities, the accomplishments, pleasures, sorrows, all of man's discoveries, his successes and failures, all understandings and misunderstandings, all greatness and all mediocrity have their origin in the life of our cells. All that is conscious or unconscious starts first in the unseen life of the cells.

The cell is tremendously active. We have already noted that its two essential attributes for life are (1) the capacity to harness and transform energy, and (2) the capacity to transmit information from generation to generation, that is, to reproduce. Whether we consider plant cells or animal cells, whether we consider that cells differ in structure and functions, whether they work in harmony with one another or against each other, as when cancer cells appear, they all labor at producing energy and transforming it. When their purpose is fulfilled they die in the process of their replication. Their life cycles differ and they specialize in different tasks; they all, however, are energy sources and transformers and they all have offspring.

In the seventeenth century, the English philosopher Robert Hooke expressed an early concept of the cell in saying that living things were made up of "an infinite company of small boxes." In the eighteenth century the French physiologists Marie François Bichat and Jean Baptiste Lamarck discovered that all body tissues were made of cells. In 1839, the two Germans, Matthias Jacob Schleiden, a botanist, and Theodor Schwann, a zoologist, propounded the cell theory of all living structures. In 1859, Rudolf Virchow, the "father of modern pathology," clarified the unique role of the cell as the harborer of life, and expressed this viewpoint in words that have remained famous: "Omnis cellula e celluli," "all cells are born from a cell."

There are some striking differences in functions of various kinds of cells, differences which are relevant to the problem of cancer and to which we will return in a later chapter. For the present these functions are discussed in very general terms. Capacity for reproduction is not limited to the living cell. Viruses can replicate and synthesize their own protein; they lack, however, the full endowment of the living cell and must therefore depend upon other cells for their life, that is, they must live as parasites of other cells. Single-celled organisms, such as bacteria, make their own generative enzymes and thus can grow and multiply on their own, without necessarily requiring the ingredients utilized by more complex living cells. Their simplicity and their rapid rate of reproduction have made them a suitable material for the study of cell growth and reproduction.

The multicellular organisms are much more complex. Their unique characteristics among the world of cells is that within the organism as a whole diverse cells have different functions; each cell, when it replicates, must also differentiate into the appropriate type of cell from which it originated. Multicelled organisms are characterized by the attribute of differentiation, as well as by growth and replication. Such cells show a curious, dramatic, and unique trait: they recognize other cells of their own kind; they assemble by families and functions; they stick together and exclude "strangers" from their midst. A kidney cell sticks to a kidney cell, a brain cell to a brain cell, a heart cell to a heart cell. This capacity for *agglutination* according to function seems to be directed by the cell membrane, but the precise mechanism of the process is still unknown.

THE CELL AS SEEN UNDER THE MICROSCOPE

Very few cells can be seen with the naked eye; most of them were first visible under the magnification of the light microscope (fig. 2–1). It is only recently, after the invention of the electron microscope and the development of molecular biology, that the molecular bases of cellular life could be investigated. Light microscopes allowed scientists to view the content of cells as small as one-thousandth of a millimeter in size. But the electron microscope is so powerful that it can enlarge cellular structures by as much as 30,000 to 40,000 times the original size; with it we can observe particles one-millionth of a millimeter in size.

Thanks to molecular biology and electron microscopy biochemists can study the functions and interrelationships between the hitherto invisible units which constitute the cell. They can thus separate cells into subcellular fractions, thereby gaining a new dimension in the understanding of cell structure and function.

The study of single-celled organisms and of cells isolated from the organs that they constitute has given us most of our knowledge of the structure and composition of cells. In brief terms, the cell is made of a membrane which surrounds a jellylike core called the *cytoplasm*. At the center of the cytoplasm is the *nucleus* which is itself separated from the cytoplasm by its own membrane, the *nuclear membrane*. The interior of the cell is composed of large and highly complex molecules, many of which are proteins serving as enzymes that stimulate cell functions, or as catalysts, which, as we have already seen, speed up and facilitate chemical reactions within the cell.

The essential compound contained in the nucleus is deoxyribonucleic acid and the major constituent of the cytoplasm is ribonucleic acid, the two nucleic acids described in chapter 1. It was mentioned there that both play a vital role in cell reproduction and protein synthesis: the DNA of the nucleus sends its instructions to the cytoplasm through its messenger, messenger RNA (m RNA); the messenger passes on the orders to the RNA of the cytoplasm. The "message," in the instance of protein synthesis, is to arrange the amino acids of

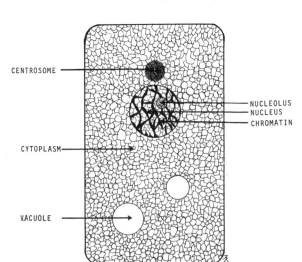

CENTROSOME

NUCLEOLUS
NUCLEUS
CHROMATIN

CYTOPLASM

VACUOLE

FIGURE 2–1. *Schematic diagram of a cell. This generalized representation shows the features that can be seen in the conventional light microscope.*

digested foodstuffs into linked polymers, the all-important proteins. The DNA is the architect, the knower; its contractor is the obedient RNA. Their association and work will be described in detail in subsequent chapters.

In addition to the cell membrane, the cytoplasm, and the nucleus, other essential structures related to cell reproduction can be observed through the light microscope. These are the *centrosomes* (centrioles) in the cytoplasm, the *nucleoli* in the nucleus, and the *chromatin strands* in the nucleus. (The chromatin strands accept dyes on staining, hence their name. They are the agents of heredity and are mostly constituted of DNA.)

After 1922 more powerful light microscopes were engineered but they were subject to certain inherent limitations in their power of resolution. The invention of the electron microscope in 1939 greatly increased the possibility of magnifying cells and other small organisms and thus broadened the ability of research workers to investigate and understand cell parts and functions (fig. 2–2).

FIGURE 2–2. *(Left) Generalized view of a cell as pictured under an electron microscope. (Right) Portion of a cell as viewed under further magnification of an electron microscope.*

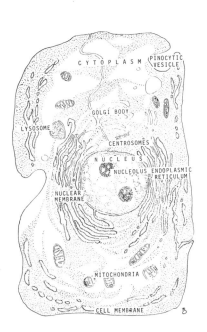
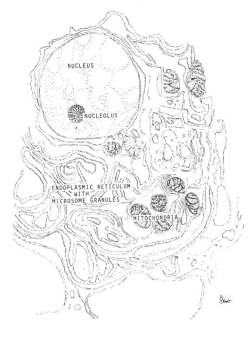

THE CELL MEMBRANE

Under the electron microscope the cell membrane is revealed to be 100 angstroms thick (one angstrom equals one ten-millionth of a millimeter, 10^{-8} mm). This membrane has the property of allowing water and chemical substances to flow through its surface and provides surface qualities to the cell which determine its behavior with respect to other cells. Two kinds of *antigens* are located on the cell's surface membrane. These are the so-called transplant antigens and immunologic antigens. Antigens are foreign substances invading cells and their action will be explained in detail in the chapter on immunology.

THE CYTOPLASM

In the cytoplasm one can clearly see the fine structures called the *mitochondria*; these have energy-producing functions in the cell, permitting photosynthesis in plant cells and extracting energy through respiration and oxidation of foodstuffs in animal cells. The electron microscope has made possible a more detailed examination of another body often associated with the mitochondria: it is the *lysosome*. The lysosomes contain digestive enzymes which break down large molecules of foodstuffs and prepare them for further oxidation and utilization by the mitochondria. The lysosomes are enveloped by a membrane which, when broken, lets the enzymes be liberated into the cell to destroy it during the process of cell division.

Close to the nucleus are the *centrosomes*, bodies large enough to be visible under the light microscope. At the time of cell division they separate and migrate to opposite sides of the nucleus; upon disruption of the nuclear membrane the chromatin strands (which have formed into chromosome rods) organize around the centrosome into spindles; these contain the cytoplasmic protein and are of the greatest importance for cell division, as we shall see later.

Another striking feature of the cytoplasm is the purposeful arrangement of most of its mass into a network of connected channels called the *endoplasmic reticulum*. This network can be separated by the ultracentrifuge and its function can then be studied. It is primarily involved in protein synthesis. Some cells which produce a high amount of protein, like the pancreatic cells, are extremely rich in endoplasmic reticulum.

Small granules named ribosomes, mentioned in chapter 1, are distributed along the endoplasmic reticulum. It is around these ribosomes that the messenger RNA wraps itself during the process of protein synthesis, when it brings the information and the direction from the DNA of the nucleus. This RNA is referred to as a "template"; it is the biological equivalent of a printing press or duplicating machine. The details about protein synthesis essential for our understanding of cancer will be dealt with later; for the moment it will be enough to indicate the importance of the endoplasmic reticulum in the synthesis of protein in the cell. The energy necessary for the chemical activity involved is provided by energy-rich phosphates, which are related to the mitochondrial function. It should be mentioned that the function of the endoplasmic reticulum is not limited to protein synthesis. It also has a role in the action of drugs on cells, including cancer cells.

The structure of the cytoplasm of the cell as revealed by the electron microscope is so diverse and beautiful that it is difficult to think of it as an area in which work is performed. Nevertheless, within it the fine structure of the mitochondria is devoted to cell respiration, oxidation, and energy transformation; the lysosomes, its associates, are elaborated for cell digestion; the centrosomes are only diffusely seen when the cell is at rest but they are clearly designed for migration toward the nucleus at the time of cell division and replication; and finally, the network of the endoplasmic reticulum is structured for the synthesis of proteins and enzymes by the cell.

All these structures, united in the cytoplasm of the cell, can be separated and studied, and conceivably could be altered by biochemical or genetic mechanisms externally imposed upon the cell. Diseases which result from deficiencies within the cell, or from abnormal messages carried in the cell, could hopefully be cured by some sort of genetic engineering. In the case of cancer the altered cell could conceivably be restored to normalcy through biological intervention, or the most delicate type of microsurgery on the cell nucleus.

THE NUCLEUS

The nucleus of the cell is bounded by a double membrane which contains many pores that permit a flow of material and information from the nucleus to the cytoplasm. Inside the nucleus are the extremely important strands of chromatin, the DNA-bearing component. When the cell is in a resting stage, that is, not involved in growth and replication, the chromatin strands are diffusely distributed. When the cell prepares for division the chromatin strands coil tightly into chromosomes. Each living organism contains a fixed number of chromosomes; the total number varies depending on the organism. A human cell has 46 chromosomes; the cells of mice have 40.

The nucleus contains the spherical bodies already mentioned, the nucleoli. These bodies are rich in RNA and are the active centers for the synthesis of RNA and protein. The nucleoli can be compared in shape and function within the nucleus to the tiny granules of the cytoplasm, the ribosomes, which are the centers for the synthesis of protein in the cytoplasm.

The structures of the nucleus bathe in an amorphous matrix called the *nuclear sap*. In recent years the qualities and functions of the nucleus have been elucidated by the use of special microscopical techniques and by biochemical methods of cellular separation such as the use of the ultracentrifuge. The nucleus is the main center for the synthesis of nucleic acids, both DNA and RNA.

The morphology and physiology of the cell nucleus is just as noteworthy as that of the cytoplasm. Its character is being explored further and is slowly yielding its secrets. The ultimate goal of research on the cell is hopefully to alter the quality of life at the cellular level, to restore the integrity of disturbed cellular activity, and to reverse the course of specific diseases caused by missing genes or enzymes— by inserting the missing gene or enzyme at the time of cell division.

3
CELL GROWTH AND DIFFERENTIATION AND GENETICS

*"Man's life is
truly a performance."*
CHINESE PROVERB

There are three great generalizations in modern biology: (1) the theory of chemical and biological evolution of life; (2) the theory of cellular structure and function as the unit of life, and (3) the theory of hereditary transfer of information from one generation to the next by chromosomal inheritance.

The origin and transmission of cancer conforms to these established principles governing the nature of living things. Cell growth, differentiation, and replication, whether it be normal or cancerous, is controlled and transferred by structures known as *chromosomes* and *genes* in conformity with the chromosomal theory of heredity.

Man has long been aware that children inherit some of the traits of their parents, like the color of their hair or the color of their eyes. Since 1860 the transmission of life with its hereditary traits has been known to occur through the union of the sperm cell of the male with the egg cell of the female. In 1868 it was found that the sperm cell consisted mostly of nuclear material and the German biologist Ernst Haeckel offered the view that hereditary traits had their origin in the nucleus of the cell. In 1865 discoveries of tremendous importance were announced by the Austrian monk Gregor Mendel, who, as a botanist, was interested in the many strange traits that appeared when plants were cross-fertilized. He experimented with garden peas for several years and ultimately became the first to establish the laws of heredity with mathematical accuracy. He observed that seeds of a given type bred true to this particular type. But when he made crosses between parent seeds different in a single trait (for instance, color) he found that the progeny had the appearance of one parent. This was the first generation cross, known as the first filial generation, the F_1 generation. In further generation crosses Mendel discovered that the characteristics from each parent were carried into the offspring. If yellow and green peas were crossed, for example, offspring would appear which would be sometimes green, sometimes yellow. The one trait, which in the F_1 generation had disappeared, now reappeared. Mendel decided that, although one trait seemed to have disappeared temporarily, both traits had been present all the time; one had had more strength than the other; he called the stronger trait *dominant* and the weaker trait *recessive*. After a great number of experiments he was able to express hereditary laws (fig. 3–1).

Mendel's discoveries were disregarded until the turn of the century, when scientific opinion became more receptive and the function of the chromosomes in the control of heredity was granted. Chromosomes could be observed under the microscope. Genes and chromosomes were found to have many traits in common, but it was obvious that chromosomes and genes could not be identical since man has only 46 chromosomes in each of his cells, yet the number of characteristics which man can inherit is much greater.

The genes, or hereditary material, are situated along the chromosomes. Each of man's chromosomes contains between 20,000 and

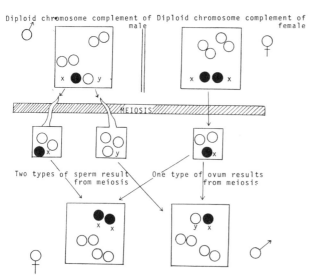

Diploid chromosome complement of male. Diploid chromosome complement of female.

MEIOSIS

Two types of sperm result from meiosis. One type of ovum results from meiosis.

Sex determined by the type of sperm entering the ovum

FIGURE 3–1. *Schematic diagram showing the pattern of inheritance as established by Gregor Mendel, the so-called Mendelian inheritance. (Adapted from James D. Watson,* The Molecular Biology of the Gene, *W. A. Benjamin, Inc., 1965, p. 19.)*

90,000 genes, the total of the human body being as many as 2,000,000. Normally genes are extremely stable and are exactly copied when chromosomes duplicate. A *mutation*, or change in a gene, occurs rarely and generally has harmful consequences. Mutations, however, are undoubtedly the basis for natural selection and for the evolution of the species. They are transmitted either as a dominant or as a recessive trait (fig. 3–2).

Among the many hereditary characteristics controlled by genes is the synthesis of enzymes, those proteins which catalyze, or facilitate, the chemical reactions taking place in our bodies. Much evidence suggests that a single gene controls the synthesis of a single enzyme. In order to analyze and to interpret all data available geneticists must work with the simplest organisms, such as bacteria and viruses. What we understand now of the molecular biology of the gene is the result of the indefatigable researches of many scientists, Kornberg, Lederberg, Watson, Crick, Ochoa, Khorana, Jacob and Monod, and others. All of these investigators utilized single-celled organisms for their research. In all probability the cancer cell will also have to be studied at the single-celled level if we are to learn the fundamental difference between a cancer cell and a normal cell, to understand its origin from a normal cell, or to convert it back to a normal cell once it has embarked on its wayward course. We must

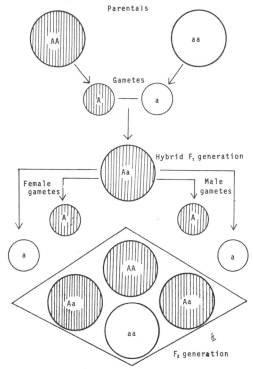

FIGURE 3–2. *The transmission of dominant and recessive traits. Shaded circles represent dominant characteristics; unshaded ones, recessive characteristics. The letter A represents the dominant gene; the letter a, the recessive gene.*

now look in simple terms at the process of cell division and cell differentiation, and at the possible distortions or the collapse of normal cell differentiation which might result in the development of the wayward cell.

CELL DIVISION

All cells differentiate, age, and die. It is in the act of dying that cells replicate, that one cell separates into two daughter cells in a process called *mitosis* (fig. 3–3). Before cell replication the chromosomes of the cell duplicate, so that each daughter cell contains the same number and the same type of chromosomes as the parent cell. This kind of cell is a *diploid* cell, ploidy being the term which describes variations in the number of chromosomes in a cell. In the case of sex cells, however, a different form of division called *meiosis* occurs. In this form the daughter cells contain only half the number of chromosomes and half the number of hereditary traits of the parent cell. These are called *haploid* cells. But when the male and female sex cells unite in the process of fertilization the total original number of chromosomes is restored, and the new cell is again a diploid cell. We shall return to meiosis in more detail later in this chapter.

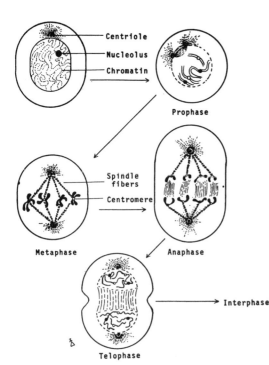

FIGURE 3–3. *The stages of cell division (mitosis). (Adapted from Herbert Stern and David L. Nanney,* The Biology of Cells, *John Wiley and Sons, 1965, p. 48.)*

MITOSIS

Cells divide at different speeds. Some of our body cells take approximately one hour to divide and reproduce. When the cell is at rest, that is, not involved in dividing and reproducing, we say that it is in the *interphase*. At this time the structure of the nucleus is not clearly discernible. The chromosomes lie in the nuclear sap in a mass of disorderly threads occupying the space of the cell nucleus. Then the activity of division begins: a group of rigidly determined events succeed one another. In the nucleus, the chromosomes gather at the center. Two small starlike bodies of the cytoplasm, the centrosomes, or centrioles, usually lying together near the nucleus, now travel to opposite sides of the cell. At this moment the cell membrane ruptures: all the rest of the mitotic process is going to take place in the cytoplasm. The cell takes an elongated shape; each chromosome doubles itself (let us remember that chemically it is composed of DNA, which has the capacity of reproducing itself); an equal number of chromosomes can now migrate to the poles of the cell. The chemical stages of mitosis are shown schematically in figure 3–4.

The first phase of cell division, called the *prophase*, is at an end. Another phase begins. For a short period, between one and ten minutes, the chromosomes lie waiting at opposite poles of the cell. The centrioles extend spindles toward the chromosomes. Each spindle attaches itself to each chromosome. Where it is hooked to the chromosome the spindle bends it in two, giving it a V shape; this point of attachment is named the *centromere*. Another phase, the *metaphase*, is now completed.

With the conclusion of the metaphase the *anaphase* begins. In the anaphase the cell begins to pinch itself in the middle, progressing to-

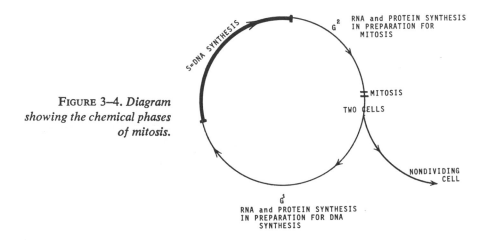

FIGURE 3–4. *Diagram showing the chemical phases of mitosis.*

ward its ultimate division. At the conclusion of the anaphase a nuclear membrane begins to develop around the chromosomes at both poles of the cell; the cell then passes over into the final phase of division, the *telophase*. In the telophase the chromosomes gradually return to the diffuse form that they assume and keep during the interphase or resting period: the spindles disappear; the cell terminates its pinching into two parts. Now the cell cycle is completed; two daughter cells are born possessing the same number and the same kind of chromosomes as the parent cell.

The process of cell division and reproduction described so far is typical of a normal cell: the two daughter cells which have emerged have not only a composition identical to that of the parent cell but also an identical growth potential prior to redividing. For a cell to remain normal it must have a normal mitosis, proceed to normal total differentiation, and achieve its life span with a continued differentiation of function. If, during mitosis, for instance, the cell division fails, a cell with two nuclei may be formed, or a cell may grow to twice its usual size but be controlled by a single fused nucleus.

Drugs such as colchicine interfere with the normal process of division and yield an abnormal cell. The cell then becomes not diploid but *polyploid*, containing an abnormally large number of chromosomes. The wayward cell, however, is abnormal in not quite the same sense: it is neither diploid, nor polyploid, but *heteroploid* (hetero = different). Often one hears reference to the rapid growth of cancer cells, but in fact a cancer cell may have a rate of growth identical to that of a normal cell. The abnormality of the cancer cell lies elsewhere, not in its frequent mitosis, but in its differentiation once division has occurred and in its differing total DNA and chromosomal content.

MEIOSIS

All the cells of our body reproduce through mitosis with the exception of our germ cells. A moment's reflection will tell us why these must behave differently.

Each human cell contains 46 chromosomes. An individual cell arises from the fusion of the male sperm cell (*male gamete*) with the female sex cell (*ovum* or female gamete). If each cell, male and female, contributed 46 chromosomes, the fertilized egg would have 92 chromosomes, not 46. Of necessity, then, each gamete, or germ cell, must contain only half the total number of chromosomes, or 23. The division and reproduction of germ cells is therefore different, showing a reduction in the total number of chromosomes during cell division. The process is called meiosis (fig. 3–5). The chromosomes replicate themselves but the cell divides into four instead of two daughter cells as in mitosis, so that each of the four daughter cells is then a haploid cell, that is, it contains half the normal number of chromosomes. The same process of meiotic division occurs in both the male and female germ cells. Of the four newborn cells, however, either male or female, only one survives. The other three are small and disintegrate. The union of the male sperm cell with the female ovum restores the cell to its full number of 46 chromosomes; half of the inherited, or genetic, material then comes from each parent germ cell. When the haploid (23 chromosomes) male germ cell fertilizes the haploid (23 chromosomes) female germ cell, a diploid cell comes into existence. This cell clearly contains 23 pairs of chromosomes, each member of the pair being of either female or male gamete origin.

FIGURE 3–5. *Shematic representation of the stages in sex cell division (meiosis). (Adapted from Stern and Nanney,* Biology of Cells, *p. 50.)*

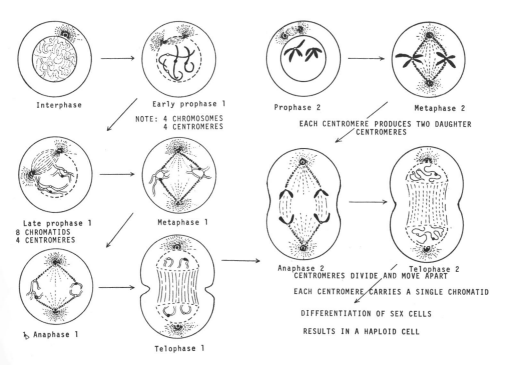

Interphase

Early prophase 1

NOTE: 4 CHROMOSOMES
4 CENTROMERES

Prophase 2

Metaphase 2

EACH CENTROMERE PRODUCES TWO DAUGHTER CENTROMERES

Late prophase 1
8 CHROMATIDS
4 CENTROMERES

Metaphase 1

Anaphase 2

Telophase 2

CENTROMERES DIVIDE AND MOVE APART

EACH CENTROMERE CARRIES A SINGLE CHROMATID

DIFFERENTIATION OF SEX CELLS

RESULTS IN A HAPLOID CELL

Anaphase 1

Telophase 1

At this juncture it is well to re-emphasize that chromosomes exist in pairs. When a haploid cell is born it contains, not *any* half of the number of chromosomes of the diploid parent, but always one half of each *pair*. Subsequently, in the union of the haploid female and male germ cells, resulting in a diploid cell, one of each of the paired chromosomes is contributed by the male and the other by the female. This explains the observation that certain genetic traits are sex-linked. The male of the species has a diploid chromosome of the XY type, while that of the female is an XX chromosome (see fig. 3–1).

In summary, meiosis reduces the parental chromosomes which permits certain traits to be carried by specific chromosomes which ultimately make a male or a female, depending upon the subsequent pairing of chromosomes during the mating process. The offspring continues to replicate and to differentiate in a diploid fashion except for its sex cells which separate as haploid cells, to return to the diploid state on subsequent fertilization.

THE DEVELOPMENT OF GENE THEORY

Mendel correctly interpreted the results of his plant-breeding experiments as indicating that various traits are controlled by a pair of "factors" which we now call genes: one factor being derived from the male parent, the other from the female parent. These genetic traits invariably followed the mathematical laws of division, multiplication and random crossover (fig. 3–6).

Mendel was also able to affirm that one gene may be dominant over another in the pair, and that some are sex-linked. The opposite version of a single trait he called "antagonistic"; today we name them *alleles*. By breeding out plants to the F_2 to F_{10} generations he showed that the dominant and recessive factors in the pair are independently transmitted and so are able to segregate independently during the formation of sex cells.

During the initial quarter of the twentieth century, genetics was largely studied with plants and the fruit fly, *Drosophila*. Thomas S. Morgan, who initiated genetic work with the fruit fly, later received the Nobel Prize for his studies in genetic mutation. The fruit fly re-

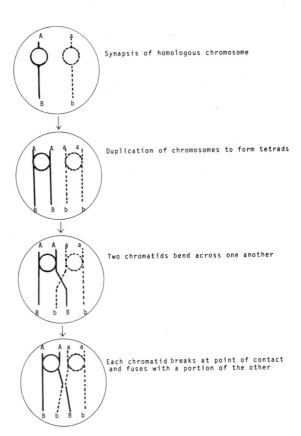

FIGURE 3–6. *Diagram illustrating the crossing-over of genes during synapsis. (Adapted from Watson,* Molecular Biology of the Gene, *1965, p. 26.)*

Synapsis of homologous chromosome

Duplication of chromosomes to form tetrads

Two chromatids bend across one another

Each chromatid breaks at point of contact and fuses with a portion of the other

produces every 14 days. It is exceptionally suited to genetic studies, owing to a curious fact that all Drosophila born in nature had red eyes; the gene responsible for red eyes was the "wild" type gene. Under laboratory conditions, however, the Drosophila often breed out with white eyes. The gene leading to white eyes was named a *mutant.* It became obvious that genes can change, or mutate, giving rise to new genes, mutant genes.

As soon as a large group of mutants became available for breeding analysis, it could be shown that two genes do not always assort independently. Examples of nonrandom assortment are demonstrated in the crossing-over of genes as shown in figure 3–6. Note that paired chromosomes break at about the same place and re-fuse at full length as the fragments cross over from one pair to the other.

The relationship of genes to chromosomes thus became established and it became possible to understand the hereditary variations formed throughout the biological world on the basis of genetic mutations. The process of genetic mutation must of necessity be a protracted one. Mutations unfavorable to organisms are rapidly discarded, and favorable mutations not only provide a slow definite source of variability but allow optimal adaptation of the organism to a changing environment.

In nature change is the exception, not the rule. Genetic information is transferred from generation to generation in almost miraculous exactitude and the transformation in forms of life is therefore very slow.

CHEMISTRY OF THE GENE

Scientists realized early that cells contained no atoms or chemicals unique to the living state. The same laws of chemistry therefore applied in the growth and division of cells as in chemical reactions within the test tube. It was known that both nucleic acids and proteins were present in chromosomes, but investigators had not elucidated the chemical composition of either. They logically assumed that the chemical structure of the gene must be copied exactly every time a chromosome divides and becomes two. They were aware that physical and chemical forces altered cell function, for experiments on the irradiation of cells showed that X-rays produced structural and functional changes in isolated cells. As early as 1927 Hermann J. Muller induced mutations in the fruit fly by exposing it to X-ray irradiation.

Still earlier, in 1909, the British physician Archibald E. Garrod had hypothesized that certain "inborn errors of metabolism" were due to the inability of the organism to form a particular enzyme. He studied a rare disease known as alkaptonuria, a condition in which the urine becomes blackened when exposed to air. In a patient affected by alkaptonuria, some normal chemical processes and transformations cannot occur—an enzyme is missing, a gene is defective, and a mutant gene has been inherited. Garrod was in effect pursuing the relationship of biochemistry to genetic variability, but the understanding of such processes was delayed for years until investigating scientists found some biological objects more suitable to genetic analysis than man.

The investigation of the control of organic characteristics by enzymes and of the control of enzymes by genes awaited the penetrating experiments on rapidly reproducing organisms such as molds, bacteria, and viruses, all of which fortunately contain nucleic acids, long recognized to be the prime chemical substances in chromosomes. The pioneering idea of Garrod then came under controlled scientific investigation, and finally E. L. Tatum and G. W. Beadle, working with a mold, *Neurospora*, proved beyond doubt that genes affect the synthesis of enzymes. For their work they won a Nobel Prize in 1958 —the concept of "one gene, one enzyme" became scientific theory, not hypothesis.

CELL DIFFERENTIATION

An egg cell is fertilized by a sperm cell. The cell which is formed divides in two, its two daughter cells into four, these four new cells into eight, and so on, until a total organism is completed. Fourteen days after conception the human embryo already has blood vessels, and the brain and spinal cord are beginning to develop. The cells have slowly begun to differentiate and to associate themselves with like cells. Brain cells have appeared. In time muscle cells, blood cells, and bone cells will appear. At the very beginning of embryonic life cells are undifferentiated—not yet organized into different tissues, organs, and functions. What determines the change from undifferentiated to differentiated cells?

One of the central and unsolved problems of biology today is how this process of cellular differentiation takes place during normal growth and development, and, as a corollary, how aberrations in the process which may lead to developmental abnormalities, or indeed cancer, come about. One attempt to portray this process graphically is shown in figure 3–7.

If we think of the infinitely complex structure and functioning of the human body, it is easy to realize that cells differ radically in their functions, that they organize and differentiate in amazingly diverse ways. There are differences between cells, both chemical and physical. These differences can be measured; they are, however, relatively insignificant. How are we then to account for the striking differences in cell functions? Again, we cannot, but we are beginning to have some idea of how differentiation occurs.

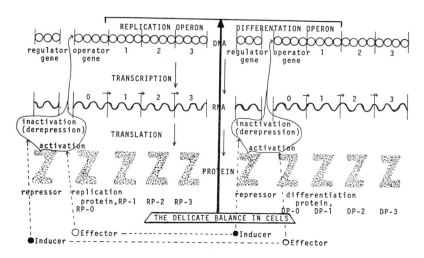

FIGURE 3–7. *The mechanisms involved in maintaining balance in cell growth, replication, and differentiation. Cancer may originate when these balances are upset. (Adapted from Henry S. Kaplan, "Some Possible Mechanisms of Car-cinogensis," in* Cellular Control Mechanisms and Cancer, *ed. P. Emmelot and O. Mühlbock, Elsevier Pub. Co., 1964, p. 378.)*

As we have already seen, all the information about cell functions and indeed about life itself is contained in DNA, the chemical consti-tuent of our genes. But each cell utilizes only the particular informa-tion which is necessary for its specific function. How? We have also noted that the "language of life" is contained in the four letters, A, G, T, C, standing for adenine, guanine, thymine, and cytosine, the four bases of DNA. A combination of three of these letters, or a *triplet*, codifies a particular function, as for example, the role of a certain amino acid in the cell (fig. 3–8). The essential information about a structure, or tissue, or organism, is imprinted along the length of its chromosomes in a code composed of triplets. The triplet code specifies one amino acid; a group of triplets specifies one amino-acid sequence, and it is called a gene. One gene controls one enzyme. A functional group of genes specifying a sequence of enzymes is called an *operon*. In the "language" of the DNA code, a triplet can be re-garded as a letter, a gene as a word, an operon as a sentence. When such "sentences" are combined into "paragraphs" or groups with a uniform purpose, we can describe them as a tissue. And when "para-

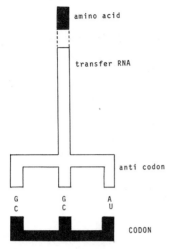

amino acid

transfer RNA

FIGURE 3–8. *Stylized representation of the way in which the function of an amino acid is coded into triplet codons for recognition and transmittal by messenger RNA.*

anti codon

G	G	A
C	C	U

CODON

graphs" join together into a "chapter" they are the equivalent of an organ. Finally the association of organs would correspond to a "book" or to a body.

In very simple terms the essence of differentiation is the choice of the activation of certain genes along the chromosomes with the repression of others. This simple concept has received experimental verification in the elegant studies at the Institut Pasteur by François Jacob and Jacques Monod, two Frenchmen who won the Nobel Prize in Medicine in 1965 for their work in differentiation.

Jacob and Monod worked with one of the simplest of living organisms, the colon bacillus, *Escherichia coli.* This bacterium contains a relatively small amount of total genetic material, is subject in its growth and differentiation to complexities similar to those of cells of higher organisms, follows the same chemical mechanisms for growth and differentiation, lives or dies in the presence of specific amino acids which can be readily identified and analyzed, survives despite an extremely high death rate, and multiplies rapidly. Indeed the progeny of a single bacterium dividing every 20 minutes without death of any of the offspring could in two days achieve a mass equal to the size of the earth! Jacob and Monod were able to show that cells contain "structural" genes and "control" genes; the control genes have the power to start and to stop the activity of the structural genes and ultimately to initiate or not initiate the formation of enzymes (fig. 3–9).

It is the interactions of multiple structural genes within a cell that determine the complexity and differentiation of the cell. The ultimate

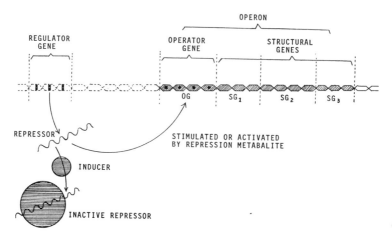

FIGURE 3–9. *Diagram showing the control of gene activation according to the Jacob–Monod hypothesis. (Adapted from André Lwoff, Biological Order, MIT Press, 1965, p. 59.)*

differentiation and complexities found in the cells of different tissues and organs is merely a detailed elaboration and amplification of the basic principles of cell organization and gene control. The common theme in cellular growth and differentiation is *gene control.* The variations of the theme include specific cellular enzymes, organization of like cells into tissues and organs, control of mitosis, aging, and death, and the balance between cellular regeneration and destruction. The coding of the cell is in its genes, and Virchow's "all cells are born from a cell" can be paraphrased as "all life forms are born from DNA."

Genes are activated or destroyed by chemical messengers voyaging within and around the cell. Extracellular or environmental factors also control the hereditary information. Thus differentiation is the result of complex intracellular and extracellular interreactions on the genes and their products, the enzymes. Tissues and organs, systems of like cells working cooperatively together, are sensitive to chemical messengers acting on them as targets: the well-established messengers which affect target tissues are called *hormones.* But recently some chemical messengers within tissue itself have been identified; these are called tissue *chalones.*

Each cell and each tissue has a specific potentiality for mitotic replacement and differentiation. In a long-lived animal any breakdown in messenger gene control mechanism (either within the cell or within a tissue) may lead to cancer. If control genes do not do their job properly in their direction of structural genes, it is possible that the ultimate deterioration of cell function and differentiation will occur and result in cancer. When there is a breakdown in tissue *homeostasis,* that is, its essential stability, a wayward cell appears. This process is carcinogenesis.

The single most important characteristic of every wayward cell, or tumor, is its abnormal growth. The primary damage is in the mechanism of cellular homeostasis, a mechanism identical in all cells of all tissues. We can liken this mechanism to rhythmic figures the molecular components of our genes weave along the thread of life under the masterful direction of chemical messengers.

4

THE TRANSFER
OF INHERITANCE

*"Life is the
co-ordination of actions."*
HERBERT SPENCER

The human mind has an innate need to organize into a coherent picture the complexities of the universe. With regard to living things man has succeeded in defining with mathematical precision a geometrical order in living structures, and in expressing in quantitative and qualitative chemical and physical terms the elements and forces which govern life.

Advances in the deciphering and ordering of the puzzle of life have been profoundly influenced by the scientific tools available to the researchers. But nowhere is the strange interplay of technological advances and geometrical and chemical ordering of biological systems better illustrated than in the deciphering of the genetic code, the molecular arrangement and distribution of the particles of life along the helical path of DNA.

ADVANCES IN BIOCHEMISTRY AND GENETICS

Before 1950, although geneticists were convinced that DNA was the main chemical substance in chromosomes, chemists knew very little about the structure of large molecules such as nucleic acids and proteins. During the 1950's, however, some remarkable new techniques were developed for molecular separation and purification. These included paper chromatography and ultracentrifugation.

Paper chromatography, a method utilizing filter paper and solvents, permits a visual display of molecular composition in a spectacular fashion. The different amino acids of the protein chain can be spread out by their varying rates of migration. Subsequent staining yields a multitude of colors over the paper and forms a design which biochemists can "read" as we read a sentence. The constituent amino acids of a protein can be carefully and beautifully analyzed. With ultracentrifugation techniques chemists are able to separate proteins by molecular weight, a feat impossible with the ordinary centrifuge. The ultracentrifuge can produce a centrifugal force 900,000 times as powerful as the force of gravity at the surface of the earth. Finally, an additional tool, X-ray crystallography, has permitted a three-dimensional view of the way molecules within proteins are linked together.

Back in the 1920's, the British biologist W. T. Astbury began making pictures of human hairs, demonstrating for the first time some geometrical order in biological structures, specifically in the hair protein, keratin. He had created the first spark of interest in structure as a function of order in biological systems. Much subsequent work was devoted to such studies.

In 1951 Linus Pauling surmised that the spatial structure of proteins was a helix, a figure similar to that of a circular staircase. This helical figuration he named the alpha helix (fig. 4–1). Shortly afterward (1953 to 1959) Max Perutz and John Kendrew in England, working with hemoglobin, the oxygen-carrying protein of our blood,

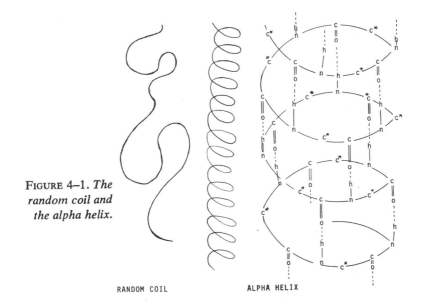

FIGURE 4–1. *The random coil and the alpha helix.*

RANDOM COIL   ALPHA HELIX

and with myoglobin, a muscle protein, and using X-ray diffraction techniques, could definitely demonstrate that proteins do assume a helical structure as postulated by Pauling.

The 1950's were an unprecedentedly rich period in discoveries for biochemistry. But during this time the geneticists too were active. They were deeply interested in large molecules, particularly nucleic acids, and they suspected that DNA and RNA were related to inherited traits in all species. They worked with single-celled organisms, both plant and animal, the chemical composition of which was by then known to be nucleic acids.

As early as 1944, a momentous discovery had been made by the biochemist O. T. Avery: he demonstrated that the hereditary properties of the pneumonia bacteria could be altered by the addition of DNA. The events leading to this discovery are worth mentioning. Pneumonia is caused by two different strains of pneumococcus, one smooth-coated, the other rough-coated. The British bacteriologist F. Griffith had found that if he injected a mouse with a mixture of live rough-coated bacteria and dead smooth-coated bacteria the mouse's tissues would show evidence of live smooth bacteria. The apparent impossibility of this situation had to be explained. It was first assumed that "something" in the dead smooth bacteria had influenced the live rough one. Avery and his associates discovered that the mysterious "something" was DNA. DNA from killed smooth pneumonia bacteria was capable of changing rough pneumonia bacteria to smooth bacteria. The transduction of bacteria through DNA was established; it had been proven beyond doubt that DNA, a synthesizable chemical, was related to genetic transmission of hereditable traits.

In 1947, Erwin Chargaff, applying chromatographic analysis, showed that there were only four *purine* or *pyrimidine* bases in DNA. Each of these bases went into a different nucleotide (the building blocks of nucleic acids). He also demonstrated that the amount of adenine, a purine base, equals the amount of thymine, another purine base, and the amount of cytosine, a pyrimidine base, equals the amount of guanine, the final pyrimidine base. These four bases—adenine, thymine, guanine, and cytosine—constitute the four different bases of the nucleotides of DNA. In addition, Chargaff showed that the amount and ratio of the four nucleotides vary from one species to another.

After the discoveries of Pauling, Avery, and Chargaff, it remained for James D. Watson and Francis Crick to consolidate them and heighten the interrelationship of chemistry and genetics with the Watson–Crick hypothesis. This hypothesis suggested that the nucleic acid molecule was a double helical structure (see fig. 1–4). The long spiral lines of the chain consisted of links of sugar to phosphate, and the crossarms, the steps of the spiraling staircase, consisted of the purine and pyrimidine bases—adenine, thymine, guanine, and cytosine. The details of the fascinating events which led to the Watson–Crick hypothesis are well described by Watson in his book, *The Double Helix* (1968).

The concept of the double helix revolutionized the analysis of genetical data and immediately suggested a way in which hereditary transmission is simple and feasible. It was suggested that one of these two intertwined strands of complementary structure serves as a specific surface, or template, upon which the other strand is synthesized.

Subsequent advances in molecular biology, gained through recent studies of bacteria and viruses, have augmented our knowledge to the point where, hopefully, this information may be applied to the elimination of diseases due to defective or altered or deficient genes. Ultimately this knowledge will bear on clinical cancer, for cancer, to the best of our present knowledge, can be included in this category of disorders in man. Diabetes, sickle-cell anemia (due to abnormally shaped and functioning red blood cells), and phenylketonuria (a cause of mental retardation) have already been proved to be due to altered or defective genes. Cancer, similarly, appears to result from a genetic change in the cell which may be either a direct mutation or an extragenomal or epigenetic defect.

But let us now seek answers to the questions which have the greatest relevance for our understanding of life, death, and cancer. How does a cell work to produce proteins and enzymes essential for life? How does a cell reproduce (or copy itself)?

HOW DOES A CELL WORK?

Since the days of Pasteur, in the middle of the nineteenth century, scientists have realized that living cells gain energy from sugar, carbohydrates, fats, and proteins. In 1897 Eduard Buchner crushed

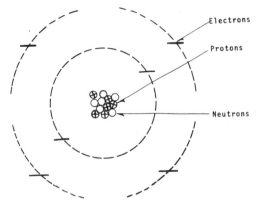

FIGURE 4–2. *Chemical properties of an element depend upon the number and arrangement of electrons around the atomic nucleus, which is occupied by protons and neutrons. Differences in number of neutrons alter the atomic weight of an element, yielding isotopes with different weights but identical chemical properties. (Adapted from James D. Watson,* The Molecular Biology of the Gene, *W. A. Benjamin, Inc., 1965, p. 117.)*

Electrons

Protons

Neutrons

yeast cells and extracted yeast juice which could carry out alcoholic fermentation in the obvious absence of live yeast cells. The subtle distinction between life and nonlife had become blurred—and all fermenting agents, whether in live or killed cells, were given the name of *enzymes.*

From 1900 to 1950 biochemists focused their attention on the problem of cells related to energy-producing reactions. During this period much was learned about the fine chemical structure of the cell and the nature of atoms and molecules within the living cell. Of the 103 known elements only six are of primary importance in the understanding of cell function. They are hydrogen, carbon, oxygen, nitrogen, phosphorus, and sulfur. Each atom of a particular element is composed of a central nucleus with a positive electrical charge, and a system of negatively charged particles, the electrons, which revolve around the nucleus at terrific speed. The concept of the atom can be traced back to the Greeks; it was Democritus (ca. 460 B.C.) who gave the name atom (indivisible) to the smallest possible particle of matter.

A single element may take different forms consisting of a collection of atoms identical in nuclear charge and number of electrons but slightly different in molecular mass (fig. 4–2). Their chemical properties do not vary noticeably but the slight difference in nuclear weight makes possible the separation of elements by different atomic weights into variants called *isotopes.* In other words, a particular element and its isotope have the same chemical composition but a different atomic weight. Isotopes are extremely important in modern chemistry and other sciences. Radioactive isotopes permit the tracking of elements

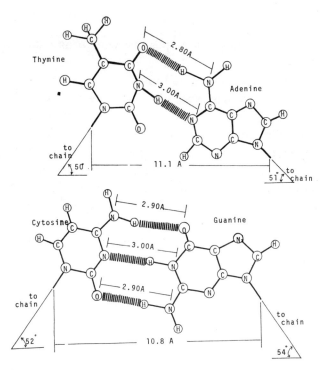

FIGURE 4–3. *The hydrogen-bonded base pairs in DNA. Adenine is always attached to thymine by two hydrogen bonds, whereas guanine always bonds to cytosine by three hydrogen bonds. All the hydrogen bonds in both pairs are strong, since each hydrogen atom points directly at its acceptor atom (nitrogen or oxygen). (Adapted from Watson,* Molecular Biology of the Gene, *p. 117.)*

in chemical reactions. As an example, radioactive carbon isotopes permit the tracing of carbon in plant photosynthesis.

When atoms are grouped together the resulting compounds are called molecules. Each molecule has a molecular weight equal to the sum of the atomic weights of its atoms. Atoms are bound together to form molecules by strong inner forces. Two atoms joined chemically are said to be bound by chemical bonds; this involves the sharing of electrons. A very strong type of bonding occurs when one or more electrons are shared by two atoms, a primary or covalent bond. These bonds, which have length and direction, give the substances bound together a physical configuration in space. But electrons are not always shared between atoms; one electron may jump from one atom to the other, giving one a positive charge and the other a negative charge—an ionic bond. Considerable energy is necessary to break these strong (covalent and ionic) chemical bonds.

There are other types of bonds between elements that are weak, not strong. The most important of these to our body chemistry is a type called hydrogen bonding. Large molecules like proteins are an aggregation of smaller polypeptide chains bound together through the mechanism of such bonding (fig. 4–3). These weak bonds can be easily broken by a change in temperature, yet restored by the return to the initial temperature. Hydrogen bonding governs the arrangement of the unique shapes and structures of the cell's chemical substances, particularly the proteins and the nucleic acids. Hydrogen bonding is all-important in the reproduction of nucleic acids: since it is weak it facilitates the separation of the two coils of a nucleic acid, permitting not only the initial separation but also the subsequent duplication and the re-aggregation of the replicated molecule with equal facility.

HOW DOES A CELL COPY ITSELF?

A cell's ceaseless metabolic activity depends upon the presence of specific enzymes and the availability of an external energy supply which comes through adenosine triphosphate, ATP. Enzymes are proteins. The number of proteins necessary for the life of the cell would be inordinately large if each different protein had to duplicate itself from the ground up. Therefore some sort of "copying surface," or "template surface," and a "code" for copying appear essential. Biologists knew that the nucleus of the cell was all-important in cell replication and reproduction, but it was only when cell division became observable under the microscope that the irregular rods in the nucleus, the chromosomes, were recognized to be the carriers of information, the blueprints so to speak, from the cell to its progeny.

A piece of hereditary information in control of a particular characteristic is located at a particular point on a particular chromosome. This is the gene. Genes control the life of the cell by directing the synthesis of enzymes and proteins. Enzymes and proteins consist of a linear linkage of some 20 essential amino acids. The concept of a template surface provides a workable scheme for cell replication and protein synthesis from the various amino acids. The template surface would merely serve to line up amino acids of proper sequence, and they could be attracted to the template surface by weak secondary forces, or hydrogen bonding.

The chemical components of genes are proteins and nucleic acids. But the nucleic acids are linked in a way unlike that of proteins. Proteins are linear links of amino acids, nucleic acids are links of nucleotides, each nucleotide being composed of a sugar molecule, a phosphate group, and either a purine or a pyrimidine base.

NUCLEIC ACID, THE REPLICATING MOLECULE

The complex interrelation of the chemical elements in DNA is shown in figure 4–4. We can see the linear chain of a sugar alternating with phosphoric acid, and the projecting bases at the sides, adenine and guanine (A and G), the two purines, and cytosine and thymine (C and T), the two pyrimidines. This spatial arrangement, first proposed by Watson and Crick, has been verified with the help of X-ray crystallography.

Watson and Crick's model explained the primary function of DNA which is to replicate. When a cell divides, the DNA in each daughter cell is identical with the DNA in the parent cell. In replication the DNA helix unwinds into two separate strands; this separation is facilitated by the weak hydrogen bonding between the paired bases;

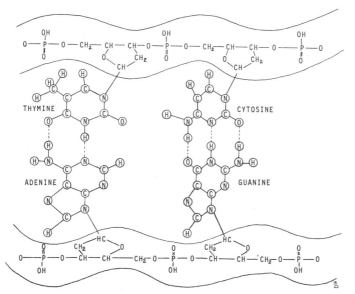

FIGURE 4–4.
Schematic diagram of the essential chemistry of DNA. (Adapted from Watson, Molecular Biology of the Gene, *pp. 133 and 304.)*

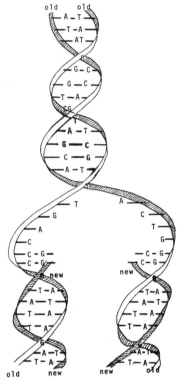

FIGURE 4–5. *Diagram showing the supposed action of DNA during replication. The older DNA carries a message (genetic code) as it unwinds. The newly synthesized DNA replicates the genetic message in the antecedent code. (Adapted from Watson,* Molecular Biology of the Gene, *p. 133.)*

each strand serves as the template on which the second half is paired off according to the Chargaff rules. Two double helices result, each being identical with the other and with the original double helix (fig. 4–5). Confirmation of this process has been secured by observation of DNA replication under the electron microscope and of bacteria growing in a synthetic medium: DNA replicates itself in exactly the manner predicted by Watson and Crick. It unquestionably performs the first function of life, namely, self-reproduction.

MESSENGER RNA, THE CARRIER OF THE GENE

We know that DNA is built along a linear sequence of bases and that proteins are built along a linear sequence of amino acids. We know too that one gene controls the formation of one enzyme. How is the base sequence in the chromosomal DNA transported into the amino-acid sequence of proteins of many different kinds? Since DNA is in the chromosomes of the cell nucleus and protein synthesis occurs within the cytoplasm, on the ribosomes, it is necessary for

DNA to do its work indirectly, through the intervention of an intermediary. This intermediary between DNA and cytoplasm, which carries DNA's message for protein synthesis, is called messenger RNA.

RNA is very much like DNA, but it differs in two ways. First, its sugar has an additional oxygen on its chain; it is a ribose sugar whereas DNA's sugar, with one less oxygen, is a deoxyribose sugar. Secondly, the bases in RNA are slightly different from the bases in DNA. Uracil (symbol U) takes the place of thymine; uracil is a pyrimidine base, and like thymine, pairs with adenine; the four bases of RNA are abbreviated A, G, C, U, instead of A, G, C, T.

There are three kinds of RNA in the cytoplasm: messenger RNA, already alluded to, ribosomal RNA, and transfer RNA. It is now possible to separate these three constituents and study them in what is called a cell-free system. When cells are crushed in a mortar the cells as such are destroyed but their constituents remain whole and active and their interactions can be observed. Protein synthesis can occur in a cell-free system with the introduction of energy in the form of high-energy phosphates.

The exact function of ribosomal RNA is unknown. But the function of transfer RNA is quite clear: we know that messenger RNA brings the instruction for protein synthesis from chromosomal DNA to the cytoplasm where it attaches itself to the ribosomes. But how do amino acids, which build up proteins, assemble in correct order? An adaptor molecule is necessary for this part of the process. This adaptor molecule is transfer RNA: on one end it hooks itself to the amino acids, on the other end to the exposed complementary bases on the messenger RNA. The transfer RNA and messenger RNA fit together like a lock and key.

There must of necessity exist at least 20 different transfer RNA's, one for each of the 20 amino acids essential for life. And in fact at least 20 different types of transfer RNA have been identified and 20 specific activating enzymes have found to attach each amino acid to a transfer RNA.

Protein synthesis can be observed with the help of the electron microscope. One sees the messenger RNA wrapping itself around the ribosomes of the cytoplasm at one end and the complete synthesized

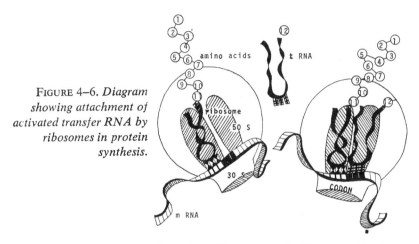

FIGURE 4–6. *Diagram showing attachment of activated transfer RNA by ribosomes in protein synthesis.*

protein being released at the other. The process is illustrated in figure 4–6.

Nucleic acids can truly be said to be the molecules of heredity in the living cell; DNA replicates itself, carries the information for the synthesis of proteins through the formation of messenger and transfer RNA. The coding of this information remains to be explained.

THE COPYING CODES

The language of life, as explained above, can be expressed in only four letters. We have already identified them to be A, T, G, and C. The emotions and feelings, the thoughts, valid or empty, which can be expressed in the language of the alphabet, are themselves the result of the language of life, of changes, mutations, degenerations, acceptances, and rejections which take place in the recesses of our cells.

Let us look at some possible arrangements of the four letters A, G, T, C, and relate them to words we understand. If we choose the three letters C, A, and T, we can assemble them thus:

—A C T, which reads act,
—C A T, which reads cat,
—T C A, which reads . . . nothing.

Suppose now that in C A T we insert G for A; the word C A T, or cat, now reads C G T, or nothing; it is a nonsense word (fig. 4–7).

What we have actually been doing by arranging the three letters

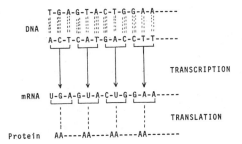

DNA T-G-A-G-T-A-C-T-G-G-A-A-----
A-C-T-C-A-T-G-A-C-C-T-T-----

TRANSCRIPTION

mRNA U-G-A-G-U-A-C-U-G-G-A-A-----

TRANSLATION

Protein AA----AA----AA----AA------

FIGURE 4–7. *Transcription, translation, and protein synthesis.*

into a meaningful or nonsensical word is a parallel of what occurs in DNA, of the way the four bases—adenine, guanine, thymine, and cytosine—assemble into triplets which are either useful and packed with meaningful information, or become erroneous, nonsensical, and ineffectual. By shifting these three letters a series of known processes recognized in the genes can be visualized. These processes can be called substitution, deletion, insertion, or the establishment of nonsense and gibberish by erroneous interchange of letters (fig. 4–8).

Much information about the language of life has been gained from the study of simple organisms—bacteria and viruses. They can be exposed to physical changes in the environment, for instance to irradiation; since X-rays can produce genetic changes in cells, these

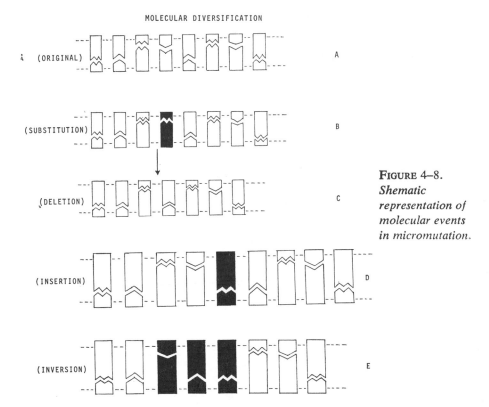

MOLECULAR DIVERSIFICATION

(ORIGINAL)   A

(SUBSTITUTION)   B

(DELETION)   C

(INSERTION)   D

(INVERSION)   E

FIGURE 4–8. *Shematic representation of molecular events in micromutation.*

changes, or mutations, can be studied and "read" in terms of new arrangements of the bases of DNA, the chemical constituent of our genes. Ultraviolet light, too, can be responsible for genetic changes, as well as certain chemicals (nitrous acid, for example, can turn cytosine into uracil). Radioactive fallout from nuclear weapons has been shown to have genetic effects, as on some unfortunate survivors at Hiroshima.

Mutations can be lethal or crippling but they can also be beneficial. Such beneficial mutations make evolution possible and in the not-too-distant future may hopefully be induced for the cure of inherited diseases.

Cracking the entire code of life would be simple if we knew the base sequence in messenger and transfer RNA. At the present time they are still unknown but scientists are coming closer to their discovery, and already they have decoded the bases of amino acids which, bound together, make up the proteins.

Transfer RNA is a relatively small molecule containing 70 to 80 nucleotide bases. Messenger RNA is longer, and genetic DNA is enormously longer, containing a million or more bases in the mammalian cell. There are a minimum of 1,500 nucleotides per gene, and 100 to 200 genes per chromosome. Because of the number of combinations possible, we are still a long way from knowing the base sequence of genes or chromosomes.

CODING FOR A SINGLE AMINO ACID

We know that the coding for the 20 amino acids essential for life resides in the four available nucleotide bases A, G, T, C. We are now going to examine why, as we have asserted before, the coding must be written in triplets of these four letters. If we conceived that one letter codes for one specific amino acid, we would obtain only four amino acids; if we had decided that two letters code for one amino acid, we would have $2 \times 2 \times 2 \times 2$, or 16 possible combinations from four different letters, thereby coding for 16 amino acids. We have not as yet reached the necessary diversity of 20 amino acids essential for life. We must then have at least three symbols for a given amino acid: a simple calculation shows that four letters taken three at a time will yield 64 different possible combinations, more than enough to specify, or code, for the 20 essential amino acids. The necessity of triplet combinations of bases has in this manner been demonstrated. It is pure mathematical logic.

With our 64 different codings for 20 essential amino acids we have in fact some 44 superfluous combinations; these combinations are called nonsense coding. Two or three different combinations can also code for the identical amino acid; scientists name this situation degeneracy within the code. It is possible that nonsense coding results in punctuation marks along the code and that ultimately the 44 superfluous combinations will provide for diversity and clarity within the code, for the beginning and ending of a human protein, for the punctuation marks and for the brevity which is essential for the coding of the 20 amino acids.

The first code deciphered for the identification of amino acids was made by Severa Ochoa when he showed that UUU (that is polyuracil) codes for phenylalanine (an essential amino acid) and that poly-UUU codes for polyphenylalanine (a peptide chain in which every amino acid is phenylalanine). Degeneracy of the code was established: UGA, UAG, UAA, were shown to be nonsense triplets, which apparently provide signals to the cell when one protein molecule is finished and another is to be started. These are the start and stop signals necessary for the beginning and ending of any given protein.

CELL-FREE SYSTEMS

The concept of a triplet code has received experimental proof in cell-free systems. We have said that a cell-free system is a mixture of the constituents of the living cell in the test tube: ribosomes, a supply of amino acids, some transfer RNA particles, activating enzymes, a supply of energy (ATP) are allowed to react and agglomerate in the test tube; then messenger RNA is added and the manufacturing of protein takes place (fig. 4–9). The ability of the cell-free system to work with an artificial messenger (a piece of synthetic RNA of known base sequence) has enabled scientists to determine the triplet coding for each of the 20 essential amino acids. The "dictionary" for amino acid and protein synthesis is now almost complete.

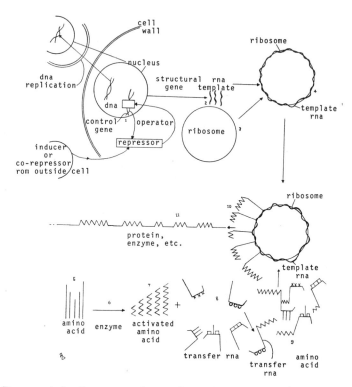

FIGURE 4–9. *Current understanding of protein synthesis by genetic replication and activation. (Adapted from Melvin Calvin, "Atom to Adam,"* American Scientist, *June 1964, p. 179.)*

5
VIRUSES, IMMUNITY, AND THE SYNTHESIS OF LIFE

*"Mysteries are not
necessarily miracles."*
GOETHE

More and more scientists have turned their attention to the study of the extremely small particles which exist on the borderline between life and nonlife. These simple forms of lifelike organisms are the viruses. Viruses can exist only as parasites on other living things. They have no ability to synthesize chemicals on their own but depend upon the metabolic function of their host for survival and reproduction. They attach themselves to human beings, animals, plants, and bacteria. In man they cause many diseases, from the common cold to poliomyelitis and possibly cancer. They definitely produce cancer in experimental animals. In the plant world, the best-known virus is the tobacco mosaic virus. As for bacteria, the viruses that attack and destroy them are called *bacteriophages.*

Viruses are very small but are still a thousand times larger than ordinary proteins and can be observed through the electron microscope. Their simple structure and rapid rate of reproduction make it possible to study mutations and the all-important process of *antigen-antibody* mechanisms within the cell. In this latter process, a cell attacked by a virus manufactures for its own protection the antibodies which will fight the viral antigens. Viruses have also been the material utilized by Arthur Kornberg in his recent work on the chemical synthesis of life, an incisive feat which he successfully accomplished in the late 1960's.

COMPOSITION AND ACTION OF VIRUSES

The two chemical constituents of a virus are the protein of its outer protective coat and the nucleic acid of its inner core, which may be either DNA or RNA (fig. 5–1). Viral nucleic acid can be isolated and subsequently injected into a host cell where it carries the code for its own replication and for the amino-acid sequences of its protein coat. This is true for RNA viruses as well as for DNA viruses and provides the only known situation in which genetic information flows from RNA to DNA instead of the usual opposite direction.

As soon as the virus invades the host cell the cell's normal pattern of replication is altered. The cell is now not only responsible for its own replication but is compelled by the virus to manufacture messenger and transfer RNA for the replication of viral DNA or RNA and the protein of the outer coat of the virus. The virus did carry the code for its own replication into the cell, but it is the host cell which must initiate and carry through the entire process of viral replication.

The viral nucleic acid may be either single or double stranded. The smallpox virus (DNA virus) has a double helical structure. The tobacco mosaic virus, the influenza virus, and the polio virus (RNA viruses) are single stranded. Whether the nucleic acid is DNA or

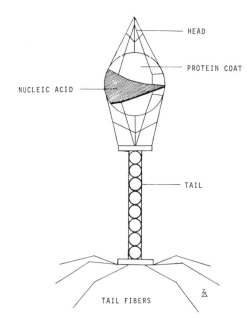

FIGURE 5–1. *Generalized model of a virus, showing the principal physical structures, the outer protein coat, and the nucleic acid core.*

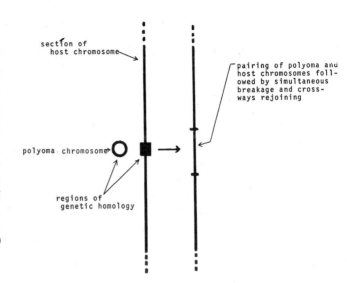

FIGURE 5-2.
Schematic diagram showing how the circular polyoma chromosome might integrate into a host chromosome. (Adapted from James D. Watson, The Molecular Biology of the Gene, W. A. Benjamin, Inc., 1965, p. 455.)

RNA, whether it is single or double stranded, the genetic information is present in the base sequences of its nucleotides. The proof that RNA is a genetic component has been gained from study of the tobacco mosaic virus: the protein shell and the RNA core are easily separated and infection of a host cell can be subsequently produced by the isolated RNA alone; the infection is identical whether initiated by pure RNA or the intact virus.

Once the virus has invaded the host cell the viral specific proteins are synthesized in exactly the same manner as ordinary proteins, but it is the viral messenger RNA molecules which attach themselves to the host's ribosomes (fig. 5-2). The types of proteins which form the coat of a virus are never found in a normal, noninfected cell, and are specific to a given virus. Exactly how the host cell releases the viral proteins is not known, but it has been shown that many bacteriophages have a gene which codes for a particular enzyme named *lysozyme*, a destroyer of the host cell's wall.

The metabolism of a cell is radically changed by viral infection and the cell becomes the servant of the parasite. This subservient relationship goes quite far since the cellular RNA never serves as template for the formation of new strands of RNA. The formation of RNA viruses requires from the host cell that it manufacture a new enzyme for this particular purpose only.

The reversal of the flow of genetic information whereby RNA viruses could induce genetic changes in the DNA of a cell defied comprehension until the brilliant work of Howard Temin in 1970. He proved that these RNA viruses possessed a new enzyme called RNA-dependent DNA polymerase. This enzyme converted the RNA of the virus into a DNA double helix. The new DNA strand then became incorporated into the genome of the host cell, changing it from a normal cell to a cancer cell. A new ray of hope emerged from this discovery with respect to the prevention or treatment of RNA-induced cancers. An antibody to this new enzyme could be produced, or the enzyme could be inactivated, thereby preventing or inhibiting the growth of the cancer. Unfortunately, this RNA-dependent DNA polymerase has now been discovered in many normal cells. It is, then, an exciting new discovery explaining the reversal of the flow of genetic information from DNA to messenger RNA to protein, but its significance and destiny remain to be elucidated.

REGULATION OF CELL DIFFERENTIATION

From a virus to a mammalian cell the degree of complexity in structure and function increases immensely. The smallest virus consists of only three to five genes, and since one gene codes for one protein, the smallest virus consists of three to five proteins. A bacterium is 10 to 100 times as complicated as a virus in genetic makeup, and a mammalian cell contains about a thousand times as much DNA as a single bacterium of *Escherichia coli.* A single bacterium can code for about a thousand proteins, but a mammalian cell might be capable of synthesizing more than a million different proteins.

Mammalian cells are far from being uniform. They are instead highly diverse, ranging from the relatively simple red blood cell (which has no nucleus) to the extremely complex brain cell. Despite our current knowledge, the mystery of the transformation of the fertilized egg into a multicellular organism has not been solved. The forces which control differentiation are still unknown. What impels the many divisions observed in the embryo to reach their complete and ultimate form? We do not know. What keeps a differentiated cell from reversing to an undifferentiated stage? We do not know. However, our current knowledge indicates that differentiation is probably linked to a specific activity at certain sites on the chromosomes. How a cell remains differentiated, or in some relatively rare instances returns to an undifferentiated state, how a normal cell becomes a wayward cancer cell, has been clarified by a concept introduced by Jacob and Monod, upon which we have already touched (see fig. 3–9). Some genes are assumed to be "structural genes" and some others "control genes." A structural gene is inactive, repressed by a repressor gene until an "operator gene" gives it the signal to function. "Cancer genes" are presumed to be present in normal cells but rendered inactive by "cancer repressor genes" and lashed into activity when "cancer operator genes" (or "cancer operons") give them the signal to go.

ANTIBODY SYNTHESIS

Investigation of the synthesis of antibodies offers promise as a means of studying cell differentiation. When a foreign substance, such as the antigen of a virus, invades the cell, the latter defends itself against this intrusion by synthesizing chemicals known as antibodies. This defense reaction is referred to as an antibody system. Two types of antibodies can be manufactured in our cells: (1) free-circulating proteins called humoral antibodies, and (2) cell-bound proteins called cellular antibodies. Figure 5–3 shows how the injection of an antigen

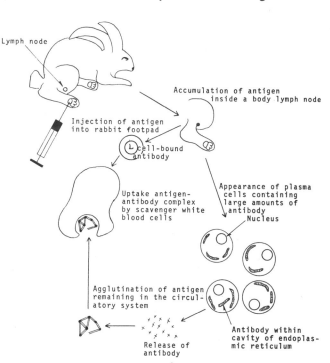

FIGURE 5–3.
Diagrammatic view of the sequence of events between the injection of an antigen and the appearance of circulating antibodies. (Adapted from Watson, Molecular Biology of the Gene, *p. 423.)*

into the hind foot of a rabbit initiates the production of both circulating humoral antibodies, and of cell-bound, or cellular, antibodies.

An antigenic substance must be at least the size of a virus to stimulate antibody production. But it is possible for a small molecule, which is nonantigenic, to become antigenic by association with a larger molecule such as a protein. Antigenicity does not reside over the entire surface of the molecule but in certain groups of atoms of the molecule which are named the *antigenic determinants,* and which nature provides in large quantities (approximately 10,000).

Much is already known about the nature of antibodies. For one thing they are all proteins. Most antibodies in man can be made to sediment in the ultracentrifuge and are classified according to their speed of sedimentation. Each antibody has two sites at opposite ends of its molecule where it combines with the invading antigens. These binding sites between antigens and antibodies are very strong and can paralyze, or inactivate, the antigen, thereby protecting the cell against its invader.

The action of antigens on antibodies is currently explained by the so-called *selective theory*: it is presumed that the contact of the antigen with the antibody-producing cell acts as a signal to the cell nucleus to produce the messenger RNA specific for the formation of antibody protein. Another theory, introduced by Sir McFarlane Burnet, proposes that each antibody-producing cell is able to manufacture a specific antibody; in other words a single-cell single-antibody theory. According to the theory, the antigen selects out its complementary cell and induces it to produce the complementary antibody. Furthermore it induces the cell to grow into a group of cells capable of producing the same antibody; such a group of cells is known as a *clone*, and the process as the clonal selection theory of antibody formation (fig. 5–4). This theory has received experimental confirmation from the study of plasma cells, which produce free-circulating, or humoral, antibodies.

FIGURE 5–4. *Schematic representation of the clonal selection theory of antibody production. (Modified from Sir Macfarlane Burnet, "The Mechanism of Immunity,"* Scientific American, *Jan. 1961, p. 11.)*

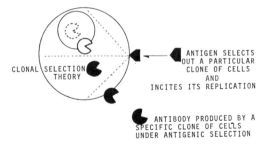

CLONAL SELECTION THEORY

ANTIGEN SELECTS OUT A PARTICULAR CLONE OF CELLS AND INCITES ITS REPLICATION

ANTIBODY PRODUCED BY A SPECIFIC CLONE OF CELLS UNDER ANTIGENIC SELECTION

An antigen may be accepted by an organism in a phenomenon known as tolerance. This situation is explained by the absence or destruction of clones of cells which would ordinarily produce antibodies for the annihilation of this specific invading antigen. When an antigen is totally rejected, the phenomenon results in a state of immunity, which is the opposite of tolerance. The explanation is the growth of a large number of clones of cells which produce antibodies capable of destroying the invading antigen.

The balance between antigens and antibodies in organisms is expressed in situations varying from total tolerance to total immunity. Here the concept of *immunological tolerance* should be introduced, for it is important in the study of cancer (see fig. 5–5). Cancer cells are abnormal cells which grow in a state of variable tolerance in the host's organism. Sir McFarlane Burnet has offered a hypothesis which explains how an organism "recognizes" self from nonself. During embryonic life the individual "learns" to distinguish self from nonself through the destruction of clones of cells which would produce antibodies against self, so that at birth the organism will have retained only those clones of cells which produce antibodies against

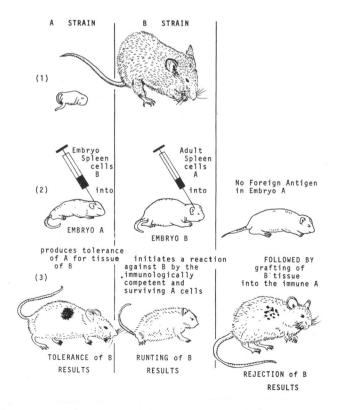

FIGURE 5–5. *Procedure followed in producing immunological tolerance by intraembryonic injection of foreign antigen. (Modified from Burnet, "The Mechanism of Immunity," p. 6.)*

A STRAIN   B STRAIN

(1)

(2)   Embryo Spleen cells B   into   Adult Spleen cells A   into   No Foreign Antigen in Embryo A

EMBRYO A   EMBRYO B

produces tolerance of A for tissue of B   initiates a reaction against B by the immunologically competent and surviving A cells   FOLLOWED BY grafting of B tissue into the immune A

(3)

TOLERANCE of B RESULTS   RUNTING of B RESULTS   REJECTION of B RESULTS foreign substances, nonself. Such a process of immunological maturation does indeed occur, as Sir Peter Medawar has shown experimentally: if an antigen is injected into an embryo before maturation the antigen is accepted as self and no antibodies are formed against it. After birth the animal retains its tolerance of the foreign substance, still accepts it as self. The animal is said to be in a state of "acquired immunological tolerance."

It would seem simple to isolate antibody-producing cells and to study them outside the body. Yet all attempts at the production of antibodies at this level have been unsuccessful. Apparently antibody production occurs only in an intact animal; it is therefore probable that an unknown substance necessary for the antigen to initiate the production of antibodies is present in the animal. It is hoped that antibodies will one day be synthesized in a cell-free system and in a single-cell system. If this becomes possible the still unknown substance could be added to the ribosomes, messenger RNA, transfer RNA, and necessary enzymes in the test tube to produce antibodies.

Let us repeat that an organism "recognizes" self from nonself early in life and that an embryo injected with a foreign protein cannot in later life form antibodies against this particular protein; it is then in a state of acquired immunological tolerance. Let us also remember that it is the balance between antigens and antibodies in the organism (in terms of strength and amount) which is at the basis of immunological tolerance.

At this point certain basic questions concerning cancer present themselves:

Does the cancer cell contain a foreign antigen or does it lack a specific antigen which would permit the normal checks and balances?

Why isn't the cancer cell, if foreign, rapidly destroyed (since it appears in adult life)?

Would it be possible to make cancer cells produce antibodies more actively by joining them with other known antigenic molecules?

Is the antibody produced by the cancer cell a humoral antibody or a cellular antibody?

These questions and others will be discussed in detail when we approach a better understanding of antigen-antibody reactions in chapter 14 dealing with immunology in cancer. For the moment it will be useful to examine the recent exciting work of correlating chemical structure with biological function, the synthesis of infective DNA, by Arthur Kornberg, Mehran Goulian, and Robert Sinsheimer, of Stanford University and the California Institute of Technology.

SYNTHESIS OF BIOLOGICALLY ACTIVE DNA

We have analyzed in the preceding chapter the chemical structure of living things and are now led to ask the next logical question: would it be possible to take these known chemicals, allow them to react together in the test tube, and obtain a biologically active, "living" product?

In the early 1960's Arthur Kornberg had already succeeded in synthesizing DNA in the test tube and had discovered the particular enzyme, DNA replicase, to catalyze the reaction. However, the DNA he obtained was not biologically active; it had the same chemical and physical structure as DNA in nature but it lacked the essential characteristics of life.

Kornberg and his associates continued with their work and in 1968 their skillful and elegant experiments were entirely successful. DNA from an infectious virus (phage X 174) was introduced into the test tube as the template, or "printing press," for its duplication; to it were added nucleotides of adenine, thymine, guanine, and cytosine—the building blocks of DNA—and the indispensable enzyme or catalyst, DNA replicase. Not only did the viral DNA copy itself but it was biologically active, or "alive," for it was infective—it could penetrate host cells and give birth to more viruses like itself (fig. 5–6).

At this point one may well ask how this achievement, however remarkable, relates to cancer or to other diseases in man. We know that some viruses (the polyoma virus for one) produce cancer in experimental animals. Following Kornberg's techniques, it is conceivable that we may be able to synthesize polyoma viral DNA. We might then be able to determine what nucleotide base sequence could convert a normal cell into a cancer cell. Control of sickle-cell disease and of diabetes could similarly be attained, since both of these diseases are known to alter or delete the DNA chain. It has been recently shown that pieces of DNA capable of replacing or repairing a defective cellular DNA can be carried into animal cells by agents such as nonpathogenic viruses.

We are reaching the stage when we will know where particular genes reside on the chromosomes, and which gene is related to a given disease. In the words of Arthur Kornberg (1968): "This is a contribution that must come from the chemist, the biologist has neither the tools nor the disposition to solve such problems and regrettably our support for the chemist has lagged woefully behind our support for the disease-oriented biologist. . . . To sum up, the synthesis of biologically active viral DNA would appear to have significance for future medical progress provided it can be translated into basic understanding of the mechanisms subserved by DNA in the genetic control of both normal and aberrant physiological functions. Such translation will depend upon our ability to mobilize resources, particularly those encompassed in the discipline of nucleic acid chemistry for the development of methods of analysis and modification of animal and human metabolic and bio-synthetic processes."

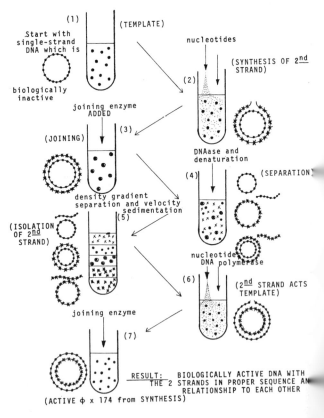

FIGURE 5–6. *Stages in the synthesis of biologically active DNA. (Adapted from Arthur Kornberg, "The Synthesis of DNA," Scientific American, Oct. 1968, p. 77.)*

6

NORMAL CELLS TO
CANCER CELLS: VIRAL
CARCINOGENESIS

*"Not versions,
but perversions."*
ST. JEROME

With the basic information which we have gleaned from the preceding chapters we are now ready to deal more directly with the subject of cancer. We can relate what we have learned about viruses and genes to experimental cancer in animals. We know that single-stranded viruses, composed of either DNA or RNA can produce cancer in animals, but there is as yet no evidence that this is true for cancer in man. Viruses are the simplest form of life, possessing only one to a few genes, and are relatively simple to study, but mammalian cells are much more complex and differentiated and, therefore, the study of cancer in higher animals and man is extremely complicated.

Cancer is one of the most intractable, variable, and incomprehensible forms of cellular derangement. A cancer is a *crab* as its name indicates. It claws at us, it hides in the sands of our flesh; like a crab it ignores straight walking, progresses sideways both in its refusal to behave in an honest, purposeful manner, and in its need to invade neighboring tissues and to shoot some of its cells far away from its point of origin, that is, to metastasize. Truly cancer is a fundamental derangement of the normal mechanisms controlling the rate of growth, division, and wandering of cells. But before we plunge into

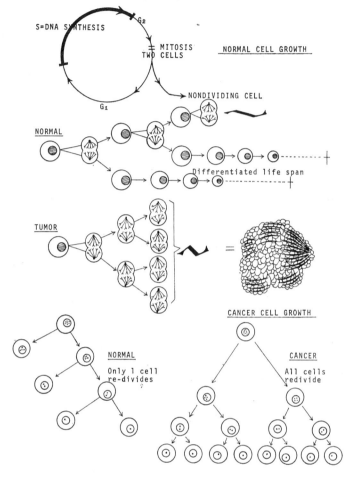

S=DNA SYNTHESIS

G_2

MITOSIS
TWO CELLS

NORMAL CELL GROWTH

G_1

NONDIVIDING CELL

NORMAL

Differentiated life span

TUMOR

CANCER CELL GROWTH

NORMAL

Only 1 cell
re-divides

CANCER

All cells
redivide

FIGURE 6–1. *Normal cell growth compared to growth of cancer cells. (Modified from Henry S. Kaplan, "Some Possible Mechanisms of Carcinogenesis," in* Cellular Control Mechanisms and Cancer," *ed. P. Emmelot and O. Mühlbock, Elsevier Pub. Co., 1964, p. 374.)*

the mysterious sea of human cancer it might be well to relate some absorbing observations on the interrelationships of genes and viruses to experimental cancer in animals. We shall thus greatly increase our chances of understanding the disease in man.

Cancer is related to abnormalities in the molecular order of cells, a subject which has been discussed in some detail in chapter 4. From a normal, useful cell, a cancer cell can be born. But whereas normal cells divide and stop dividing after a certain fixed time, cancer cells do not. They do not "know" when their division is to be stopped and they proliferate in an anarchistic fashion (fig. 6–1). What complicates the matter is that we have very limited knowledge of what tells a normal mammalian cell to stop dividing. Bacterial cells and viruses keep on growing until they exhaust their sources of food and energy but mammalian cells must live in balance. The balancing factors are not definitely known: they may be immunological in character; they may be the regulator genes mentioned in chapter 3. Despite our uncertainty about these processes, information is gained every day and hopefully we shall soon know enough to reach a better understanding of the mechanisms and life of the cancer cell.

GENERAL BIOLOGICAL NATURE OF CANCER

As soon as cells become cancerous they lose their ability to control their growth and division. Not satisfied with uncontrolled growth they can penetrate the blood and lymph streams which become dangerous underground rivers for carrying the illness in our bodies. Thus cancer cells can emerge in parts of the organism at a distance from their point of origin. They are said to metastasize, and the sites of distant spread are called metastases.

A cancer cell grows by forming a continuous mass of cells called a *tumor*. Cancer cells have different degrees of affinity for each other, which accounts partly for their propensity to metastasize. An *invasive* cancer cell is a cancer cell that has a great predilection for spreading rapidly and uncontrollably.

Even though our knowledge about the division of normal cells is limited, we do know that they stop growing when they touch each other if placed on a solid surface such as that of a glass slide. This mechanism of growth control is called contact inhibition (see fig. 1–2). Cancer cells, however, growing in the same conditions, do not stop proliferating; they have lost contact inhibition. While normal cells grow on solid surfaces in single layers, cancer cells show less affinity for the solid surface and grow in irregular masses several layers deep.

This loss of the ability of one cell to control its relation to its neighbor, this loss of contact inhibition, manifests itself in the capacity of the cancer cells to disseminate. Normal cells stick to one another and have a "home" of their own. A kidney cell stays in the kidney and a lung cell in the lung. Cancer cells may be said to belong nowhere, to have no proper residence, no "home." This characteristic is extremely puzzling if we compare the chemical composition of both normal and cancer cells, for they have the same components, although in slightly different amounts and relationships. For instance the DNA content of a cancer cell is greater than that of a normal cell. But cancer cannot be explained on the basis of these chemical differences at the present time. Perhaps when we know the entire sequence of the nucleotide bases in a single mammalian cell and in a single cancer cell we may be able to define the differences in chemical terms.

Cancer can be induced experimentally in animals by external agents called carcinogens. Once a cell has changed from normal to cancerous its succeeding generations are cancerous too; this is true at the cellular level only, for a mother cannot (except in unusual circumstances) transmit cancer to her child.

We know that cancer cells remain generally cancerous. The transformation is permanent, yet theoretically reversible. But we do not know why or how cells become cancerous. There are, however, three main hypotheses about human cancer, the outgrowth of experimental and clinical observations.

1. Cancer is due to an accumulation of somatic mutations.

2. Cancer is due to viruses.

3. Cancer is an instance of a generally irreversible de-differentiation within the cell.

It is not possible at the present time to study either normal or cancer cells at the molecular level, as is done for viruses and bacteria. Much can be learned, however, from the study of viruses as causes of experimental cancer in animals.

VIRUSES AND CANCER IN EXPERIMENTAL ANIMALS

No human cancer has been shown to be related to a virus, except possibly the Burkitt lymphoma, which is endemic in some parts of East and South Africa. However, as early as 1908, Wilhelm Ellerman and Bernard Bang of Copenhagen postulated the existence of a tumor virus when they transmitted a type of leukemia in chickens by inoculation of cell-free filtrates. In 1920 F. Peyton Rous was able to transmit a fowl sarcoma by the same means. The sarcoma had developed spontaneously in a Plymouth Rock hen. For years it was believed that viral tumors occurred only in fowl until in 1932 R. E. Shope found small tumors under the skin of the paws of a wild rabbit.

He transmitted tumors to both domestic and wild cottontail rabbits by cell-free tumor extracts; it was thus demonstrated for the first time that a mammalian tumor could be caused by a virus.

Then in 1942 J. J. Bittner found that a breast tumor in the mouse was attributable to a virus. This tumor could be transmitted "vertically," that is, from mother to offspring, through the milk of the mother. He initiated a group of precise foster-nursing experiments with two inbred strains of mice, one cancer-free and the other cancer-prone. He found that if the suckling young of the cancer-free strain were nursed by a cancer-prone mother they developed mammary tumors; if cancer-prone young were nursed by a cancer-free mother they developed no mammary tumors. Later the actual virus was identified with the help of the electron microscope and it was proved beyond doubt that the viral particle was transmitted through the maternal milk.

In 1957, Sarah Stewart, Bernice Eddy, and others isolated the polyoma virus from mice. As its name implies the polyoma virus can cause a variety of tumors in mammalian species. As a result of these discoveries we now regard viruses not only as particles that will kill cells as they multiply within those cells, but as specific particles of new genetic material which, once introduced in the cell, may initiate cancer.

GENERAL NATURE OF VIRAL TUMORS

Most tumor-producing viruses are likely to produce cancer in newborn animals rather than in wild animals of adult age. The newborn laboratory animal has an immune system that is not fully developed, a tolerance that is great, and a resistance that is low to the introduction of foreign substances, or foreign antigens. Two types of transmission are possible: vertical transmission from generation to generation through the female ovum or through the milk of the mother (as in mouse mammary cancer), and horizontal transmission (far less common) by cross-infection from one individual to another.

Tumors produced by viruses are comparable to all other tumors, but viral tumors have an antigen specific for each particular virus, whereas chemically induced tumors have antigens that are different for each tumor, even if produced with the same chemical. This specific antigenicity of viral tumors has been an invaluable research discovery aiding the study and identification of viruses capable of inducing cancer.

Viral cancer may be initiated by either DNA or RNA viruses. The best-known DNA virus, the polyoma virus, produces a variety of tumors when injected into a newborn animal. The best example of RNA virus is the Rous sarcoma virus. Each type will be discussed separately since they probably act differently in producing tumors. It has recently been shown that in DNA viruses the DNA commonly has a ring form; this structure may be responsible in part for the virus's *oncogenic* (cancer-producing) quality, for ringed viruses may be more readily integrated into the cell, being more resistant to destruction by cellular enzymes.

When infected by a tumor-producing virus a cell undergoes a morphological transformation observable in tissue cultures; the cell grows out as a clone of cells lacking contact inhibition and the number of abnormal cells is in proportion to the dose of virus injected.

THE POLYOMA VIRUS

The polyoma virus is a DNA virus which normally grows in rodents. As noted above, it can initiate a variety of tumors when injected into newborn animals. It is a small spherical virus which contains enough DNA to code for only five proteins at most. Since it codes for only five proteins and since one protein represents one enzyme which is coded for by one gene, it would contain only five genes. The length of the DNA chain in nucleotide units is thus small enough so that we could optimistically hope to work out the entire sequence of the nucleotide bases in these five proteins within the next few years. In the polyoma virus one gene must code for temperature dependency of the virus, another for its ability to produce thymidine-kinase, a newly identified enzyme, and a third for the viral antigen which gives it its immunological specificity. The coding for cancer transformation must reside then in a very short segment of the viral DNA chain, and at least for the DNA virus, we should reasonably soon be able to know the sequence of the nucleotide bases which renders the virus capable of inducing cancer in experimental cells.

A cell invaded by a polyoma virus has two possible fates: the most common is its destruction through the multiplication of the virus; the other is its transformation into a morphologically distinguishable cancer cell. The characteristics of such transformed cells are increased growth potential, lack of contact inhibition, and the ability to form tumors on subsequent transplantations. This kind of transformation is called a neoplastic transformation (neoplastic indicating new form).

A neoplastic transformation is caused by the DNA of the virus. The viral gene becomes incorporated into the DNA of the transformed cell. Experimental evidence has demonstrated that its action is only transiently required. In the transformed cell the function of the viral gene is abolished at 39° C and present at 31° C; it is possible to turn off or turn on the function of the mutated gene by altering the temperature from the higher to the lower state. If the cell is first transformed at 31° C and the temperature then raised to 39° C the cell remains transformed, which shows that the mutated gene's action need only be temporary for the transformation of the cell, or, in other words, for its incorporation into the genome of the cell. This also indicates that one of the genes of the virus codes for temperature dependency.

Tumors induced by the polyoma virus possess a specific antigen which elicits the production of antibodies by the invaded cell. Adult rodents will develop antibodies against the tumor-producing virus and tumors are thus relatively rare in nature in adult animals. But tumors can be induced easily in newborn laboratory animals because these newborn animals are immunologically immature and accept the foreign virus in a state of immunological tolerance. For the host to survive it must establish its immunological defense, by producing a specific antibody against the DNA core of the virus which contains a "transforming principle." The newborn laboratory animals develop tumors from the action of the "transforming principle" since they are immunologically immature, and unable to produce the necessary antibodies.

After its transformation, the invaded cell contains a viral chromosome—also called a *provirus*—integrated into one of its chromosomes. Part of the secret of cancer may reside in this provirus, and one part of the answer to the riddle of cancer may be the identification of this provirus and of its effects upon the cell.

Since the polyoma virus is so small and its DNA codes only for three to four proteins at most, it should not be too difficult eventually to find the exact differences between the composition of a normal cell and that of a transformed cancer cell. The genes coding for temperature dependency and viral antigenicity and specific enzyme production (thymidine-kinase) are already known to be distinct from the remaining three or four genes, any or all of which can code for the production of cancer. With the aid of amino-acid analyzers and computerization of data, it is hoped the entire code of DNA viruses will soon be established and the cancer-producing gene identified.

ROUS SARCOMA VIRUS

We know that not all cancer-producing viruses contain DNA. The Rous sarcoma virus (RSV) which produces sarcomas and *leucoses* in chickens is a single-stranded RNA virus, member of a group of viruses collectively named myxoviruses. The Rous sarcoma virus contains 40,000 nucleotides, is six times larger than the polyoma virus, has 10,000 amino acids, and codes for 25 different proteins. When infected by a single RSV particle a normal cell is almost immediately transformed into a cancer cell; this fact makes the RSV particle extremely interesting from the standpoint of the relationship of RNA to genetic replication to cancer.

The RSV infected cells grow in tissue culture on glass surfaces, proliferating and piling up to form masses of cells that show evidence of a loss of contact inhibition characteristic of cancer cells. In the early 1960's Harry Rubin discovered that when single cells are infected by single RSV particles the induced cancer cells do not release any virus; they have become nonreproducing cells, and the infecting virus has seemingly vanished into the cell in rendering it cancerous. He then found that these tumor cells can produce RSV particles if they are super-infected with a related virus which he called the Rous *associated* virus (RAV), or Rous *helper* virus (RHV) (fig. 6–2). The addition of RAV to a transformed cell resulted in the production of both RAV and RSV particles within 24 hours (fig. 6–3). This led him to the conclusion that RSV is a defective virus,

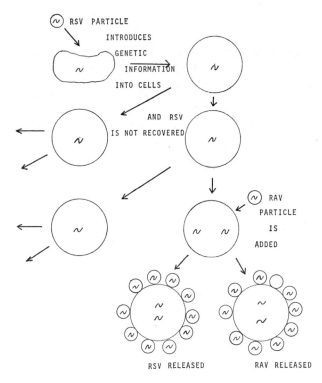

FIGURE 6–2. *An infection by a single Rous sarcoma virus (RSV) particle introduces RSV genetic information into a normal cell. The cell is transformed and the RNA genome is replicated each time the cell divides. (Adapted from James D. Watson,* The Molecular Biology of the Gene, *W. A. Benjamin, Inc., p. 463.)*

and that it requires a helper virus such as RAV for its reproduction. Specifically RSV is defective in the production of its protein coat and needs the cooperation of RAV for the synthesis of this coat. It thus needs RAV to become complete; on its own it is only capable of replicating its inner RNA core. The completion of the RSV virus which can occur only with the help of the RAV virus is accomplished by the pinching out of a portion of the cell membrane of the infected cell.

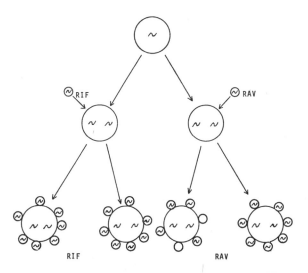

FIGURE 6–3. *Stages in conversion of a nonproductive RSV cell into virus-producing cells by the addition of helper viruses. (Adapted from Watson,* Molecular Biology of the Gene, *p. 465.)*

What has become known about RNA viruses could conceivably be related to human cancer. It is possible that human cancer could be produced by viruses, but that the offending viruses, being defective, would be identifiable, complete with their outer protein coat, only when an associated helper could also be found. The search to find the offending cancer virus may require the isolation first of the appropriate associated virus. A most encouraging development in this regard is the recent discovery of the technique of cell fusion, or cell hybridization. By the use of this technique under appropriate experimental conditions the genes of one cell can be forced to fuse with the genes of another cell, producing a hybrid. Newly discovered hybridization techniques for the study of sections of nucleotide bases in the DNA of cells may soon enable us to isolate the cancer section of the DNA chain, that is, the small portion of the DNA chain which codes for the process of neoplastic transformation.

NEW DIRECTIONS IN VIRAL CANCER RESEARCH

The investigations of the viral induction of cancer have not yet given us much understanding of the changes cells undergo when they become cancerous. Nor do we know when cancer cells become entirely autonomous after their conversion to the neoplastic state by DNA or RNA viruses. But these investigations can lead the imaginations of research workers into new pathways in the fullest sense of what William Blake once wrote: "To the man of imagination nature is imagination itself."

One can speculate about a number of important questions:

Is the striking feature of the Rous sarcoma virus—its inability to manufacture its own protein coat, that is, its defectiveness—related to its high carcinogenic capacity?

How do other viruses, which are not defective, produce cancer?

Does the RNA of the Rous sarcoma virus produce mutations in the DNA of the cell nucleus it invades? We may recall that here there is a unique instance of a flow of information from RNA to DNA instead of vice versa.

Has the membrane of a cell infected by an RSV particle a role in inducing cancer? The defective virus's coat is made of a portion of the invaded cell's membrane, yet this ability to form an outer coat on the viral particle and concurrently to kill the cell takes place in certain viruses only with the intervention or association of a helper virus. It is possible that a cell attacked by a viral particle has its cellular membrane so altered by the entrance of the viral DNA into the cell that the cell is thereby released of normal contact inhibition and becomes a cancer cell through loss of normal cellular membrane function.

What can be learned from the antigenicity of a viral cancer cell? We have seen that cancer-producing viruses possess specific antigens which elicit the production of antibodies by the infected cell but that the RSV particle, although able to produce cancer on its own, is weakly antigenic. Only when associated with a helper virus does RSV obtain its outer protein coat and thereby become highly antigenic.

Will the identification of antigens produced by viruses enable us to discover the offending viruses in human cancer?

Will the discovery of helper viruses and the subsequent identification of defective viruses permit the development of vaccines against viral cancer?

It must be emphasized that at the present time no human cancer is known to be produced by a single virus. Recently, however, many tumors detected among children in certain parts of Africa (Burkitt lymphoma tumors of the lymph nodes) have been strongly suspected of being due to a virus. These tumors are very similar to those of Hodgkin's disease and to lymphoblastomas in general (other types of lymph gland tumors which occur in man) as well as to leukemias. It is well known that leukemias in animals are due to a virus and it is likely that leukemias and lymphoblastomas will be the first human tumors in which a virus will be isolated. At the present time, however, one cannot say that the viruses are specific causes of any tumor in man, and one must also realize that these viruses can be nonpathogenic passenger viruses, in association with cancers which are produced by other causes.

In any case, the relationship of viruses to human cancer remains one of the fruitful and fertile fields of current research in cancer. Since the action on an infected cell by DNA viruses is not the same as that of RNA viruses, different methods of investigation will be required. It might be possible to detect DNA viruses through the antigens they produce. It might be possible to detect RNA viruses through their associated helper viruses, or through cell hybridization techniques. It would be extremely helpful if we could obtain cell transformation by viruses in tissue culture from mammalian cells, thus establishing the cancer-producing potential of viruses for human cells. Some of the cellular changes induced by small viruses which code for cancer are already known. They include:

Proteins of the viral particles (two or three polypeptide chains),

Tumor antigen,

Ts — a function for replication of viral deoxribonucleic acid (DNA),

Induction function for replication of cellular DNA and synthesis of cellular enzymes,

Modification of thymidine kinase,

Helper function for adenovirus replication.

Recently, Dr. Maurice Green and others have begun to link viral genes to human cancer by new testing techniques. Their methods may soon enable us to know how viral genes are grafted into the host's normal genetic makeup (fig. 6–4). A time may thus be envisioned when malignant transformation, or cancer, may be linked to certain proteins specific for tumors, proteins synthesized in the cell by the command of the viral genes. The continued study of these parasites of living cells may break their code, which dictates the synthesis of only 5 to 20 proteins. Within the comparatively short length of the DNA chain reside the gene, or genes, coding for neoplastic transformation and antigenic specificity. It is far simpler to break the code of a viral cell and decipher the portion of the DNA chain encoding for cancer and cell differentiation than to struggle needlessly and prematurely with the mammalian cell which is a thousand times greater in the length and complexity of its DNA chain.

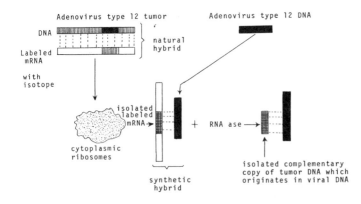

FIGURE 6–4.
*Identification of viral genes linked to cancer.
(Modified from K. Fujinaga and M. Green,* Scientific Research, *Sept. 1966, p. 44.)*

PART TWO

THE CLINICAL PROBLEM

7
THE HISTORY
OF CANCER

"Science, ever since the time
of the Arabs, has had two functions:
one, to enable us to know things,
and, two, to enable us to do things."
BERTRAND RUSSELL

In his story "The Doctor" Chekhov tells of a little boy who is dying of a brain tumor. His description of the mother's grief and of the atmosphere of doom surrounding her is compelling. Chekhov uses simple words, which, better than any ornate prose, express the emptiness and despair in the mother's heart. "The doctor went slowly back to the drawing-room. There it was by now dark, and Olga Ivanovna, standing by the window, looked like a silhouette. Not a sound floated in from the outside as though the whole world, like the doctor, were thinking, and could not bring itself to speak. Olga Ivanovna was not weeping now, but as before, staring at the flower-bed in profound silence." Earlier the doctor had told her, "We must look the hideous truth in the face. . . . Such cases never recover."

This was written in 1887. In 1884, for the first time, a brain tumor had been removed by a British surgeon, Sir Rickman John Godlee. If the skills and techniques employed by Dr. Godlee, or even more advanced ones, had become widely known in Russia in 1887, perhaps the little boy of Chekhov's story could have been saved, perhaps his mother could have been spared her ordeal. This history of medicine presents us constantly with such tragic eventualities; it mirrors the human condition with its struggles, discoveries, errors, failures, and successes. The history of cancer, in particular, is the story of human struggle against tremendous odds, of slow advances, of many setbacks, and of some successes.

When there was no knowledge of anatomy, of physiology, of pathology, or of the nature of illness there could be no knowledge of how to treat it. The doing was blocked by the absence of knowing. Illness appeared to be a magical interference with life and was treated magically. With the development of observation and the very beginning of experimentation, ill health was attacked in an empirical manner, on a primitive trial-and-error level. When the knowledge of anatomy, physiology, and pathology increased, sounder foundations could be established for the diagnosis, treatment, and cure of illness. The discovery of the microscope, of asepsis, and of anesthesia brought greater possibilities for correct diagnosis, and greater safety and comfort in the treatment of patients.

After the first experiments using controlled biological studies in animals, the discovery of X-rays and radium, and with the advent of biochemistry, research on the nature of cells and the effects of heredity and environment on cellular processes emerged and began to make great progress. As a result of the discovery of bacteria and viruses, of recent findings in immunology (the study of the natural resistance of the body to illness), and of new theories on the nature of life and the structure and function of the cell, we have been able to move from the darkest ignorance to more and greater clarity, increased knowledge, and therefore augmented power to prevent and control cancer. That the path is not at an end, that there is more to be studied and discovered, one cannot deny. But already much has been accomplished.

Today one cancer patient in three is being saved from cancer. According to recent figures given by the National Health Education Committee it was only a few years ago that one out of four or fewer patients were being saved, so that "there is a gain of lives saved of some 47,500 patients each year" at the present time. However, the same committee reported in June 1967 that "a hundred uranium miners have died of lung cancer and perhaps a thousand more will die because they have for too long breathed radioactive dust in poorly ventilated mines." In the same report we could read that hundreds of men forty years of age and younger had died of lung cancer after smoking two to four packs of cigarettes a day for fifteen years.

After reading such reports, we may be tempted to echo the opinion that cancer, in spite of medical progress, is a disease of civilization, and that it increases with advances in our technology. And yet it is a very old disease. Several million years ago a dinosaur could be a victim of bone cancer, as fossilized remains discovered in Wyoming have shown. Perhaps other forms of cancer existed in those remote times, but bones are the only vestiges of extinct animals and therefore give a record of bone cancer alone.

Cancer in the ancestral species of man is more than a million years old. Some traces of it have been found in an anthropoid unearthed in Java in 1891. In antiquity the oldest evidences of cancer are Egyptian and Indian. Bone cancer is identifiable in some mummies discovered in the Great Pyramid of Gizeh. The Edwin Papyrus (2500 B.C.), the Leyde Papyrus (1500 B.C.), and the famous Ebers Papyrus (1500 B.C.) describe symptoms of cancer and primitive forms of treatment, such as the use of the knife. From the Hindu epic, the *Ramayana*, we learn that arsenic pastes were administered as long ago as 500 B.C. as a treatment for cancerous growth. Hippocrates (about 400 B.C.) describes many forms of the disease, among them cancer of the breast, uterus, stomach, skin, and rectum. From him we have inherited the term carcinoma (Greek *karkinos*, crab—the great veins sometimes surrounding the malady were compared to the claws of a crab). But treatment in those days was crude, employing caustic pastes and cautery, although Hippocrates had the wisdom to advocate *no* treatment for what he called occult cancer and which would nowadays be called deep-seated cancer.

Hippocrates enunciated the humoral theory of disease, which was to form an integral part of medical history for centuries. According to him there were four humors—blood (from the heart), phlegm (from the head), yellow bile (from the liver), and black bile (from the spleen). If the four elements were not properly balanced, bodily health would be impaired and illness would appear. Hippocrates believed that the black bile was mainly responsible for cancer. His theory of humors, although erroneous, demonstrated clearly his certainty that illness originated from natural causes, in contrast to beliefs in the magical, diabolical, or divine interference with human health.

Approximately four centuries later, in the first century A.D., the Roman physician, Aurelius Cornelius Celsus, was the first to operate on cancer, and during the operation to *ligate* blood vessels. He knew about the invasion of distant sites by original cancer cells. He described the appearance of secondary tumors after the primary one had been removed, and he was aware that certain tumors were painless and silent until they grew large enough to ulcerate.

Two great personages in the medical world of the second and third centuries A.D. were Leonides of Alexandria, and the Greek Galen, who practiced and taught medicine in Rome. Leonides greatly improved the technique of ablation of the breast, mastectomy; he used a scalpel, and with the help of cauterization, prevented hemorrhage and destroyed possible remnants of cancer. He was a clinician as well as a surgeon and was the first to describe retraction of the nipple in cancer of the breast.

Galen advocated the black bile theory of cancer, and his considerable influence blocked discoveries about the nature of the disease until after the Renaissance. Nevertheless he was the first to correlate psychosomatic problems and emotions with an understanding of cancer. In his treatise on tumors he wrote that melancholic women are more prone to breast cancer than sanguine women, a view which, obviously much modified, is supported and extended by psychological research into cancer today. It is also of interest to note, since one may wonder how primitive surgery without anesthesia could be tolerated by patients, that Galen prescribed poppy-seed infusions for the soothing of pain. Morphine is the modern derivative of the poppy seed and is used extensively for the alleviation of pain and suffering in cancer.

Arabian physicians of the twelfth century, Avenzoar and Averrhoës, used esophageal sounds to diagnose cancer of the throat and to improve feeding of patients whose esophagus was obstructed by cancer. Their clinical description of stomach and esophageal cancer is accurate, but they were greatly handicapped by the fact that the Islamic religion forbade both dissection and surgery.

During the Middle Ages, all scientific learning went into an eclipse, medical learning included. Even the "father of surgery," Guy de Chauliac (1300–1368), brought nothing new to the treatment of cancer. Galen's thoughts were still an influence and continued to be so in the practice of the later surgeon, Ambroise Paré (1510–1590). Another surgeon of the Renaissance, Fallopius (1523–1562), preferred caustic pastes to surgery in the treatment of cancer. It is perhaps worthy of note that there has been a return to the use of caustic pastes, as in the method of chemosurgery advocated by Dr. Frederic Edward Mohs in certain cases of face, head, and neck cancer.

The modern era of cancer surgery really began with the breakthrough of the accomplished German surgeon, Fabricius Hildanus (1560–1634), who excised axillary lymph nodes in the treatment of breast cancer. The difference between benign and malignant tumors was clarified shortly after Hildanus's time by Marcus Aurelius Severinus. In the eighteenth century the first cancer hospital was founded in Reims, France. At that time cancer was considered to be contagious and persons sick with various forms of the disease were avoided like lepers. It is easy to imagine that the new hospital must have presented a haven to the unfortunates whom everyone shunned and abandoned. Regrettably, it was possible to accommodate only a limited number of patients.

Eventually the French surgeon, Henri Ledran (1685–1770), rejected the humoral theory of cancer. He showed the path through which the illness spreads along the lymph stream and the appearance of metastases, as in cancer of the breast when a secondary involvement appears in the lungs. He also advocated surgery as the only treatment for cancer and discarded all pastes and ointments.

Discoveries were made in many directions during the latter part of the eighteenth century. The first experiments on animals were begun. Occupational cancer, in the form of scrotal cancer of chimney sweeps, was described (1775) by Percivall Pott. He noted that chimney sweeps were in the habit of taking off their clothes to perform their work and that prolonged irritation from contact with soot often produced cancer of the scrotum. Advances in pathology came through the work of John Hunter, René Laënnec, and Marie François Bichat, who espoused a concept of cells as basic units of tumors. The French gynecologist, Joseph Récamier, who spoke of generalized cancer, described invasion of the bloodstream by cancer cells. It was he who coined the term metastasis to describe the establishment of secondary cancer centers in the body as a result of the transportation of cancer cells by lymph and blood.

Bichat was able to affirm that the basic unit of tumors was the cell even though he did not use a microscope. Johannes Müller, in Germany, advanced the knowledge of pathology by an extensive study of diseased tissues with the help of the microscope, and his student, Rudolf Virchow, who became the eminent pathologist of the nineteenth century, brought this knowledge to its logical culmination when he was able to declare "every cell is born from another cell." Although it was known that all tumors, benign or malignant, were constituted of cells, their origin was not yet clear. As late as the middle of the nineteenth century, a great physician like Alfred Velpeau in France was still influenced by the old humoral theory of disease and of cancer as being caused by black bile. Virchow dispelled these false beliefs with his cellular theory of cancer.

The modern understanding of cancer stems from the work of Louis Pasteur and Joseph Lister in the late nineteenth century. Pasteur discovered that bacteria existed in the air and that since, as he maintained, lifeless matter could not produce life, all infection was due to a proliferation of micro-organisms. Lister opened the door to modern aseptic surgery in the treatment of cancer with his insight of the problem of asepsis and antisepsis. Deaths due to infection following surgical operations were gradually eliminated.

Toward the end of the nineteenth century in Germany, Christian Billroth, Alexander von Winiwarter, Wilhelm Freund, Themistokles Gluck, and others began to perform cancer operations with better success and on a larger scale than ever before. Hysterectomy and laryngectomy became possible. At a time when the uninformed public believed in the incurability of cancer, Winiwarter showed that out of 170 patients who received surgical treatment for breast cancer eight (4.7 percent) survived and were in sound physical health three years or more after successful surgery. The scope of surgery was rapidly extended by the control of infection and by improvements in anesthesia and management of shock. Godlee, Harvey Cushing, and others opened the field of neurological surgery in the treatment of brain tumors and these operations soon became comparatively safe.

Early in the twentieth century the American surgeon, William Halsted, enunciated his classic surgical principle in the treatment of cancer, namely, that the lesion, together with the regional lymph nodes, should be removed in an attempt to prevent metastases. This principle is best illustrated in his radical mastectomy operation for cancer of the breast. His method is still widely practiced today. High standards in the surgical treatment originated by Halsted have been extended until today cancer in any area of the body is accessible to the benefits of surgical therapy; indeed operations of enormous scope and magnitude are possible through ensuing advances in our understanding of asepsis, anesthesia, the metabolic responses of the body to surgery, and the control of shock.

The increasingly rapid improvement of the treatment of cancer through surgery within a single century may be exemplified by comparing the experiences of three U.S. presidents, Thomas Jefferson, Ulysses S. Grant, and Grover Cleveland (Marx, 1960). Jefferson's constant abdominal pains in his old age are assumed to have been caused by cancer, but nothing could be done to help him. Grant had a cancer at the root of his tongue which was inoperable at the time; he was given sedatives in the form of cocaine and morphine, but no other form of treatment was then (1885) available. (During his illness he was writing his memoirs, work that demanded a tremendous efort. Dictation had become impossible, for cancer had invaded his vocal cords, and he went on with his writing without the help of a secretary, displaying great courage and endurance.) Only thirteen years after his death radium was discovered by the Curies and shortly thereafter an entirely new field of treatment for this particular cancer became a reality.

By 1893, however, when Grover Cleveland was found to have cancer of the left upper jaw, surgery was possible. The president was taken aboard a private yacht which was equipped with an operating theater; within a short time he underwent two operations in circumstances of great secrecy, due to the political and economic situation, for the country was in a difficult financial crisis. This surgery, which cured his cancer, went unknown to the public and indeed remained a secret for the next fifteen or twenty years, until the president's death from unrelated causes. The surgeon who performed the operations, Dr. John Erdman, of New York, died only a few years ago.

Until the brilliant discoveries of Wilhelm Roentgen and Pierre and Marie Curie, surgery remained the only successful treatment for cancer. In 1895, Roentgen discovered some unknown rays which were to become very important in the diagnosis and treatment of cancer. As he was working in his laboratory, experimenting with a vacuum tube through which an electric current passed, he noticed that a nearby piece of paper coated with barium platino-cyanide was giving out an unexpected glow. He placed different materials between the vacuum tube and the treated paper and found that some substances stopped the glow while others did not. He had the proof that certain rays emanated from the vacuum tube, and that denser materials interrupted them but lighter ones did not. The rays are sometimes known as roentgen rays, but more often by the name he gave them, X-rays.

Three years later, the two great French scientists, Pierre and Marie Curie, made another outstanding discovery when they found a new element in the ore pitchblende, which had already yielded uranium. This element they named radium. They found that the radiations emitted by radium are much more intense than those which uranium was already known to discharge. Unfortunately, Pierre Curie died in an accident only a few years after the discovery of radium. Nevertheless his remarkable wife continued their work and as a result received two Nobel Prizes and was the first woman to teach at the Sorbonne and the first woman to be admitted to the French Academy of Sciences. She was also the first victim of the study of radium, which kills as well as heals; she developed anemia from protracted exposure incident to her long years of research with this radioactive element.

Both X-rays and radium can be dangerous and doctors and researchers have had to learn how to protect themselves from prolonged contact with radiations. But as the first cures by roentgen rays and radium were effected, the first deaths from exposure to radiations occurred too. A patient with an epithelioma of the cheek was cured after X-ray treatment. In the same period a man employed in a factory making roentgen tubes developed an ulcer in an arm, the arm had to be amputated, and he finally died after a recurrence of the ulceration in the axilla. The first treatment of cancer with radium was accomplished in a case of carcinoma of the face; the cancer healed.

But meanwhile, one of the pioneers in radium therapy fell a victim to his work: the surgeon, Robert Abbe, died of anemia like Marie Curie after long exposure to radiations.

Many lives have been saved and will be saved by radiation therapy. Many lives are saved by the utilization of X-rays for the diagnosis of cancer. It is right that we pay tribute to those who died in pursuing the selfless researches that led to these indispensable tools. Among many others is the French physician, Jean Bergonié, who, with L. Tribondeau, gave us the Law of Radiosensitivity. Bergonié died in 1925 from cancer caused by X-rays. First his fingers, then one of his arms, had to be amputated. He finally developed pulmonary metastases, which ultimately caused his death.

The Law of Radiosensitivity first expressed how cancer cells, which reproduce in volume at a higher speed than normal cells and which do not possess the latter's elective functions, are more affected by radiations than normal cells. "The greater the reproductive activity of the cell, the less definitely fixed their morphology and functions, the more intense the action of X-rays upon them." Because of the formulation of the law, it is possible to use X-rays in such a way as not to harm healthy tissues. Bergonié did not die in vain.

The twentieth century has seen further dramatic improvements in the understanding and treatment of cancer. To surgery and irradiation, the current mainstays in the treatment of cancer, has been added a third promising avenue of therapy, *chemotherapy*. Whole families of drugs have been discovered which have remarkable influences on the growth of cancer cells and on the mechanisms whereby cells replicate, transmit, and translate genetic information. These new drugs not only influence the cancer cells themselves, but have many effects on bodily processes in the individual harboring cancer. It is conceivable that we may soon be able, not only to destroy or to attenuate the cancer cell itself, but also to strengthen the bodily processes involved in resistance to, and destruction of, the cancer cell within the tumor-bearing host. But these new adjuncts in the treatment of cancer are at the very forefront of our knowledge and will be discussed in detail in later chapters. For the moment we shall have to note our current inability, despite surgery, irradiation, or chemotherapy, to cure cancer in a high proportion of cases, and to emphasize the importance of early diagnosis in achieving successful treatment by present therapy.

Much of the current success in early diagnosis is due to increasing public awareness of the warning signs of cancer. This is largely because of the efforts of the American Cancer Society in publicizing the warning signals. Thanks to their energetic campaign men and women are better educated today than formerly about cancer and they know that certain signs require an examination by a physician. They also know that time is important, that they must not postpone a visit to the doctor if suspicious signs appear. Every time a women sees her gynecologist for a Pap test, every time she reports a lump in her breast to her doctor, every time a man or woman tells his physician about a sore which refuses to heal, a persistent bleeding, a change in an ordinary mole or wart, reports constant indigestion, or difficulty in swallowing, or persistent cough or hoarseness, a change in bowel habits, they help not only themselves but others as well. The habit of caution, the knowledge of danger signals is being spread throughout the community; prompt reporting to a physician decreases the possibility of advanced cancer in the individual and protects society as a whole.

Many years have passed since Chekhov wrote the dramatic story of a mother's desperation in the face of a hopeless illness. Great progress has been made since then in the treatment of cancer. It seems fitting to end with another story that is not fictitious but may appear undramatic and even commonplace in the light of today's knowledge. It is only one example of how lives are saved every day almost routinely, and how cancer is fought successfully when it is discovered at an early stage.

While she was taking her morning shower, a woman discovered a small lump in her right breast. She was a physically and mentally healthy person, was not alarmed, and knew that it was unwise to conceal what she herself had found. That very day she saw her physician, who told her that the lump was very small, that it might disappear within a week or so, but that if it did not she must come again to have it excised and examined under the microscope. Here our patient made a mistake of a kind that needs to be guarded against. Since she felt well, the initial reassurance of the doctor was misinterpreted and she neglected to return. A few weeks passed. Then the doctor called, reminding her of the necessity of a second examination. The concern of the doctor prompted her to go in immediately. The lump had not disappeared and she was informed that she must undergo surgery for the removal of the tumor and possibly a mastectomy (removal of the breast) if the biopsy showed positive signs of cancer. She received the news calmly. Once in the car on her way home, she felt tears come to her eyes. She was more surprised than frightened: Why should I be so weak? she wondered. Surprise overwhelmed her. She was stunned. There was a 50 percent chance that the tumor might be malignant her doctor had said. He had been direct, frank, matter-of-fact in a kindly way. At the moment of their conversation she had sensed only the necessity of the operation. Now strong emotions possessed her, more violent as the minutes passed. She thought: How little one knows about oneself. Is it the uncertainty which is frightening? Is it the inner compulsion to present a dignified composure? Is it the struggle to remain proud and calm in view of possible physical deformity? Her husband comforted her. A drink, a good meal, a laugh at her sensitivity, all contributed to a return of inner peace.

The next day, upon entering the hospital, she was nervous again. The efficient, friendly air of the hospital, the sunny soft evening, a light, amusing book reassured her again. A sympathetic talk with her doctor, then a sedative, brought a quiet, peaceful sleep. In the morning she was ready, without fear or unpleasant anticipation. A smile returned to her face as she was wheeled to the operating room. The preoperative medication had made her relaxed and comfortable. The anesthetists pierced the skin of her arm with a needle and quickly she slipped away from the world and from herself.

When the woman awoke in the recovery room, she felt pain but drifted back to unconsciousness in the next instant without noticing that the clock on the wall had indicated the passage of several hours; far too much time had passed for the performance of a simple biopsy. But she was beyond caring one way or the other. All she wanted was sleep and freedom from pain. Later when she had regained consciousness in her room she realized that several hours had passed, that she was having far more discomfort than she had anticipated from a simple biopsy, but she did not want to know the truth. Shortly the doctor appeared and explained that the tumor in her breast had indeed been cancerous, that a radical mastectomy had been performed, that everything had gone well, and that she would recover.

The words penetrated her consciousness slowly. She understood them as soon as she was physically ready to hear them. The doctor was clear and gentle. The truth now came flooding in. She was conscious enough to understand that it was better to know than to be left wondering and worrying alone in the night ahead. She looked at her husband who was too moved to speak, and she smiled. She had decided to show calm and equanimity. She had just decided that she was an adult and must not feel sorry for herself. She had just decided that she was one of the lucky ones, whose condition had been discovered in time for a practically certain recovery.

From this reaction and some of her former ones we may conclude that this woman was a rather nervous person, an easy prey to emotions. Her decision to show a façade of courage and equanimity may not have been the most realistic of decisions, not even the best in the circumstances. It is better to admit and accept sorrow and shock as such rather than to deny them. One need not give in to excessive emotions, but discussing them with others without too much pride is probably the healthiest approach.

A beautiful and rapid recovery ensued, despite the woman's somewhat unsuccessful attempts to control her complex emotional responses to her physical deformity. The sense of physical well-being gradually overcame her anxieties and painful reflections. A few weeks after the operation she could swim again. A month later she could play tennis and was astonished at the ease with which she could use her right arm. Good muscular command gave a great boost to her morale. She felt part of the world again, able to return to former activities, to forget herself, and to lead a perfectly normal existence.

A simple story? Yes. Nothing dramatic about it. Many of us will recognize ourselves in this patient. Even her mistakes, her shortcomings, are of a simple order. Almost everyone makes them. None of us is very different in our responses to illness or disease. The only marvelous aspect of such a commonplace happening is that something like it occurs every day, that countless patients are protected from cancer invasion around the clock all around the world.

8
ENVIRONMENTAL CARCINOGENESIS

*"There is nothing
in the whole world
which keeps its form."*
OVID

It must be remembered that cancer is a disease of the whole organism. It possesses attributes ranging from unrestricted growth to invasiveness. The disease also displays metastasis, transplantability, autonomy, lack of contact inhibition, and a number of other disturbed biochemical characteristics. Therefore many phenomena have to be investigated to reach an understanding of environmental carcinogenesis. These include the cancer-producing properties of certain chemicals, the effects of radiations, the influence of hormones on cell growth and differentiation, and the control mechanisms which govern the cell. However, it can be said that the very beginning of the cancer process is a change within the cell, or a mutation.

Living organisms not only grow and differentiate, but they change and they transmit their change to the progeny. All these manifestations of life take place in the molecules which constitute our cells. In this book we have approached some of the intricacies of molecular biology and we have considered genetic change, the process of mutations called mutagenesis. Yet the road from mutagenesis (changes in the chromosomes) to carcinogenesis (development of cancer cells) is neither straight nor clearly defined. Certainly not all cellular mutations can be equated with cancer nor do they necessarily lead to cancer, nor are they inevitably irreversible.

It is true that many agents that are mutagenic, that is, responsible for cellular mutation, are also carcinogenic, capable of inducing cancer, but a direct correlation between mutagenic and carcinogenic potentialities remains to be established. We know that if a mutation occurs within the cell it may initiate cancer. Let us consider this eventuality. First, for a mutation to happen an agent foreign to the cell constituents is needed. We have already discussed the changes that can be brought about in cells by viruses. In chapter 12 we will describe the cellular changes produced by X-rays. A number of agents then are capable of producing cellular mutations and sometimes ultimately cancer. These agents are listed in the following tabulation and various cellular mechanisms are shown in figure 8–1.

(1) CHEMICAL AGENTS
    a. Exogenous
        Aromatic polycyclic hydrocarbons and related heterocyclic compounds (with substitution of nitrogen, oxygen, or sulfur for carbon)
        4-nitroquinoline oxide
        Aromatic amine
        Azo compounds
        Urethane (ethyl carbamate) and closely related compounds
        Alkylating agents
        Polymers
    b. Endogenous
        Hormones, especially estrogens
        Cholesterol

(2) PHYSICAL
    a. Ionizing radiations
    b. Ultraviolet radiations
    c. Burns
    d. Other wounds

(3) GENETIC
    a. Gross and visible chromosomal abnormalities
    b. Genetic defects not visible cytologically

(4) VIRAL
    a. Leukemia and lymphosarcoma viruses in mouse, fowl, and cattle
    c. Mammary tumor virus in mouse (Bittner)
    d. Kidney tumor virus in frog (Lucke)
    d. Vibroma virus in rabbit (Shope)

At first the cancer may be dormant. The processes of cell growth and differentiation are only mildly at variance with their normal state. But if the initiation process is followed by another process, due to the influence of another agent, the neoplastic cells grow from a

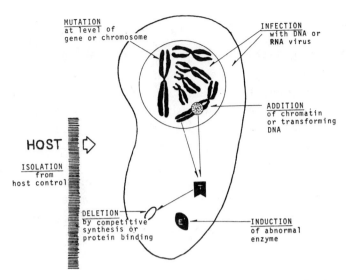

FIGURE 8–1. *The various pathways of oncogenesis (production of cancer) shown in relation to their effect on the cell or parts of the cell. (Modified from E. J. Ambrose and F. J. C. Roe,* The Biology of Cancer, *Van Nostrand, 1966, p. 50.)*

dormant to a visible state; the cancer process has been promoted. Finally, the process may progress and become irreversible. At this stage the cancer cells can be studied by epidemiologists, classified by pathologists, and contained temporarily or permanently by surgeons, radiotherapists, or chemotherapists.

We can thus distinguish three steps in the development of cancer:
1. Initiation (or the first change)
2. Promotion (from the dormant to the visible stage)
3. Progression (leading to the irreversible state).

The first stage, or initiation, could be a phenomenon of the cell surfaces, resulting in the loss of contact inhibition between cells, and leading in turn to unrestricted growth. Contrary to popular opinion, cancer cells do not grow faster than normal cells. This erroneous conception may have its origin in the fact that when a cancer cell divides both daughter cells retain their capacity to divide and are freed from normal control mechanisms.

All normal cells have a finite life span. The normal cell divides in two at a constant rate, then the two daughter cells into four, and so on, but along the road of reproduction some of the cells die at a constant rate equal to the rate of reproduction. Balance is therefore maintained. But not so for cancer cells. They do not have a finite life span. Nor do they die in the same proportion as those that reproduce. Uncontrolled growth, or geometric, not linear, reproduction occurs, the outstanding characteristic of cancer cells (see fig. 6–1). The volume of the growing tissue continuously increases, and balance in number and volume is not maintained. In this first step toward cancer the transformed cells have escaped the controls and balances which govern normal cells.

Cancer is generally regarded as an irreversible change in the cell, but if we consider the three stages of cancer development we must somehow modify this statement. Once a neoplastic cell has reached the stage of progression, the third stage in carcinogenic growth, it is a cancer cell forever. But before that stage the neoplastic transformation may be reversible. The first step, initiation, or mutagenesis, does not necessarily lead to cancer; if the second stage (promotion) fails to take place, the third and definitive stage will not be attained. In other words the initial change in the DNA of the cell may not be permanent or irreversible. This concept of reversibility explains the well-established observation of *regression* in certain tumor growths.

The hypothesis of reversibility of neoplastic transformation is most tenable for chemical and physical carcinogenic agents, far less so for virus-induced cancers. This is because tumors induced by chemical and physical agents tend to have a very long latent period, with a slow evolution of autonomy and progression; contrariwise tumors of viral origin may have an explosive course, with little or no latent period, and a highly malignant behavior from the moment of neoplastic transformation.

If we think of the process of neoplastic transformation in terms of the interaction in the cell of DNA, RNA, and protein, we could say that the primary change, or initiation, occurs in the base sequences of DNA; the second step, promotion, and the third step, progression, would be expressed in the perpetuation of the change as DNA replicates itself. In terms of the Watson—Crick model, initiation would be a "mistake in incorporation," and promotion and progression a "mistake in replication."

As we have noted, the language of DNA can be expressed in four letters, A, G, T, C, the initials of its four nucleotide bases. Every function of the cell is written with a combination of three of these four letters, each triplet coding for one amino acid. When messenger RNA brings an order to the ribosomes of the cytoplasm for the formation of a given amino acid, the code is written in the form of a triplet. All cell functions are ordered by codes and combinations of codes of this sort, and therefore it is logical to assume that disrupted cell functions are the outcome of the disruption in the writing of these pieces of information or in their wrong translation. We could say then that the primary change, or initiation, occurs when, under a disrupting influence, the triplet word is written erroneously. The second and the third steps occur when DNA replicates itself according to the erroneous code.

The mistake in replication would occur in the following manner. In the ordinary replication of the DNA double helix a particular base always pairs with another particular base, as adenine with thymine and guanine with cytosine. If one of these bases has been altered or destroyed, obviously the pairing will be altered too and the replication of DNA will express the perpetuation of this alteration. Ultimately when messenger RNA brings its message to the cell cytoplasm, the message will be wrong and the end result, or cell function, will thereby be altered.

The three stages of carcinogenesis may also be explained in terms of the functioning of genes, or regulation of genes, as described in the Jacob and Monod theory. Normal cells obey definite laws, cancer cells evade them. The essence of Jacob and Monod's explanation of the lawlessness of cancer cells lies in the distinction between structural genes and control genes. The structural genes preside over all the specialized functions of the cell; the control genes, or regulator genes, regulate the action of the structural genes by blocking or releasing their activity. A structural gene responsible for a particular function, let us say cell replication, is inactive, repressed by a repressor gene until an operator gene gives it the signal to function. Translating this theory into the explanation of the behavior of the cancer cell we can conceive of a "cancer gene" existing even in normal cells; this "cancer gene" is held inactive by "cancer repressor genes" but rendered active by "cancer operator genes." Under the influence of chemical, physical, genetic, or viral agents the cancer operator gene takes over and inhibits the cancer repressor gene. It codes then

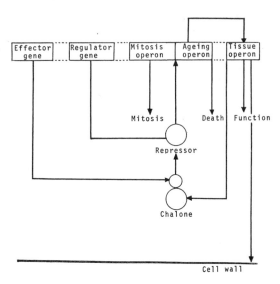

FIGURE 8–2. *A conjectural model of the mechanism controlling mitosis, aging, and function in a tissue cell. The mitosis and aging operons, together with their regulator and effector genes, must be common to all types of tissue. (Modified from W. S. Bullough,* The Evolution of Differentiation, *Academic Press, 1967, p. 122.)*

for the replication of cancer cells and for all the abnormalities characteristic of the cancer cell (fig. 8–2).

Cell differentiation presumably occurs by a blocking out of the function of all triplet words, or codes, except those necessary for this particular function. Cell replication would occur by a blocking out of the function of all codes except those necessary for replication. Thus replication and differentiation can be viewed as reciprocal processes: when one function is released the other is suppressed, a kind of game of genetic teeter-totter. This, too, applies to cancer. If, for instance, the reciprocal relationship of reproduction and differentiation is destroyed (perhaps by alteration of a control gene), the cell no longer differentiates but is free to reproduce without inhibition exactly as the cancer cell does.

The Jacob–Monod hypothesis provides a variety of explanatory mechanisms for derangement of cell growth, replication, and differentiation. It offers a simple explanation for the clinically observed phenomena of initiation, promotion, and progression.

CHEMICAL CARCINOGENESIS

It is probable that a high proportion of human cancer, perhaps 60 to 70 percent, is due to environmental causes. Cigarette smoke, atmospheric pollution, and various other materials in our environment contain certain hydrocarbons which can produce cancer. For centuries some meats have been conserved in salt and it has been found that the nitrates present in meat cured in this way can also be carcinogenic.

As noted in chapter 7, Percivall Pott, the famous English surgeon of the eighteenth century, was the first to discover a clear-cut relationship between pitch, tar, soot, and skin cancer. In the 1920's Sir Ernest Kennaway, working in the same London hospital as Pott before him, isolated the precise chemical in pitch and tar responsible for skin cancer: a polycyclic hydrocarbon. At that time, the techniques available for isolating polycyclic hydrocarbon compounds were slow and difficult, but today it is possible to identify such compounds in a single afternoon by mass spectrometry and chromatography.

The study of chemical carcinogenesis is now one of the most important and interesting aspects of cancer research, but the exact mechanisms of action of chemical carcinogens on the cell are not yet clearly defined. It is known, however, that they influence first the nucleic acids of the cell, DNA and RNA, and then through messenger RNA, the cellular proteins and enzymes.

Chemical carcinogenesis is generally a two-stage process which can be described as consisting of, first, initiation, and second, promotion. An example of this double process is to be found in the relationship of croton oil and polycyclic hydrocarbons to skin cancer. Croton oil alone rarely produces skin cancer but if a single dose of a polycyclic hydrocarbon is applied to the skin of an experimental animal and if this is then followed by an application of croton oil, skin cancer frequently occurs: the polycyclic hydrocarbon acts as an initiator and the croton oil as a promoter of the cancer process. Observations of this type are pertinent to human cancer since we know that our natural environment contains a number of chemical carcinogens. It is logical to assume that even a low level of these chemicals might serve as initiating agents, and that association with promoting agents could result in cancer. The common environmental carcinogens are alkylating agents, nitroso compounds, lactones, azo dyes, and polycyclic hydrocarbons. Let us briefly review the mechanism of action of these substances on cells. Since all manifestations of life, including its aberrations, take place in the recesses of our cells, the ultimate solution to the cancer problem will depend upon the eluci-dation of the changes in the cells invaded by carcinogens. The two probable steps in establishing a mutation are: (1) a primary change in a base of the DNA template, either an alteration, deletion, or sub-stitution, and (2) replication of the altered base pair in the formation of subsequent DNA molecules. The first step leads to the second but the perpetuation of the change depends upon the second stage, for the double helix formation is essential for the transmission of the genetic message.

Each of the groups of chemical carcinogens listed is discussed be-low in terms of its probable action.

ALKYLATING AGENTS

During the past 10 years experiments have verified the carcino-genic properties of nitrogen mustards and other alkylating agents. In studying the action of alkylating agents on nucleic acids in vitro it has been found that both for DNA and RNA the primary reaction takes place at the level of the base guanine. The toxic action on the cell thus impairs the functioning of DNA as a genetic template. The influence of alkylating agents on the cell is very direct: it occurs dur-ing interphase (the "rest" period before cell division) and the resulting damage to the cell appears during mitosis; the cell either dies or un-dergoes malignant change. Some repair mechanisms, however, exist with the cell, and reversibility of the initial change is possible. How these repair mechanisms operate, obviously a very important ques-tion, cannot be answered at the present time.

NITROSO COMPOUNDS

We have said that meat conserved in salt contains large amounts of nitrates. Nitrates are also widely used in the curing of pork and in the prevention of formation of gas in meat. Nitrates have long been known to have toxic effects on blood pressure and the carrying of oxygen by hemoglobin. In 1956 P. N. Magee and his associates pro-duced malignant primary hepatic tumors in rats by feeding them a nitroso compound, *nitrosamine*. In 1961–1962 N. Koppang and his colleagues in Norway produced severe diseases in ruminants by feed-ing them a diet of herring preserved with sodium nitrates. Many nitrates and nitrosamines are carcinogenic agents in experimental animals; they can produce tumors of the liver, esophagus, tongue, gut, bladder, kidney, and lungs. For years a widely distributed fungus, *streptomyces,* has been known to be a contaminant of human food, and recently an antibiotic isolated from a particular streptomyces has been shown to contain a nitrosamine capable of inducing kidney tumors in rats. In 1963, G. L. Laqueur and his colleagues found a carcinogenic agent in the cycad plants of the tropics and subtropics which seems to have biochemical and biological actions identical to those of nitroso compounds.

This is not to say that one should not cure meats or make antibiotics from streptomyces. Nevertheless potential carcinogenic agents do occur in our natural environment. Certainly the relation of these agents to carcinogenesis must be investigated. We have no proof that man is susceptible to nitrosamine carcinogenesis but there is no reason to believe he is not.

The action of nitroso compounds on cells is less direct than that of alkylating agents: in fact nitrosamines generate alkylating agents in the body and the induction of tumors is the consequence of cellular alkylation as discussed in the section on alkylating agents.

LACTONES

It has been discovered recently that a lactone can induce sarcomas in rats at the site of injection and that skin tumors can also be produced after repeated local applications. The cancer-producing qualities of lactones result from chemical reactions with cellular constituents, but the exact mechanisms of these reactions are unknown.

AZO DYES

If rats are fed over long periods of time with certain azo dyes they often develop liver tumors. These tumors are specific for the rat and for the liver. The azo dyes have been shown to bind to both the nucleic acids and the proteins of the cell, so their mechanism of action may be a dual one.

One explanation of the action of azo compounds on cells hinges on immunological mechanisms: damage to the cell proteins could result in the loss of recognition of those antigens which disrupt normal cell growth. Another theory proposes that the damage to cell proteins essential to the control of growth results in a subsequent unchecked cell growth.

POLYCYCLIC HYDROCARBONS

It was only as recently as the 1920's that Sir Ernest Kennaway found pronounced carcinogenic properties in some polycyclic hydrocarbons which were soon identified to be the active substances in cancer-producing pitch. The brief period of research since then has led to the discovery of a host of polycyclic hydrocarbons which are powerfully carcinogenic. Like all carcinogens, polycyclic hydrocarbons react in the cell both with nucleic acids and proteins.

Chemical carcinogens initiate cancer by altering the DNA of the cell, producing a deletion, inversion, substitution, or dimerization (fig. 8–3). The ultimate alteration of enzymes and proteins within the cell induced by carcinogenic chemicals suggests the possibility of controlling cancer by the substitution of the enzyme itself into the altered cell. At the primary level of DNA the initial alteration of the cell DNA could possibly be repaired by the elimination of the genetic change or by its reversal.

FIGURE 8–3. *Changes in DNA brought about by chemical carcinogenesis (A) and radiation carcinogenesis (B). (Adapted from Peter Brookes, "Quantitative Aspects of the Reaction of Some Carcinogens with Nucleic Acids,"* Cancer Research, *Sept. 1966, 26: 1995.)*

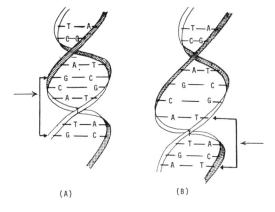

(A)

(B)

CROSS-LINKAGE OF GUANINE

THYMINE DIMERIZATION

RADIATION CARCINOGENESIS

In 1935 Jacob Furth showed that X-rays could induce leukemias in mice and during the following years many workers conducted more studies on radiation carcinogenesis. These studies have shown that irradiation of cells by X-rays, ultraviolet light, and other physical sources can be broadly categorized into two mechanisms:

1. *Direct mutagenic effects*—an immediate physical or chemical event at the molecular level, within the fraction of a second.

2. *Indirect mutagenic effects*—an alteration of a normal balance within the organism and a subsequent neoplastic transformation in the cell through loss of normal resistance or control.

DIRECT EFFECT OF IRRADIATION ON CELLS

Physical particles, such as X-rays, gamma rays, fast electrons, alpha particles, and ultraviolet particles, carry high amounts of energy and when they strike a cell a direct change occurs in the cell's chemical bonds. We have said that an immediate event occurs within the cell but it would be more accurate to say that more such events are necessary for the cell to be inactivated by irradiation. Here is why. If a dose of X-rays, let us say 1,000 units, produced one mutation, 2,000 units should produce two mutations and the cell's response to irradiation could be expressed graphically in a straight line; in reality, however, the line is not quite straight but presents a bend at its end. The analysis of such a sigmoidal curve has shown that two to six events take place in the cell for its inactivation, the shoulder in the curve indicating the action of possible repair mechanisms within the cell. Examples of the action of these repair mechanisms or their failure are illustrated in the protection given by various drugs against radiation damage, or conversely, the rendering of cells more susceptible to irradiation if the irradiation dose is administered in an environment rich in oxygen.

The nucleus of the cell is far more responsive to radiations than its cytoplasm and in the nucleus itself the RNA is the macromolecule affected. It is therefore logical that the function of the cell most sensitive to radiation is the reproductive one since it is engineered by the nuclear DNA.

Studies utilizing viruses have been greatly helpful in the elucidation of radiation effects on cells. Viruses may be either double-stranded or single-stranded, and they can be used in experiments either whole or deprived of their outer protein coat. Whatever virus is employed, whether it is intact or not, makes little difference; in all cases it is the nucleic acid core which is radiosensitive.

INDIRECT INDUCTION OF CANCER BY RADIATIONS

Dr. Henry Kaplan and his associates at Stanford University (from 1950 to 1970) have done the most to elucidate the mechanism of irradiation induction of cancer in mice. He has essentially proved that the induction of cancer by irradiation is an indirect, not a direct, mutagenic effect. Lymphatic leukemia of the thymus in mice can be induced only if the thymus is irradiated following irradiation of the mouse's entire body. Many workers interested in the induction of leukemias in animals had shown that irradiation of the upper part of the body alone, including the thymus, of course, did not induce leukemia. This paradox was explained by Kaplan who found that the induction of leukemia in mice required irradiation of the bone marrow, spleen, and thymus, and not the thymus alone.

When the upper part of the body alone was irradiated the spleen and bone marrow cells acted as protective agents against the induction of cancer. When the bone marrow and the spleen were also irradiated their protective capacity was annihilated and the mice developed thymic tumors. Kaplan also demonstrated the indirect induction of leukemia in mice in another manner; he injected the irradiated host mouse with the normal thymic cells from an *isogenic* mouse (a mouse from an identical genetic strain): a striking event occurred: the isogenic grafts (which had never been exposed to irradiation) began to develop tumors. Therefore, a substance, or hormone, or unknown element, in the irradiated animal, indirectly converted the normal thymic graft into a malignant lymphoma.

More research was necessary before the unknown element could be identified. Leukemias in mice finally were related to leukemogenic viruses. In 1950 Ludwik Gross had first shown that cell-free filtrates, or extracts from spontaneous leukemias in a certain strain of mice could, if injected into mice from another strain, induce leukemias in this strain. The experiment was successful only if the injected animals were newborn mice that were immunologically immature, and thus unable to reject the foreign viral antigen (see chapter 5). Subsequently, in studies with the electron microscope, the virus particles could be clearly seen and since then a host of viruses have been identified as producing certain leukemias in mice.

As a result of years of exacting studies by Kaplan and others we have come to understand the general pattern of indirect irradiation carcinogenesis. A virus is the actual cause of leukemias in mice; the virus persists in the tissues of naturally infected strains throughout life (in a state of immunological tolerance) without sufficient strength to induce cancer; mice injected with thymus extract from isogenic animals develop leukemias only after being exposed to total body irradiation, a process which weakens or cancels their immune response (fig. 8–4). The primary, or initial cause of the cancer is the virus, but the triggering action can be attributed to X-rays; these two phases of one process can be compared to the inducing and promoting phases of chemical carcinogenesis already discussed above.

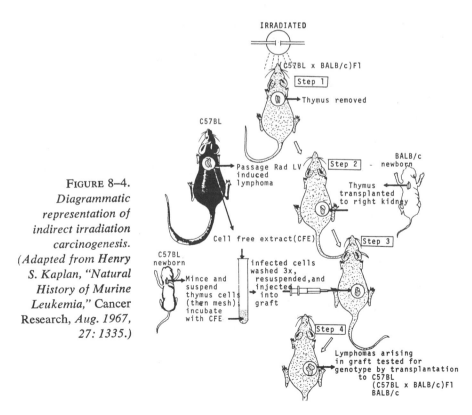

FIGURE 8–4. *Diagrammatic representation of indirect irradiation carcinogenesis. (Adapted from Henry S. Kaplan, "Natural History of Murine Leukemia,"* Cancer Research, *Aug. 1967, 27: 1335.)*

CONCLUSION

From observations on radiation carcinogenesis we can perceive obvious direct implications for man. The amount of irradiation in our environment must be diligently controlled. The indirect induction of cancer by radiations also has implications in man, particularly with respect to human leukemia. We do not know whether leukemias in man are of viral origin or not but it is quite possible that leukemia viruses exist ordinarily in man in a state of immunological tolerance and that their leukemogenic potential may be evoked by various physical and chemical hazards in the environment.

The carcinogenic effects of irradiation have been shown for a variety of cancers in man. Sarcomas occur from ingestion of radioactive isotopes, such as those deposited in the long bones of radium dial painters; pulmonary carcinomas in underground mine workers result from exposure to alpha radiations in high concentration from radon in the air of underground mines. In addition it is possible that polonium, existing in low doses in tobacco, is a carcinogenic agent in cigarette smoke.

Patients treated by irradiation for ankylosing arthritis of the spine and the survivors of the Hiroshima and Nagasaki atomic blasts show an increased or excessive incidence of leukemia. Breast cancer is more frequent in women undergoing multiple fluoroscopic examinations in the treatment of pulmonary tuberculosis. A single X-ray film of the abdomen of a pregnant woman produces significant increases in the incidence of cancer, including leukemia, in the child. The risk of radiation carcinogenesis to the population as a whole is clear, but the boundary between safe and unsafe levels is still unclear. More epidemiological studies in man are necessary before a definite assessment of the dangers of radiation can be made. Nevertheless, radiation levels in our environment must be scrupulously controlled now and in the future.

ENDOCRINE CARCINOGENESIS

The idea that tumors arising in organs whose growth and functions are under humoral control might be influenced by the state of the endocrine glands of the host was first proposed by G. T. Baetson in

1896, and it is now established that certain cancers are "hormone-dependent," or, better, "hormone-sensitive."

It might be well here to give a brief résumé of the action of the endocrine glands. Endocrine glands produce secretions called *hormones*. As their name implies, endocrine glands discharge their hormones within the body through the blood and the lymph streams. The pituitary, also called hypophysis, a small gland at the base of the brain, is the master gland. Other endocrine glands (thyroid, adrenals, gonads or sex glands, and breasts) are under the dominance of the pituitary whose hormones stimulate their functions; but in turn the end organs produce their own hormones directly and the resultant feedback inhibits the production of further stimulating hormones by the pituitary. In other words, under normal circumstances, there is a state of balance, or *homeostasis,* between the master gland, the pituitary, and the endocrines. Derangement of this particular functional relationship (hormone excess or deprivation) interferes with harmonious endocrinal mechanisms.

Baetson, in experiments with mice, was able to obtain remissions in a few cases of breast cancer by removal of both ovaries. Later, in 1932, A. M. Lacassagne, in an experiment which has become classic, induced mammary cancer in mice by the administration of female sex hormones (*estrogens*). In 1939, Charles Huggins obtained good remissions of cancer of the prostate in man by removal of the testicles, the main source of male sex hormones (*androgens*) controlling the activity and growth of the prostate gland. For his comprehensive studies on the treatment of prostatic carcinoma Huggins received the Nobel Prize in Medicine in 1966. The joint prize winner, Dr. F. Peyton Rous, the discoverer of viral carcinogenesis, could then write: "The significance of this discovery far transcends its practical implications; for it means that thought and endeavor in cancer research have been misdirected in consequence of the belief that tumor cells are anarchic" (Rous, 1967). In the mid-1940's Sir Harold Dodds and his co-workers found methods for preparing active synthetic estrogens which could be administered by mouth and Huggins showed that remissions in prostatic cancer could be obtained by the taking of these hormones rather than by castration.

In short, prostatic cancer in men can be influenced by the administration of female sex hormones or the interruption of the production of male sex hormones by castration. Conversely, breast cancer in women can be influenced by the administration of male sex hormones or by the surgical removal of the ovaries (oophorectomy), with the subsequent annihilation of female sex hormone production. Unfortunately secondary adrenal hyperplasia occurs and the adrenal hormones begin to substitute for and replace both estrogenic and androgenic hormones, following removal of either the testicles or the ovaries.

In 1945 the chemical nature of adrenal hormones was well enough understood so that for the first time life could be maintained in man following the removal of the adrenal glands. Huggins and others attracted worldwide interest with the use of oophorectomy and adrenalectomy in the management of breast cancer in women.

The mechanism of hormone action in the development of cancer is still poorly understood but in general terms there can be both a direct action of the hormones in inducing cancer or an indirect, permissive action of the hormones in promoting and favoring the growth of a tumor. These actions are discussed in the following subsections.

EXPERIMENTAL ENDOCRINE CARCINOGENESIS

1. *Direct Action of Hormones.*—Some pituitary tumors can be induced in mice by obliteration of the thyroid after irradiation, thyroidectomy, or prolonged administration of a drug stopping the production of thyroxine hormone. Pituitary tumors in mice can appear following gonadectomy at an early age. A whole host of experiments involving endocrine manipulation indicate that the reduced function of a target organ alters its reciprocal relationship to the pituitary, causing ultimately neoplasia, or cancer, of the target organ. The sequence of events seems to be as follows: the endocrine imbalance produces hypersecretion of the pituitary, which in turn provokes overstimulation of the target organ, and ultimately neoplasia. Yet hopefully the neoplastic transformation could be prevented if a normally functioning hormonal state were to be restored.

A strong indication that hormonal imbalance is essential to the development and maintenance of the tumor is shown by the fact that such endocrine-induced tumors cannot be transplanted.

2. *Indirect Action of Hormones.*—The response of mouse mammary glands to carcinogenic hydrocarbons is most remarkable. It is characterized by the rapid development of breast tumors. Since this type of breast tumor was discovered in mice by Huggins it is named Huggins' tumor. Such tumors develop regularly in female rats, not in males, unless the males are castrated or have isogenic ovaries grafted into them. The cancers produced by chemical carcinogens are unquestionably hormone-dependent, for excision of the ovaries or of the hypophysis produces profound regressions of the cancerous condition. It seems that a given target tissue, such as the breast, has a specific affinity for a particular chemical carcinogen, and that an estrogen is required for the chemical carcinogen to have an effect on the target tissue.

Carcinogenic hydrocarbons have a strong resemblance to estrogens, and it is possible that they compete for the same active binding sites in the target cells. The main difference between the two is their initial capacity to injure the target cell: hydrocarbons produce mammary cancer more readily than estrogens; an estrogen-induced carcinoma requires a prolonged exposure to the estrogen for the cancer to develop. But the process of mammary cancer induction by chemical carcinogens and estrogens is in all probability the same.

As previously noted, the neoplastic transformations which are endocrine-dependent could probably be prevented by changing the hormonal environment of the host. Another hopeful clinical possibility has emerged from a recent discovery that there are localized sites of hormonal action in target tissues. Some tissues, those of the uterus and vagina for example, contain a unique component which has a striking affinity for estrogens and specific binding sites have been determined in the uterus and vagina of rats. These sites have been named estrogen receptors. Subsequently this identification of receptor sites in normal tissues led to the identification of receptor sites in rats' mammary tumors due to polycyclic hydrocarbons. If such binding sites can be determined in human tissues, it may become possible to decide with accuracy whether a given breast cancer will be benefited by oophorectomy or adrenalectomy or by other methods of hormonal alteration. Such a program has already been initiated and the early observations are promising. As Elwood G. Jensen (1966) has said:

"The surgeon who strives for perfection
Needs some basis for patient selection.
He would like to be sure
There's a good chance of cure
Before he begins the resection."

Such a day may soon be with us if it becomes possible to identify endocrine receptors in specific cancers in women.

ROLE OF THE PITUITARY

In the 1950's Jacob Furth found that the pituitary produces hormones needed for the initiation and growth of mammary tumors in mice. Mammary tumors in animals, whether produced by chemical carcinogens, radiations, or a virus, are all susceptible to these hormones. In such cases the hormones are promoters and not initiators of the carcinogenic process. The mammary tumors regress after oophorectomy and hypophysectomy and are stimulated by administration of estrogens or of pituitary hormones. Isolation of these hormones and the possibility of measuring their level in man will bring a better understanding of breast cancer and of the effects of ablation of endocrine glands in the containment of these tumors.

These experimental facts are many and rich in their implications. What, then, are the therapeutic and clinical conclusions which seem valid for human cancer?

CLINICAL ENDOCRINE CARCINOGENSIS

Two main approaches present themselves to the clinician in studying clinical endocrine carcinogenesis.

1. The search for humoral factors which will offer prognostic information about certain tumors, notably breast cancer.

2. The effects of endocrine ablative procedure on certain selected human cancers, notably breast and prostatic cancers.

Since the endocrine dependency of tumors is pretty well limited to those of the breast and prostate, the evidence of endocrine effects will be presented primarily for these two tumors. Our main focus will be on breast cancer, for this tumor is now the commonest malignant tumor of middle-aged women and the leading cause of death in white women between the ages of 39 and 44 in the United States.

Estrogens can cause breast cancer in laboratory animals. No direct evidence for the induction of breast cancer in women by estrogens exists, but much indirect evidence indicates that estrogens have a crucial importance in the growth of human breast cancer and on the survival of the patient.

It is generally conceded that tumors grow by a doubling of each cell, or in a geometrical progression. One cell divides into two, two into four, four into eight, eight into sixteen, and so on. If it is assumed that a tumor must reach about the size of a small cherry (1 cc) to be clinically observable, the process would probably represent 30 doublings of a single cell. Thus a long period of development would have passed unobserved before the tumor reached a clinical critical size. Since, in human breast cancer, the doubling time takes between 23 and 209 days the length of the period before clinical detection might well be as long as 5 to 10 years.

Removal of the ovaries in young women suffering from breast cancer may have rather dramatic effects on regression of growth of the tumor. Large amounts of male hormones (androgens) may have similar effects, for in at least half of the patients with breast cancer female hormones (estrogens) are necessary for the tumor to grow. (Curiously, large doses of estrogens tend to produce regression of breast cancer in elderly women over 70.) Unfortunately the estrogens cannot be measured in the blood; however, their end products can be detected in the urine; hopefully it will be possible to make accurate measurements directly from the blood in the near future.

Androgenic end products can also be found in the urine of women suffering from breast cancer (androgens are present in women's adrenals). It is even possible that abnormalities in androgen excretion *precede* the onset of breast cancer and obviously it would be of great importance to detect their appearance in the urine of women as an early indicator. Certainly in future studies it will become possible to determine which women are most likely to develop breast cancer and which are most likely to respond to treatment. The long developmental period before breast cancer becomes clinically detectable will undoubtedly become shorter as better means of recognition and control are devised. At the present time, however, we have no way of predicting which woman is apt to develop breast cancer and what endocrine environment is most favorable or unfavorable to the establishment of a human breast cancer.

ENDOCRINE ABLATION THERAPY

About 40 percent of cancers of the breast in women and cancers of the prostate in men are hormone-dependent to various degrees. It is impossible to cure cancer by endocrine ablation; the effects are purely palliative. The alteration of the hormonal environment of the patient restrains the rate of growth of the cancer, nothing more. It is never curative.

Between 25 and 35 percent of premenopausal women with advanced or disseminated breast cancer respond to oophorectomy. Palliative effects of the surgery last for variable periods, but generally from 10 to 14 months. The best response is for women who have had a long free interval between the initial mastectomy operation and the appearance of metastasis. There is no absolute answer to the timing of oophorectomy but it probably should not be used as an adjunct immediately at the time of operative treatment of the initial breast cancer. It is better reserved for the treatment of recurrence of the disease which makes the need for it obvious. At the time of recurrence the patient's response to ovarian ablation can then be evaluated. This response is of great help in the assessment of subsequent endocrine ablative therapy for this particular person.

Removal of the adrenals is a relatively new technique in the treatment of mammary cancer. After removal of the ovaries estrogenic end products can still be found in the urine of the oophorectomized women; these end products arise from the adrenals, and since today life can be maintained after total removal of the adrenals, adrenalectomy, as suggested by Huggins in 1945, has become a form of treatment for advanced or disseminated breast cancer.

Not all patients will have a favorable response to this procedure. Here, too, a long free interval between the removal of the tumor and removal of the adrenals is essential for good results. In addition, if the patient has already had a good response to oophorectomy she will be more likely to respond well to adrenalectomy. Yet only 40 percent of patients show a favorable response to removal of the adrenal and this lasts on the average only about a year; the results are better in rather young women who are still hormonally active.

Removal of the pituitary (hypophysectomy) has been suggested as an alternative in the control of mammary cancer. The results of hypophysectomy are almost identical to those of adrenalectomy, but it is a more difficult surgical procedure to employ and the postoperative therapy is somewhat more complicated. The pituitary can be excised surgically, destroyed either by the proton beam of the cyclotron or by yttrium-90 needle implants, or be removed by *cryogenic* surgery (surgery under very low temperatures). Clearly the delicate choice between different methods of treatment, the decision in favor of or against oophorectomy, adrenalectomy, or hypophysectomy, are matters of personal decision and not purely clinical questions. These choices can be resolved only by each patient and each surgeon facing these difficult questions, for alleviation of suffering, not cure of cancer, is their goal and the goal, once achieved, is of temporary duration, a matter of a year or two at most.

Let us repeat that endocrine ablation is not curative but only palliative. The effects are of a rather short duration and successful in only 25 to 35 percent of the cases. The medical history of the disease in each individual patient determines the result of endocrine ablation therapy rather than the particular method employed. Fortunately the joy of living is not lessened appreciably by ablative procedures, and they are, in selected cases, useful adjuncts in the total treatment of certain cancers.

HORMONAL THERAPY

Both breast cancer and prostatic cancer benefit from the administration of hormones to patients with advanced stages of these diseases.

Androgens are most effective in the treatment of breast cancer and estrogens in the treatment of prostatic cancer. The administration of androgens is more successful in younger women but 20 percent of all women with advanced breast cancer show objective remissions of their tumors after such treatment. A curious fact, already mentioned, is the regression of breast cancer in women over 70 (20 percent of the cases) after the administration of estrogens. Here again there is a possible correlation of response to hormonal therapy with a disease-free interval after mastectomy.

Hormonal therapy, unfortunately, has quite unpleasant side effects. Estrogens produce loss of appetite, nausea, vomiting, abdominal distress, diarrhea, increase in libido, pigmentation of the nipples and of the skin, and edema of the breast and sometimes of the whole body. Androgens produce hoarseness, drowsiness, vomiting, ruddy complexion, increase of libido, and edema.

CONCLUSIONS

Clearly, in the face of the clinical evidence, what seems to be needed are better discriminants in deciding which patients will respond to endocrine alteration. It is not possible to propose an answer to this question at the moment. Yet 30 percent of the treated cases do respond to hormonal therapy, whether endocrine ablation or hormonal administration. Experimental studies on many fronts are under way now, which are outgrowths of the methods described in the foregoing section on experimental endocrine carcinogenesis. When it is possible to grow breast cancer tissue in isolated cell systems, to study systematically the response of these cells to hormones and to the alteration of their hormonal environment, a great step forward will have been accomplished.

CHROMOSOMAL ABERRATIONS IN CANCER

One of the oldest theories of cancer is that the disease results from abnormalities acquired through mutations in the chromosomes of the cells. Most cancer cells do show abnormalities in their mitotic pattern (pattern of division) and in their chromosomal pattern. With the current understanding that DNA is the repository for genetic information (which ultimately confers upon the cell its distinctive characteristics) the study of chromosomes has assumed increased importance.

It must be emphasized, however, that changes in the cellular DNA do not necessarily mean a discernible change in the chromosomes. The primary change in cancer could still be in the genes without any gross change in the chromosomes. Chromosomal abnormalities in cancer may be secondary phenomena rather than primary phenomena, mere epiphenomena resulting from the abnormal growth of the cell.

What changes do occur in the cell chromosomes in relation to cancer? We know that there are a certain *number* of chromosomes in normal cells, that the chromosomes are grouped by pairs, and that they have specific shapes for any single pair. In human cancer and leukemia any of these chromosomal characteristics may be altered. A cancer cell may contain an abnormal number of chromosomes, or chromosomes grouped in an abnormal way, or chromosomes with an abnormal shape.

The human cell contains 46 chromosomes, the human germ cell 23. For that reason the normal cell is termed a diploid cell and the germ cell a haploid cell. Of course when two germ cells unite through fertilization the total number of chromosomes becomes 46 and a normal diploid chromosome number is restored.

Cancer cells are not diploid, but may be (1) anaploid (with no constant number of chromosomes); (2) hypoploid (with less than the normal number of chromosomes); (3) heteroploid (with more than the normal number of chromosomes); or (4) tetraploid (with twice the diploid number). Sometimes, however, cancer cells have 46 chromosomes, the normal number, but these chromosomes are grouped in an abnormal way. In a preceding chapter we have described mitosis, or cell division: at a certain time, after the chromosomes have doubled, they migrate to either pole of the cell in equal number; there they group in pairs according to length and shape. This grouping of chromosomes within a normal cell is called *karyotype,* from the Greek *karyon* meaning nucleus. A normal karyotype is shown in figure 8–5.

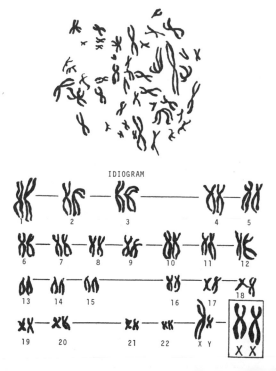

IDIOGRAM

FIGURE 8–5. (*Top*) A typical chromosome "spread" as viewed under a microscope. (*Bottom*) Arrangement of chromosomes according to characteristics (*karyotype*). Male chromosome X-X; female chromosome X-Y.

Cancer cells often present abnormal karyotypes, that is to say their chromosomes are not grouped according to the usual assemblage of lengths and forms, but the chromosomal groupings and arrangements have some abnormalities which can be clearly detected.

CHROMOSOMAL CHANGES IN LEUKEMIA

Abnormal mitosis, which is expressed in an abnormal chromosomal content of the cell, was linked to malignancy as early as 1912, by Theodor Boveri. It was not until 1961, however, that Peter Nowell and D. A. Hungerford demonstrated the presence of an abnormal chromosome in chronic granulocytic leukemia. This abnormal chromosome is known as the "Philadelphia chromosome." It is the invariable accompaniment of chronic myelocytic or granulocytic leukemia. The number of chromosomes is normal but one of them is abbreviated, with its arms shortened (fig. 8–6). It is not known whether the deleted section is translocated into another unit in the karyotype, or completely absent.

In acute leukemia there is no constant number of chromosomes; a state of anaploidy therefore exists. This stage regresses as treatment restores the cell count to more normal levels.

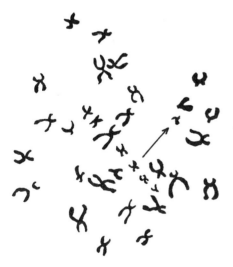

FIGURE 8–6. *Chromosome pattern in chronic granulocytic leukemia. The so-called "Philadelphia chromosome" (arrow), characteristic of the disease displays a shortened arm. (Adapted from Avery A. Sandberg, "The Chromosomes and Causation of Human Cancer and Leukemia,"* Cancer Research, *Sept. 1966, 26: 2074.)*

CHROMOSOMAL CHANGE IN CANCER

Whether primary or metastatic, cancer cells may be anaploid, hypoploid, heteroploid, or tetraploid. In other words they do not contain the usual, normal number of chromosomes. When occasionally they do, as in the pseudo-diploid cell, the 45 chromosomes that are present are fuzzy, ill-defined, and abnormally shaped.

No two cancer cells have a similar karyotype, even when the tissue of origin is the same. Then, too, many abnormal chromosomes are found in cancer cells, and cancer cells have an astonishing diversity of chromosomal characteristics.

There is no evidence of a cause-and-effect relationship between cancer and chromosomal abnormalities. At the present time changes in the chromosomes must be viewed as a secondary phenomenon, while the initial cause of malignancy is malfunction of one of the genes in the chromosomes. It is supposed that the secondary changes in the chromosomes give the cancer cell a growth advantage over a normal cell, permitting it to grow independently of the normal cell controls.

In conclusion, the chromosomal abnormalities of cancer cells are worthy of detailed studies: at the present time techniques are being developed which will make possible refined studies of identifiable segments of chromosomes. Hopefully new specific therapies for particular types of malignancy will be the outcome of such studies. When the functions of chromosomes can be related to their various genetic segments, more light might be shed on the causes and treatment of human cancer.

GENERAL SUMMARY

Jacob and Monod have studied the control of genes by their environment in bacterial systems. As we have seen their scheme is applicable to neoplasia—the development of abnormal and ultimately cancerous cells. In bacterial cells there is a reciprocal relationship between the induction and repression of a function. One gene (operator gene) controls the synthesis of one enzyme. The genetic message is accepted by messenger RNA (transcription), then the specific protein or enzyme is manufactured (translation). The induction of this function can be repressed (repressor gene) and there is a reciprocal relationship between induction and repression.

The same concept applies to the control of neoplasia: here replication is related reciprocally to differentiation. When one function is taking place the other is inhibited (see fig. 3–9).

This delicate system of balance is altered when carcinogens invade the cell. Radiations, environmental chemicals, hormones, and any process upsetting template stability (the stability of the messenger RNA), could influence replication and differentiation of the cell, and ultimately promote carcinogenesis. These mechanisms of cancer induction are now being critically studied at the molecular level since the theories are becoming amenable to direct experimentation. Inherent in such theories are, as we have already mentioned, the phenomena of regression or reversion of malignant cells to a nonmalignant state.

It is possible to explain most of the defective controls in cancer by alteration of messenger RNA in the neoplastic cell. Crucial experiments must be done to map out the portions of the genes responsible for replication and differentiation; to establish the nature of the altered messenger RNA; to determine whether messenger RNA can be restored to a normal state; therefore, to demonstrate whether the malignant process can be reversed, first in experimental animals, and ultimately in the human patient.

9
THE STATISTICS OF CANCER

"There is no more common error
than to assume that, because
prolonged and accurate mathematical calculations
have been made, the application of the result
to some fact of nature is
absolutely certain."
A. N. WHITEHEAD

Many patients with cancer have an excellent chance for arrest of the illness. One and a half million who had cancer five or more years ago have had it arrested. The struggle against the disease becomes more intense every day and millions of dollars are being spent; in 1970 this nation spent $200,000,000 for cancer research alone.

Yet it is true that some 52,000,000 Americans now living will some day have cancer and even today every sixth death in the United States is caused by cancer. About 208,000 persons were saved from cancer in the year 1970 in the United States; but about 330,000 died of the disease in the same year and it is estimated that about half these deaths could be prevented by earlier detection followed by appropriate therapy. In addition many cancers could be prevented entirely by the elimination of their causes, for example, those cancers related to environmental hazards, ranging from cigarette smoking to breathing polluted air, and cancers produced by chemicals.

The magnitude of the cancer problem is reflected in the figures reported by the National Institutes of Health in 1963; in that year the

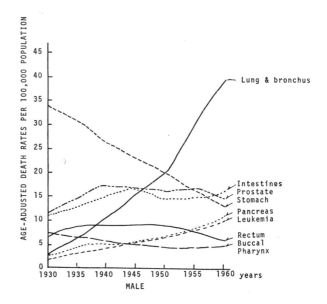

loss in goods and services resulting from cancer was estimated at a billion dollars. The cost of hospital care, physicians' services, personnel services, and supplies was estimated to be $920,700,000. Today, of course, these costs are even higher.

One of the most important unsolved problems relating to cancer is the relative influence of heredity and environmental factors on the disease. Few cancers are hereditary; among these are a cancer of the eye in children (*retinoblastoma*), tumors of the nerve cells (*neurofibromatosis*), and a particular intestinal cancer derived from intestinal *polyposis*. Some cancers (gastric, pulmonic, mammary, and uterine) are not truly hereditary, but are related strongly to racial, ethnic, and environmental factors. The analysis of the effects of climate, altitude, air pollution, humidity, temperature, the amount of solar and other radiations, and viruses can therefore yield useful statistical information. Of special interest are the relationship of human migrations to specific cancer types, the relationship of cultural and anthropological data to cancer, and the relationship of ethnic and geographical factors to cancer.

Today the cancer biologist is beginning to use statistical methods for the detection of clues in the causation of cancer; in the study of a

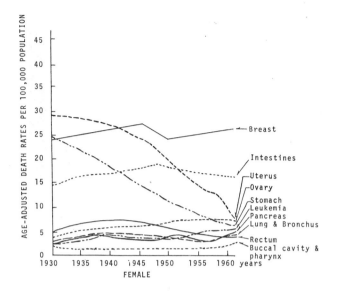

FIGURE 9–1. *Death rates per 100,000 population from cancer in selected body sites of white males and females, United States, 1930–1960. (Figures adjusted to the age-distribution of the total population of the U.S.) (Source:* Cancer Facts and Figures, *American Cancer Society, Inc.)*

problem of such magnitude no method of gathering relevant data should be neglected.

Figure 9–1 shows the incidence of fatal cancer by body sites and sex. Note that since 1941:

—more men than women have died from cancer (the main reason for this is the rising rate of lung cancer among men; it is now 10 times higher than it was 30 years ago).

—cancer remains the leading cause of death in women 30 to 54 years of age (with breast cancer producing the highest death rate).

—deaths from uterine cancer have dropped in recent years, presumably due to early detection through the use of the Pap tests initiated by Dr. Papanicolaou.

CHANGING PATTERNS OF CANCER AND MORTALITY

In the United States the cancer death rate is definitely rising. In 1900 only 3.7 percent of all deaths were attributed to cancer, in contrast to 16 percent in 1965. The majority of patients who die of cancer are between the ages of 45 and 65. Among adults the most common cancers are cancer of the breast, the cervix (narrow end of the uterus), lungs, colon, and stomach. Leukemia is responsible for about 50

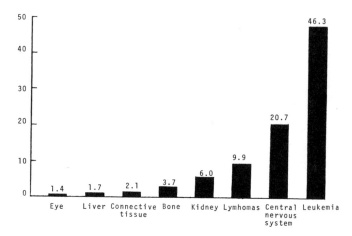

FIGURE 9–2. *Cancer deaths among children less than 15 years of age for selected body sites, United States, 1962. (Data from Statistical Research Section, Medical Affairs Department, American Cancer Society, Inc.)*

percent of the deaths of children under 15 years of age (fig. 9–2). Other cancers that are common in children are brain tumors, lymphomas, and tumors of the kidney.

During the past decade studies in epidemiology complemented by studies of mutations in cells have implicated exposure to radiations as the major cause for the increase of leukemia among children. We have already mentioned the importance of prenatal exposure to diagnostic X-rays and chromosomal aberrations such as the "Philadelphia chromosome." These are related to the genesis of childhood leukemia.

GEOGRAPHY AND CANCER

Changes in civilization, advances in industrialization, are related to cancer, as numerous demographic or geographical studies carried out during the past ten years have demonstrated. Figure 9–3 shows some of the highlights of the geographical distribution of cancer. A few of these are summarized in the following paragraphs.

Oral cancer, including cancer of the lips, is rare in the United States (3 to 4 percent of all cancers) but prevalent in India (up to 70

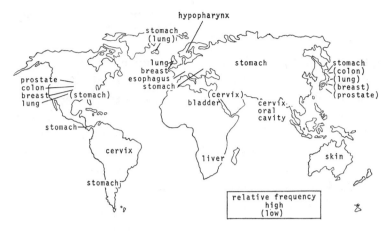

FIGURE 9–3. *The geography of cancer.*

percent of all cancers) where betel nut chewing is customary. Oral cancers in general are related to the use of tobacco and alcohol, improper oral hygiene, and the ingestion of nitroso compounds.

Cancer of the esophagus, prevalent in lower socio-economic groups, is rare in Europe and the Americas, but frequent in Japan, and most frequent in the Transkei Bantu region of South Africa (some nitroso compounds may enter the preparation of bush teas), and present in groups of Swedish women who have vitamin deficiencies and long-standing anemia. As we can see, cancer of the esophagus varies widely in geographic distribution. It is related to the use of alcohol and tobacco, betel chewing, and the ingestion of excessively hot foods and drinks.

Cancer of the stomach is very common in Russia and Japan and may be linked to the presence of carcinogenic hydrocarbons in broiled meats, in smoked fish and meats, and in highly salted food. It is low in the Americas, perhaps because of the increased consumption of dairy products and fresh fruit in these parts of the world.

Cancer of the colon is most frequent in English-speaking countries. No socio-economic gradient is recognized. Countries which have a low incidence of cancer of the stomach show a high incidence of cancer of the colon. Predisposing factors are ulcerative colitis and multiple polyposis. Curiously, cancer of the colon is more common among women than among men, while cancer of the rectum is more common in males.

FOOD AND CANCER

In chapter 8 the relationship of nitroso compounds to cancer was discussed. A number of plants containing powerful carcinogenic chemicals are still used as food by the native residents of some countries: for example the cycad plant is utilized in Guam for the preparation of flour. Long ago the zamia root (member of the same ancient cycad family) was utilized by pre-Columbian American Indians for the preparation of a stew called *softee*; this starchy stew was a substitute for the scarce wheat flour and was made into breads, cookies, and crackers. The Indians learned, however, that without proper preparation the zamia starch could be a fatal poison; they altered their method of preparation by following the usual peeling, grinding, and grating of the plant with a thorough washing of the flour obtained and thereafter a long drying in the sun.

OCCUPATION AND CANCER

After Pott's observation of the relationship of scrotal cancer to soot (chimney sweep's cancer) numerous other carcinogenic substances were discovered. In 1873 Richard von Volkmann related skin cancer to the application of crude coal tar. Paul G. Unna, in 1894, related skin cancers in farmers and sailors to constant exposure to ultraviolet light. And Ludwig Rehn, in 1895, could link the appearance of bladder cancer in dye workers to the effects of certain aniline dyes. In 1929 Harrison S. Martland related a high incidence of bone cancer among radium dial painters to the radium emanations, and in our generation the relationship of asbestos, fluorspar, and smoking to lung cancer has been clearly established. The influence of smoking on lung cancer is particularly important and will be dealt with in detail later on.

OTHER ENVIRONMENTAL FACTORS IN CANCER

We have already mentioned that nutritional deficiencies, hot foods, and alcohol are influential in the development of cancer of the alimentary tract, and that a long-term iron deficiency disease (Plummer–Vinson's syndrome) is associated with a high incidence of cancer of the upper alimentary tract in some Swedish women.

Circumcision in infancy virtually protects against cancer of the penis, suggesting that poor penile hygiene, phimosis (tightness of the foreskin of the penis) and smegma (the thick secretion found under the foreskin) may contribute to the development of cancer of the penis.

Early coitus and multiple marriages are related to cancer of the cervix, which is rare among nuns and virgins, but common among prostitutes.

Pregnancy is not directly related to cancer of the cervix, when considered independently of age in the first marriage. Cervical cancer is much less frequent in populations where the males are circumcised since smegma may be carcinogenic for the cervical epithelium as well as for the penile epithelium.

Curiously, obesity and short feminine statures are correlated with cancer of the endometrium, the mucous membrane lining the uterus. It is possible that particular female body types are predisposed to certain cancers.

CHANGING TRENDS OF CANCER

Changing trends of cancer among adults are not always understood. As an example, the rate of cancer of the pancreas is rising, for unknown reasons. But cancer of the stomach, which is becoming less frequent, may be linked to nutritional factors early in life; Japanese people who, in their country of origin, have a high incidence of stomach cancer, see the risk diminished when they have emigrated to the United States where they have partially changed their eating habits. For unclear reasons residents of urban areas are more likely to develop cancer of the colon and the rectum than residents of rural areas; this type of cancer is also more prevalent among certain ethnic groups (for instance, among Jewish people) and less among others (Japanese, Finns, Poles, and Russians). Leukemia is frequent in Israel, Denmark, the United States, and Japan; its rising incidence is linked to exposure to radiations. As an example, a recent report of the Atomic Energy Commission indicates an increase in leukemia of exposed Japanese survivors to the atomic bomb explosions. Whether or not relatively low doses of diagnostic X-rays, or radiations from natural sources, are leukemogenic, is not clear.

Among other changes in cancer incidence one of the most striking is the increase in lung cancer among males (23 percent of cancer deaths in males, 5 percent in women). This change has been linked to cigarette smoking and the inhalation of tobacco smoke. Current evidence shows that the relationship of cigarette smoking to lung cancer is so great that it far outweighs other possibilities (air pollution, urban residence, family history, and occupational exposure, with the exception of the exposure of miners to fluorspar, uranium, and asbestos).

Although breast cancer (before menopause and in the middle years of life) is the single most important cancer among women, its incidence and survival and mortality rates have been stationary for a number of years. There is a tendency in patients with breast cancer to undergo the natural menopause at a later age, which suggests that the menopause acts as a protection against breast cancer. Prolonged nursing seems to diminish the risk of breast cancer, provided the experience of lactation in a lifetime exceeds 36 months. Japanese women, who have in general a longer lifetime experience of lactation than American women (as well as an earlier menopause), show a lower mortality rate from breast cancer.

Cancer of the prostate, the commonest cause of death by cancer in sites in the male genital organs (mostly in persons over 75), is more frequent among Negroes than among whites, more frequent in married men than in single men, but curiously higher in widowed or divorced men. Studies on the sexual and reproductive behavior of different marital and ethnic groups are currently being undertaken in an effort to understand this aspect of prostatic cancer.

TRAUMA AND CANCER

Trauma is a form of irritation. The environmental and occupational cancers previously discussed are evidences of multiple repetitive traumas. To understand then what links trauma to cancer it might be well to remember the concept of carcinogenesis as consisting of the two-step process, initiation and promotion. Thus repetitive traumas could serve as a promoting agent, stimulating a latent neoplastic process to reach a critical size, and thereby to become detectable by clinical methods. Men living in environments abundantly supplied with chemical and physical carcinogens may have cancers augmented or aggravated by chronic traumas. There is no substantial evidence that this type of trauma, acting by itself, can generate cancer. This, of course, is not to deny the occasional occurrence of cancer super-imposed on burn scars, poorly healing ulcers, chronic draining si-nuses from osteomyelitis, or chronic ulcerative colitis of the rectum, but in all these situations the trauma acts as a promoting rather than an initiating agent.

The association of chronic irritation and cancer has led to the pop-ular notion that a single injury may cause cancer. Indeed the medical literature contains numerous case reports purporting to show a causal relationship between a single trauma and subsequent discovery of a malignant tumor at the site of the sustained injury. But if one con-siders the tremendous number of operations done over the past 50 years and the magnitude of such traumas as those involved in driving medullary rods down bones or inserting false femoral heads in femurs, and if one relates these operations to the unheard-of appearance of cancer following such major surgical procedures, one must be con-vinced that a relationship between a single trauma and cancer is rare or indeed nonexistent. Critical analysis of clinical cases has reduced the number of authentic cases to insignificant proportions. Among the stock of records that modern society has provided us with is a huge number of war wounds and thousands of injured patients treated for trauma over 10-year periods following automobile ac-cidents. In these massive records no evidence has shown that a single trauma sustained by healthy tissues and followed by healing is a pri-mary cause for cancer. As James Ewing, the famous pathologist, has said (1928): "Traumas reveal more malignant tumors than they cause."

SMOKING AND CANCER

In the early part of the sixteenth century explorers returning from the New World brought tobacco to Spain and England. The intro-duction of tobacco was in response to man's search for contentment; indeed pipe smoking, tobacco chewing, and the use of snuff were reputed to have medicinal action. But since the earliest times smoking has also been condemned as a foul-smelling, loathsome custom, harmful to health. The centuries-long controversies became particularly intense after 1930, when the production and use of tobacco, especially of cigarettes, reached enormous proportions and increasing deaths from lung cancer were becoming evident.

The denunciations against smoking voiced by many reputable scientists are based entirely on statistical studies of masses of population. In the U.S. there were fewer than 3,000 deaths from lung cancer in 1930, but 18,000 in 1950 and 41,000 in 1962. This extraordinary increase is true for lung cancer only, and certainly parallels the rising consumption of tobacco. No doubt smoking is implicated in lung cancer but statistical methods alone cannot establish the proof of a cause-and-effect relationship.

The most complete and reasonable estimate of the association between smoking and lung cancer has been expressed by the Surgeon General's office of the U.S. Department of Health, Education, and Welfare in a volume published in 1964 and entitled "Smoking and Health."

"Cigarette smoking," it says, "is a health hazard of sufficient importance in the United States to warrant immediate appropriate action.

"Cigarette smoking is causally related to lung cancer in man; the magnitude of the effects of cigarette smoking far outweighs all other factors. The data for women, though less extensive, point in the same direction.

"The risk of developing lung cancer increases with the ratio of smoking and the number of cigarettes per day and is diminished by discontinuing smoking.

"The risk of developing cancer of the lungs for the combined groups of pipe smokers and pipe and cigar smokers is greater than for nonsmokers but much less than for cigarette smokers. The data are insufficient to warrant a conclusion for each group individually." (See fig. 9–4.)

All studies agree that the more heavily one smokes, the longer one smokes, and the earlier one starts smoking, the more likely one is to become a prey to lung cancer. The only inconsistent factor was the

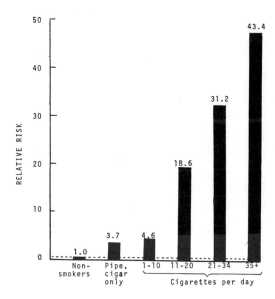

FIGURE 9–4. *Risk of incurring lung cancer among nonsmokers and various groups of smokers. (Source: E. L. Wynder and D. Hoffman, "Current Concepts of Environmental Cancer Research,"* Medical Clinics of North America, *May 1966, 50: 638.)*

discovery in one study that the proportion of lung cancers in female nonsmokers was distinctly higher than among the controls.

Let us now briefly examine some of the criticisms of the statistical types of analysis.

The Surgeon General's report on "Smoking and Health" has been extensively criticized in Congress and objections elsewhere have been clearly voiced. It has been said, for instance, that the overall death rates for all participants of seven respective studies were lower than one would expect, indicating that the studies involved a population healthier than the United States population as a whole. Among the other criticisms were the following:

1. The cause of cancer is unknown and cancer strikes many sites in the body in which there is no relationship to smoking.

2. Ten percent of lung cancer victims never have smoked and 95 percent of heavy cigarette smokers never contract cancer.

3. Prolonged exposure to concentrated cigarette smoke and tar has never been shown to produce lung cancer in experimental animals. At best smoke is a promoter rather than an initiator of the cancer process.

4. Lung cancer is rare among women, the ratio being 6 to 1 higher for men. Nevertheless smoking among women has increased since

1930, yet curiously there has not been a corresponding increase in the number of cancer deaths from lung cancer among women.

5. Cancer of the windpipe (trachea) is rare, yet this area gets the greatest exposure to tobacco smoke.

6. Cancers of the lungs occur in at least half the cases in the periphery of the lungs, yet studies on the dispersion of smoke in the lungs have shown the smoke concentration to be least in the periphery of the lungs.

7. Heavy smokers of cigarettes should contract lung cancer at a much earlier age than nonsmokers, yet the data do not substantiate this.

8. British men smoke only half as many cigarettes as American men but have twice the incidence of lung cancer.

9. The most potent cancer-inducing chemical in tobacco smoke, benzopyrene, is present in larger amounts in cigars and pipes yet there is little correlation between cigar and pipe smoking and lung cancer. Perhaps this is because the inhalation of cigarette smoke is far greater than the degree of inhalation in pipe and cigar smoking.

10. Cigarette smoking has increased 200-fold since 1915 but the incidence of lung cancer has not increased in that proportion.

11. There is also a definite correlation between cigarette smoking and coronary heart disease in males, indicating a possible genetic susceptibility to tobacco rather than a specific causal relationship between the habit of smoking and the correlated illnesses.

What conclusion, then, can be reached on the basis of the evidence displayed by the studies on smoking and cancer? Clearly there is an indubitable association between smoking and cancer but a causal relationship may still be questioned. The genetic pattern of any given individual may largely determine whether he will be susceptible to cigarette smoke. There is growing support today for the idea proposed some 30 years ago that a person's peculiar constitution creates his craving or noncraving for tobacco and that some people's bodily chemistry makes them more receptive than others to cancer of the lungs.

When Charles Lamb wrote, "For thy sake, tobacco, I would do anything but die," he expressed a psychological and social drive that is now well recognized. Smoking may relieve mental stress but a price must be paid for it. No matter how one twists the problem there is no denying that deaths from all causes are much higher among smokers than among nonsmokers. Warnings and admonitions, however, do little to deter people from smoking. Even the most casual observer knows that thousands of people smoke, yet that relatively few die of lung cancer. It is difficult for such an observer to feel personally threatened and even as careful a study as the Doll report (1964) on mortality and smoking among English physicians shows that the maximum risk rate (considering that no direct cause-and-effect relationship is involved) is only two chances per thousand of dying of lung cancer.

The advertising business spends $200,000,000 annually on its campaigns and presents smoking as sexually alluring, or as related to athletic prowess, popularity, or datability, thus encouraging a casual observer to acquire the habit. Then, too, economic objections to non-smoking are raised, since 6,000,000 people are involved in the tobacco industry, and 3,000,000 derive income through retail sales, 700,000 farm families have tobacco as their principal cash crop, and the U.S. exports $500,000,000 worth of cigarettes yearly (1967).

Yet a country as large and as prosperous and resourceful as the United States could surely absorb the shocks involved in altering the consumption of tobacco. Some approaches have been tried but they have largely failed. The current major approaches to elimination of the use of tobacco are:

Prohibition of sales to minors.

Taxation on each pack of cigarettes.

Regulations requiring that warnings of the possible damage to health be on the cigarette package.

Regulation or even prohibition of cigarette advertising.

Programs of counteradvertising stressing the health hazards of smoking.

Programs of education at elementary, high school, and college levels.

Clinics and other therapeutic tools designed to help people stop smoking.

People smoke as much as ever. How can the excess deaths related to cigarette smoking be avoided? Continued education is essential and doctors should set the "good example" by organizing antismoking clinics and gaining a better understanding of the mental attitudes of smokers, as well as by taking the necessary prevention steps among themselves.

THE NEED FOR CLINICAL INVESTIGATIVE PROGRAMS

It is beyond the general scope of this work to delve deeply into statistics but a general knowledge of the subject is essential if we want to pursue even a moderate analysis of the cancer problem.

The statistical method consists of two processes: (1) the collection of data, and (2) the analysis of data. But the first process influences the second, for the collection of data must be designed in such a way that precise and relevant answers can be obtained. Data collection today is so simple that mountains of facts are gathered with little or no purpose and what is gained in information is often lost in understanding. As an example of a lack of coordination of data, there is increasing evidence that cancer involving the lung in women is frequently a metastasis from cancer of the breast or the genital organs rather than the primary cancer. The methods of recording data on this important subject do not reflect this fact and are therefore not reliable.

The last 50 years have seen the average life span for all subdivisions of the population rise significantly. In contrast to life expectancy in 1900, which was 48 years for white males and 51 for females, life expectancy is currently 68 years for white males and 74 years for females. Because of this lengthened life span the total number of deaths by cancer, particularly lung cancer, has increased by many millions during the past half century; the inherent biological characteristic of cancer to develop in older age groups therefore results in a higher incidence of cancer simply because people live longer.

These considerations, and others, must be taken into account when any statistical study of cancer is undertaken. Planned clinical investigations are also necessary if the collection of data is to be of truly practical interest in the fight against cancer.

Although clinical investigations lack the precision and elegance of laboratory research they must not be disparaged. Many meaningful facts can be gathered from planned clinical experiments if they follow some basic guidelines, such as those outlined in the following questions:

Does the study involve substantial problems and is the information really worth securing?

Is the study properly designed to yield unambiguous answers?

Has the study already been performed satisfactorily elsewhere?

Is the experiment ethically defensible, that is, is the course of treatment proposed by the investigator ethically justified in the light of our current knowledge about the natural history of cancer?

Let us take the example of breast cancer and see what answers must be sought to obtain optimum solutions to this problem. There are 60,000 cases of breast cancer each year in the United States, with an annual mortality of 25,000. During a lifetime of 74 years one woman out of 20 will develop cancer of the breast. What is the best treatment? Radical surgery? Simple surgery? Should the regional lymph nodes be removed? Should X-ray therapy be given routinely, preferably, or just in selected cases? Should drugs be used alone, or in conjunction with other therapies? Should endocrine ablation be practiced, and if so, when? Such questions can only be answered by planned clinical investigation. All methods of treatment have been tried in the past but because of the lack of correlation retrospective studies have failed to answer the above questions. All data show that it is difficult to demonstrate improvements in the therapeutic results of breast cancer, regardless of methods of treatment; the incidence of cancer of the breast has remained stable and unchanged during the past 30 years. If the current treatments were curative, after 5 to 10 years women treated for breast cancer should die at the same rate as women of the same age in the normal population. However, recent studies show that, even after 20 years, the first cause of death is still cancer of the breast and at the same excess rate as in the early years (fig. 9–5). What is achieved for women treated for breast cancer by current methods? Only planned clinical experiments can give us the clues we are still looking for (Shimkin, 1967).

All clinical investigations must follow a number of rules insuring maximum objectivity. Two or more groups must be compared, treated by two different modalities: radiotherapy and surgery, or a carefully defined combination of both, or perhaps two different radiotherapeutic techniques. The group cases must be assigned at random, if the laws of chance are to guarantee an ultimate comparability. The groups must be comparable as to age, sex, socio-economic background, clinical staging, extent of the tumor, and associated illnesses. It is obviously impossible for individual physicians to gather significant information on a large enough scale or to plan programs of this nature; for these reasons data from clinical investigations must be gathered through a uniform procedure and on a national basis, and patient material must be collected on a random selection basis sufficient to yield meaningful statistical answers.

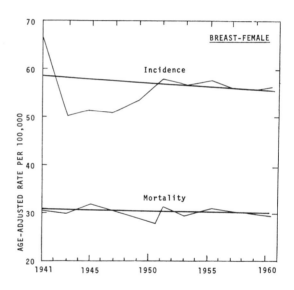

FIGURE 9–5. *Incidence of, and mortality from, cancer of the breast, New York (excluding New York City) 1941–1960. The trend lines show that mortality closely parallels incidence for all age groups even though differences among particular brackets tend to mask this. (Source: M. B. Shimkin, "End Results in Cancer of the Breast," Cancer, July 1967, 20: 1039.)*

10
EARLY DETECTION
AND PREVENTION
OF CANCER

"Before thou fight,
seek thee a helper; Before thou art sick,
seek thee a physician."
BEN SIRA, BOOK OF WISDOM

The natural history of cancer as a clinical disease suggests that the best approach to its containment would be first, prevention, and second, early diagnosis and proper treatment. As early as 1925 a National Committee on Cancer headed by the distinguished pathologist James Ewing concluded that "early diagnosis is so important that cancer detection clinics must be established in the United States." Yet today the desirable goals of prevention and early detection have not been reached. The Presidential Committee investigating the cancer problem in the U.S. in 1965 could state: "Each premature death from cancer is a personal tragedy. Each preventable death is a national reproach. Each year more and more such deaths are occurring, for the pace of science is bringing them more within our reach but the pace of application allows them to slip through our grasp."

Let us briefly review the natural history of cancer. First there is an interaction between some inciting factors and stimuli (chemical, physical, nutritional, or biological) and the patient's organism. This is a latent, dormant period, when nothing seems to be amiss. Then a change begins to appear in the tissues, in a localized site, and one speaks of cancer "in situ" (in place). The tissue changes are quite identifiable in the laboratory but the patient is still well, showing no clinical symptoms of illness; he is *asymptomatic*. Finally the clinical horizon is reached, the cancer is localized to an organ, signs and symptoms are identifiable, and the disease becomes discernible. At this time regional spreads may occur at a variable pace. Remote metastases ultimately appear: a chronic stage of the illness is now the patient's lot, with death as the outcome—if the patient is not treated or if the treatment has been rendered too late. But if the initial stimuli (varying from ultraviolet light or simple light, to the chewing of betel, to smoking, to exposure to nitroso compounds, environmental hazards, and so on) are investigated and controlled many cancers will undergo remission and become nonexistent.

SCREENING

There is no better example of the value of cancer detection than the results of mass screening programs for cervical cancer organized in British Columbia, Canada, in 1950. To date about 75 percent of the female population has been examined and cancer of the cervix has declined significantly. At the present time no simple general screening test for cancer is possible and the search must of necessity, be painstaking and on an organ-to-organ basis. Lung cancer cannot be detected without a complete X-ray of the chest; early cervical cancer cannot be revealed without a Papanicolaou smear; early rectal or colonic cancer, without a proctoscopic examination; or early oropharyngeal cancer, without an examination of the larynx by means of a laryngeal mirror. Except for the Pap test, which is so simple that it is part of the routine of a general examination for the majority of doctors, these tests are not and often cannot be given by individual physicians. Taking a complete medical history and running a complete physical examination of the patient by a physician takes at least one hour and a half. The examination must be done yearly if it is to be meaningful. In a population the size of the United States, individual screening tests defy the present ability of doctors to conduct them and of patients to pay for them. The maintenance of health, or the prevention of illness, must therefore become a concern of the community, of the state, and of the nation; the treatment of disease can remain the responsibility of the individual physician, on a patient-to-doctor basis.

The establishment of centers for cancer screening on a community, regional, or hospital basis would appear essential for the early detection of most malignancies. The establishment of these diagnostic centers will require a new and enlightened approach by both physicians and community leaders.

PUBLIC EDUCATION

Public education plays a key role in cancer prevention and early cancer detection. Accurate information must be spread about cancer and particularly about the hopeful prognosis on many forms of cancer when detected and treated at an early stage (see fig. 10–1).

The American Cancer Society in its public education program gives seven warning signals of cancer:

1. Unusual bleeding or discharge from any body orifice
2. A sore that does not heal
3. A change in bowel or bladder habits
4. A lump or thickening in the breast or elsewhere
5. Persistent hoarseness, cough, or blood spitting
6. Indigestion or difficulty in swallowing
7. A change in a wart or a mole.

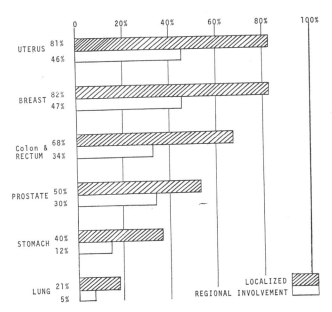

FIGURE 10–1. *Five-year cancer survival rates for selected body sites as a percentage of normal life expectancy. (Source:* End Results and Mortality Trends in Cancer, *National Cancer Institute.)*

The importance of being aware of these signals and acting on them is well illustrated in the results of breast self-examination which has been extensively publicized by the American Cancer Society in its teaching films and through the mass media. Ninety percent of breast cancers are detected by patients themselves in probing for lumps with their own fingers. Verification of the nature of the lump and its appropriate treatment, of course, requires medical supervision.

Until the screening of large masses of people is thoroughly developed on a sound and practical basis, regular medical examinations, at least on a yearly basis, are a wise and essential practice. Careful studies of routine physical examinations, however, show that less than half of the doctors involved give a complete physical examination unless specifically asked to do so by the patient. (The extreme specialization of medicine accounts in part for this fact.) Only about 50 percent of the doctors include a proctosigmoid examination (of the rectum and lower colon) as part of a routine procedure. Only about 20 percent do a laryngeal mirror examination. We have mentioned that pelvic examinations with the adjunct of a Pap smear are done commonly, with 80 percent of the doctors practicing it routinely during a general physical examination. A routine physical examination for early detection should include then:

(1) Examination of the pelvic organs by the Papanicolaou smear technique.

(2) An oro-pharyngeal examination of the larynx.

(3) A routine chest X-ray.

(4) A proctosigmoidoscopic examination.

Doctors themselves fail to give wholehearted support to yearly physical examination for they do not practice it amongst themselves. A study discloses that only about 30 percent of doctors received a physical examination during the year preceding the study and that only 30 percent have had four or more such examinations within the past 10 years. This lukewarm response of doctors to routine physical examinations accounts in part for the failure of the general public to be responsive to programs for early cancer detection.

Mass screening programs should remain the hope of the future, a future not too remote if support for such programs becomes widespread. U.S. statistics for 1970 show that 104,000 of the current

320,000 deaths by cancer per year could be averted by earlier detection and treatment. Cancer detection centers exist in Missouri and Minnesota. The work done in these centers has disclosed that cancers (of the breast, colon, rectum, and uterus) detected and treated early demonstrate at least a 20 to 25 percent improvement in the 5-year survival rate over the national average. The figures for the Minnesota detection center for 1948 to 1967 are shown in table 10–1.

TABLE 10-1

Relationship of examinations to cancers detected at
the Minnesota cancer detection center, 1948–1967

Sex	Number of patients	Number of examinations	Cancer detected	Ratio of cancers to examinations		
				Initial	Recheck	Per patient
Male	6,447	34,108	307	1/69	1/130	1/21
Female	7,201	35,104	260	1/91	1/154	1/28
Total	13,648	69,212	567	1/79	1/141	1/24

In a 20-year period, 13,648 persons had a total of 69,212 annual examinations, an average of five or more per person. Altogether 567 proven cancers were found. The yield from the examinations was between one case per 100 to one case per 150 examinations performed. The yield from routine chest X-ray on asymptomatic persons was two lung cancers per 35,104 examinations. If one such examination costs approximately $10, a total of $350,000 was spent on chest X-rays for the actual detection of two cancers, hardly an argument in favor of routine X-ray examinations of the chest in yearly physical examinations for patients over 45 years of age.

Many other studies are available. In a group of 1,000 asymptomatic persons (no bowel bleeding or change in bowel habits) examination of the rectum and sigmoid by proctosigmoidoscopy discovered no frank cancer but revealed that 5 percent of those examined had benign lesions due to polyps which could easily be cured and thus theoretically prevent the development of cancer in these polyps.

In another group of 1,000 patients, 30 percent had some type of symptoms (bleeding, pain, change in bowel habits); 10 percent had polyps, and one per 150 had frank cancers. When one realizes that 70 percent of all cancers of the colon and rectum are within reach of the proctoscope the value of such a simple examination procedure for the early detection of cancer of the rectum and sigmoid becomes apparent.

The effectiveness of Pap smears for detection of uterine cancer is well established. The rate of initial detection on a first examination is a modest 2.1 percent per 1,000. Pap smears should be done yearly for low risk women and every three to six months for women in high-risk cervical cancer groups, notably women in lower income and socio-economic groups. These include Negro, Puerto Rican, and Mexican and Latin American women, the latter group (women of Mexican or Latin American origin) showing a 20 to 35 percent per 1,000 rate of detection.

Routine mammography (breast X-ray) is a worthwhile procedure for the detection of breast cancer. It is true that 95 percent of breast lumps are detected by self-examination. Yet in asymptomatic women, between 1 to 1.5 breast lesions per 1,000 studies can be found on routine mammograms. In a 10-year mammographic survey on 1,121 women over 35 without symptoms of breast disease who reported for breast X-ray at an interval of 6 months, 36 cancers in 33 women were found (bilateral lesions having been present in three of the group). This early detection (the diameter of the lesion being below the size detectable clinically) put these women in a favorable situation for treatment. Another favorable factor was that 70 percent of the women did not have metatasis to the regional lymph nodes. Since the study yielded a rather high incidence of cancer in 1,121 women the usefulness of mammography is potentially comparable for early breast cancer detection to that of the Pap smear for early detection of cervical cancer. However a large-scale scanning program utilizing mammography cannot be implemented until a sufficient number of trained radiologists and paramedical personnel is available for such programs.

Mammography is certainly indicated for:

any patient with carcinoma of one breast who has a 10 to 15 percent chance of developing carcinoma in the other breast,

any patient with discharge in the nipple,

any patient with a strong family history of cancer,

patients with *dysplasia* of the breast (abnormality of development)

and *cystic mastitis* (inflammation of mammary glands),
persons with large breasts for whom clinical examination is notoriously difficult for the detection of early small lesions.

In more deeply seated organs of the body (brain, kidney, liver, and pancreas) the diagnosis of cancer is difficult by current techniques. Some promise is offered by the use of radioactive isotopes for scanning lesions of these organs. Certain radioactive isotopes are now known which will localize in internal organs, and even concentrate in a given organ; abnormalities in the configuration of an organ will generally indicate destruction of a segment of the organ. This technique is not specific for the diagnosis of cancer but indicates a lesion the nature of which must be discovered by subsequent examinations.

At present it is quite apparent that the proper procedure for cancer detection should include:

(1) Complete history and physical examination
(2) Special examination procedures, e.g. use of laryngeal mirror and proctosigmoidoscopy
(3) Rectal and pelvic examinations, including Pap smear
(4) Complete blood count and urine test
(5) Chest X-ray
(6) Mammography
(7) Radioactive isotope screening for the deeper organs.

If these procedures are beyond the capabilities of the individual physician we must change our focus on patient care. Health centers should be established not only for the screening of cancer but for all health hazards, cardiovascular diseases, renal diseases, and the like. We should make maximum use of the current advances in technology, automation, and the training of paramedical personnel to conduct the majority of examinations. Many procedures could be automated, and any abnormalities uncovered could then be referred to physicians for individual analysis. In this manner the physicians' time could be devoted to treatment and they could focus their attention on the patient and his medical needs.

Time and effort will be required for the attainment of these goals, but health and the preservation of health concern the whole national community and deserve a larger place in community affairs. The goal is to bring the patient to the doctor in time. No matter how difficult it may be to organize health centers, the rewards, medical as well as social and economic, appear so great that no effort should be spared to bring them into being.

GENETIC COUNSELING AND POPULATION GENETICS

Cancer is an increasing threat to the life and health of children. The seeds of cancerous traits are commonly sown before birth through a change in a single gene or even an inconspicuous change in the growing embryo which may, for instance, have been exposed to X-rays. Drugs, too, may initiate or promote cancerous traits. Every physician nowadays thinks twice before ordering abdominal radiographs on pregnant women or before prescribing novel drugs which may have a beneficial effect on the adult but might damage the embryo.

Many physicians are urging the creation of centers for the diagnosis and treatment of childhood cancer and the initiation of genetic counseling, with the hope of preventing childhood cancer by rapid dissemination of information about the factors involved in the heredity of cancer. But information must be brought to the public without engendering excessive concern about cancer. For it is a well-known psychological fact that fear, apprehension, and anxiety are strong deterrents to the prevention and early diagnosis and treatment of cancer.

The types and behavior of cancer in children differ markedly from those in the adult. Leukemia has already been noted as the most common type of cancer among children by far. Tumors of the central nervous system, including retinoblastoma of the eye, account for 20 percent of childhood cancers. Tumors of the sympathetic nervous system (neuroblastoma of the adrenals) and of the kidney (Wilms' tumor) also account for 20 percent of the malignancies in children.

Sadly, less than 20 percent of children's cancers can be arrested, in contrast to an overall arrest rate of 40 percent for adults. The main reason for this unfortunate situation is that childhood cancers are usually generalized diseases in more than 65 percent of the cases, so that surgery and irradiation cannot be very effective therapies.

Cancers of which children are the victims have a wide diversity of causes. Leukemia illustrates this diversity of causation for, at least by one classification, there are four different leukemias in childhood: familial, associated with Mongolism, idiopathic (of unknown causation), and radiogenic (related to radiation exposure in embryonic life or early infancy).

Some cancers of childhood are definitely due to genetic disorders. The following tabulation lists some of the known interrelationships between heredity, carcinogens, and cancer.

	Proved	*Not proved*
DISEASES RELATED TO HEREDITY	Polyposis coli Retinoblastoma Xeroderma pigmentosa Neurofibromatosis Gardner's syndrome Basal cell nevus syndrome	Leukemia Myeloma Macroglobulinemia Hemangioblastoma Melanoma
DISEASES RELATED TO NON-LIVING CARCINOGENS	Aniline dyes Coal tar Hydrocarbons Radiation Ultraviolet light Tobacco? Other chemicals (arsenic, etc.)	Smog Multiple trauma Ethanol Steroids
DISEASES RELATED TO LIVING CARCINOGENS		Leukemia virus Burkitt lymphoma Myeloma virus Adenovirus Cytomegalic virus Pleuro-pneumonia like organisms

Many "cancer families" have been identified by geneticists through the accurate mapping of family trees over several generations. These "cancer families" have a high frequency of cancer in many sites and cancer tends to appear among them at an early age.

Parents who have suffered the loss of one child from cancer naturally wonder whether it is safe to have more children. This raises the question of genetic counseling and all its profound implications. Genetic counseling should never be used in a manner capable of arousing fear of cancer but as the most delicate theoretical weapon.

What is known of genetics and cancer can serve to reassure healthy parents with an affected child: it is safe for them to have more children, unless they are clearly a "cancer family." It is particularly safe for them to have more children if the affected child reached school age. On the other hand parents with two affected children should be warned that a new child in their family would face the risk of being affected by cancer too. Persons who have survived operations for embryonic cancer in their own childhood, who have survived retinoblastoma or Wilms' tumor should probably make the decision not to have children.

The parents of a Mongol child should be informed that leukemia is frequent in such children. The chances of having a second Mongol child are statistically insignificant, however, and they need not worry about their other non-Mongoloid children developing leukemia. On the other hand if the parents already have two or more affected children (either with Mongolism or with leukemia) their chances of having a third or fourth child suffering from these abnormalities are distinctly greater.

A LOOK AT THE FUTURE

The disturbing presence of childhood cancer should alert us all the more to the need for cancer prevention, early detection, and early treatment. Public education is of paramount importance if these goals are to be attained. The potential effects of early cancer detection on cancer mortality are shown in a table of projected cancer deaths for the State of California in the early 1970's.

Cancer education has two prime objectives:

1. Spreading accurate information about hopeful prognosis for many forms of cancers.

2. Persuading the bulk of the population to participate in preventive screening programs or at least to consult a doctor for symptoms which may appear trivial but are warning signals of *early* cancer.

Public education requires an understanding of group behavior. Positive advice is needed, not negative admonitions. It is well-known

TABLE 10–2
Estimated Effects of Early Cancer Detection
on Cancer Mortality in California
(Breslow Table)

Body sites	Deaths Expected per year, early 1970's, based on 1950–1960 trends	Deaths avoidable through application of present knowledge
All Sites	30,000	7,500
Lung	7,500	3,750
Stomach	1,600	—
Colon-Rectum	4,000	800
Pancreas	1,800	—
Breast	2,700	600
Uterus (cervix and corpus)	1,100	850
Ovary	900	150
Prostate	1,300	150
Kidney and Bladder	1,400	400
Leukemia	1,700	—
All Other	6,000	800

that the implied threats of even well-meaning propaganda arouse fear and anxiety which in turn awaken defense mechanisms freezing people into inaction. What then happens is the exact opposite of what was expected.

Every medium of education has its strong and weak points. Newspapers, films, pamphlets, television, and personal contacts, all can play a useful role in cancer prevention. It is not surprising that television seems to be the most influential medium since it almost offers the closeness and intimacy of person-to-person contact. It is even less surprising that the very best results seems to be obtained from doctor-to-patient contact; man needs a climate of intimacy, trust, and even secrecy, to be most receptive to ideas that may subtly threaten his own preconceptions or fears. At the present time, when mass screening is not yet prevalent in the struggle against cancer, doctors may be the most persuasive agents in preparing the general public to accept these new procedures.

Mass screening is more readily accepted by higher income groups, who are more apt to have free time and are unafraid to lose income from absence of work. But time is important to everyone. A total screening in a short period of time would therefore be more acceptable to all concerned than a lengthy screening with multiple individual tests which demand repeated visits to a clinic. Some parts of a total screening (such as anal and rectal examinations) are distasteful to everybody. It should be the physician's role to "sell" these unpleasant but necessary examinations to the public and to make physically disagreeable procedures psychologically acceptable.

At the moment mass-screening techniques are still tedious, excessively time-consuming for patients and doctors alike, and inordinately expensive. But this is purely because of the inadequacies and shortcomings in the existing structure of health care. The focus is still on the treatment rather than on the prevention of illness. The necessary change of focus from treatment of disease to its prevention cannot be the work of doctors alone, and techniques must be devised for improving the delivery of health care to all members of our society. Surely the prevention of deaths from cancer is worth the planning involved.

Among the revolutionary methods essential for this purpose is the use of mobile doctors' offices. These mobile offices would recruit patients at their place of employment, thus replacing the traditional visit to a doctor's office. They would serve a region or community, traveling to all major working areas.

A large number of supplementary and paramedical health personnel could be employed, with only one physician present in a group of health workers.

The medical history of every patient would be taken by paramedical help, then recorded on computerized records. Questions could be phrased so that yes and no answers would be punched by the patient, and the shadings of affirmative and negative answers could be graduated from 1 to 5.

The majority of physical examinations would be conducted by nurses or paramedical personnel. They would give X-rays of the chest and breast, obtain blood, urine, and stool samples. The doctor would be available for consultation and employment of specialized techniques, including laryngeal mirror, proctoscopic, rectal, and pelvic examinations.

The laboratory analyses would be performed on the spot by current automated techniques. All results from X-rays, laboratory analyses, physical examination, and history would be scanned by a computer and any patient with an abnormality then detected could go to a medical clinic or to his personal physician for additional studies. To save time and personnel these records could be televised to the clinic or doctor's office and no doubt other techniques of practical interest will be available in the future to speed up and simplify screening of masses of population for cancer and other diseases. The saving of time alone would rapidly justify the cost of this new type of health program.

Truly a revolution in health care is essential if we are to preserve the health of our society. An enlightened nation will soon require the preservation of the health of all of its members. The prevention of cancer, and its appropriate treatment, can only be achieved through new approaches, perhaps similar to, or stemming from, those outlined above.

PART THREE

THE TREATMENT OF CANCER

11

THE SURGERY
OF CANCER

"Surgery does the ideal thing–
it separates the patient
from his disease."
LOGAN CLENDENING

When a growth endangers your life, remove it: what simpler concept could exist for the cure of cancer than an operation which extirpates the disease? As early as 2500 B.C. the Hindus employed this direct principle and eradicated cancerous lesions of the skin by means of cautery. Today with our ability to control infection with antibiotics, to prevent shock with blood or blood substitutes, to administer anesthetics safely during prolonged operations, successful procedures in the operating room range from the simple ablation of small skin cancer by cautery to the most complicated cancer surgery by the most refined techniques.

The fundamental justification for the use of surgery for the cure of cancer rests on the premise that an operation can remove every last surviving cancer cell from the patient. Such a premise is questionable, for many cancer cells do not conform to this precept. Not only do they behave as autonomous growths locally but they also show a propensity for spread and metastasis through the blood and lymph streams. Blood-borne metastases, unless solitary, are beyond surgical control. But this is not necessarily true for metastases incident to the carrying of cancer cells by the lymph. Lymph nodes in the vicinity of the cancer sites, the regional lymph nodes, may filter out the cancer cells reaching them, and can almost invariably be excised by modern surgical techniques with little detriment to the patient.

Patients can survive surgical procedures of formidable, even mutilating, magnitude but cannot be assured of absolute cure of their cancer. Surgery must be regarded, then, in terms of the functional form life will assume after completion of the operation. The quality of life becomes as important as life itself in the surgical treatment of cancer.

The ideal organ with which to evaluate the effects of surgery in the treatment of cancer is the breast. We have noted before that it is the most common site of cancer in women, and that such cancers are the leading cause of death in white women in the United States in the age group 39 to 54. No other disease kills as many mothers. Breast cancers are even more frequent in unmarried, childless women. A hereditary factor makes it more common in families. Some social factors are important, for breast cancer is more frequent in persons of lower economic status. It seems that a previous oophorectomy (removal of the ovaries) reduces the incidence of the disease. Recently the question has been raised as to whether the use of oral contraceptives has an influence on breast cancer. This has not been determined, but, on the other hand, there is little likelihood that the prolonged used of contraceptives to avoid pregnancy, lactation, and nursing is a factor in *reducing* the incidence of breast cancer.

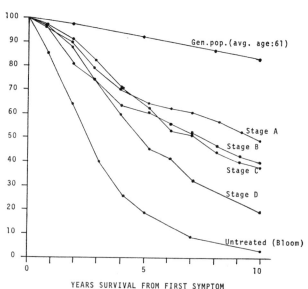

FIGURE 11–1. *Survival rates of 460 EFSCH patients treated with radical mastectomy (1940 to 1952), compared with survival rates of 250 untreated patients. Survival rates are progressively lower for operations performed at later stages. (Source: J. S. Spratt and W. L. Donegan,* Cancer of the Breast, *Saunders, Philadelphia, 1967, p. 119.*

YEARS SURVIVAL FROM FIRST SYMPTOM

The best outlook for the individual patient occurs when the cancer is diagnosed early before there is any involvement of the regional lymph nodes. The 5-year survival rates of localized breast cancers are 80 to 85 percent as compared to 45 percent or less when the regional lymph nodes are involved (fig. 11-1). Programs of education and screening by mammography or even more effective techniques are, therefore, among the most urgent tasks of preventive medicine. The two factors which influence to the greatest extent the results of treatment in cancer of the breast are:

1. The size of the lesion at the time treatment is initiated.

2. The presence or absence of involvement of regional lymph nodes at the time treatment is commenced.

The smaller the lesion, the more favorable the prognosis. The absence of regional lymph-node involvement improves the 5-year survival rate tremendously, by as much as 40 to 80 percent or more over a 5-year period. The importance of early diagnosis in carcinoma of the breast cannot be overemphasized; the earlier the diagnosis can be made the smaller the size of the invaded area and the smaller the likelihood that the regional lymph nodes will be involved (fig. 11-2).

PROBLEMS IN SURGICAL THERAPY

We cannot explore the benefits gained from the surgical treatment of cancer without equal consideration of some of the controversies inherent in this approach to the cure of cancer. Late in the nineteenth century the leading European surgeons developed safe techniques for treatment of breast cancer by surgery. The breast, and the contained cancer, could be removed with essentially no mortality. But

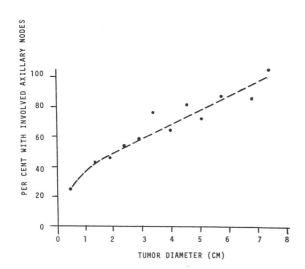

FIGURE 11-2. *The relation of tumor size to the degree of lymph-node involvement. (Source: Spratt and Donegan,* Cancer of the Breast, *p. 63.)*

recurrences of the cancer in the operative area within a period of
five years were reported by such surgical masters as Billroth and von
Bergmann in 60 to 80 percent of their cases. To reduce the incidence
of such recurrences Professor William S. Halsted, of Johns Hopkins
University, devised a surgical procedure which lowered the frequency of local recurrence to between 10 and 20 percent. The basic
techniques emphasized by Halsted were (1) wide removal of the
breast and (2) in continuity, without breaking or crossing the lymphatic channels in the underlying muscles (the pectoral muscles),
massive excision of the regional lymph nodes in the axilla (under the
arm). (See fig. 11-3.)

The main pectoral muscle, the *pectoralis major,* is a muscle on
the chest wall immediately beneath the breast. It covers the axilla
and runs through the arm, adding strength to the pulling of the arm
against the chest wall. The presence of this muscle is not essential to
the good function of the arm, and Halsted wrote: "Why should we
shave the under-surface of the cancer so narrowly if the pectoralis
major muscle or a part of it can be removed without danger and
without causing subsequent disability, and if there are positive indi-

FIGURE 11–3. *Schematic diagram of the portions of the breast involved in the radical mastectomy of Halsted. (The breast is removed together with the pectoral muscles and axillary nodes in
this surgical procedure.) (Modified from Spratt and Donegan,*
Cancer of the Breast, *p. 63.)*

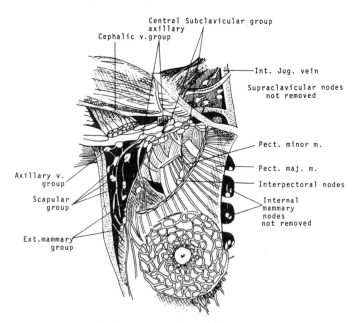

cations for its removal?" Halsted then proceeded to explain why he favored this procedure, saying: "The pectoralis major muscle, entire or all except its clavicular portion, should be excised in every case of cancer of the breast, because the operator is enabled thereby to remove in one piece all of the suspected tissues.

"The suspected tissues should be removed in one piece, (1) lest the wound became infected by the division of tissues invaded by the disease or of lymphatic channels containing cancer cells, and (2) because shreds or pieces of cancerous tissue might readily be over-looked in a piecemeal extirpation."

Halsted's insistence that all cancerous tissue should be removed in one piece and that the axilla should be meticulously cleaned out, has become the central tenet of present-day surgery for cancer of the breast. The radical removal of the pectoralis major and of the re-gional lymph nodes do not result in any significant weakness of the arm, but in about 10 percent of the cases there is a rather pronounced swelling of the arm named *surgical elephantiasis* (elephantiasis chi-rurgicae), due to the accumulation of fluid and difficulty in the drain-age of the lymph from the arm. This lymphedema is massive in a very few cases (about 3 to 5 percent), but some swelling of the arm occurs in 70 percent of the patients who have undergone Halsted's opera-tion, the classical radical mastectomy. Edema is more apt to occur if the patient has received postoperative irradiation therapy. The condition can usually be treated reasonably effectively through the provision of elastic sleeves, Ace bandages, or pressure dressings but can remain troublesome to some women for a lifetime.

On the debit side of a radical mastectomy is a significant defor-mity of the chest wall resulting from both the loss of the breast and the extensive removal of the pectoral muscles. The use of the arm is rarely significantly impaired; rather there remains a psychological burden to many women, a feeling of loss of femininity. This burden would not be excessive if surgery could truly be said to cure breast cancer, but does it? The concept of "true," or actual, cure must be explored, for cancer is not always an autonomous growth, restricted to the site of its appearance, nor can it always be checked and annihi-lated. It has an innate tendency to spread, and metastases are not easy to detect.

The concept of true cure really depends upon the degree of lymph-node involvement and dissemination of the disease through the bloodstream, both of which may require months or years to become apparent. The usual standard in assessing results in the treatment of cancer is the arrest of the disease for a period of five years, the 5-year arrest rate. Notice that this is quite different from a cure, and that we do not speak of a 5-year cure rate, but in terms of the 5-year arrest rate, the 10-year arrest rate, and so on. The word cure is rarely used in assessing end results of the treatment of cancer. If this appears to be too pessimistic a view, it is nonetheless a realistic one. Let us remember that descriptions of the treatment of cancer deserve the same objectivity that discussions of the scientific knowledge about cancer merit.

At the beginning of this chapter we noted that the 5-year survival rate in breast cancer is as high as 85 percent if the axillary lymph nodes are uninvolved at the time of surgery but a much lower 45 percent when the axillary nodes contain tumor cells at the time of the initial surgery. This fact has been observed for the last 50 years. Unfortunately, in at least 25 percent of all cases lymph nodes other than the axillary lymph nodes are invaded by cancer too when one is dealing with a cancer of the breast. The *internal mammary chain,* situated within the chest, along the breast bone, is apt to contain cancer cells if the tumor is located in the inner quadrant of the breast, or, particularly, if the axillary lymph nodes are already involved with tumor; and the *supraclavicular lymph nodes,* above the clavicle, are commonly the site of cancer spread once the axillary lymph nodes have become the repository of cancer cells. Figure 11-4 shows the total possible lymphatic spread to the adjoining lymph nodes from cancer of the breast.

FIGURE 11–4. *Total possible spread (in percent) to adjoining lymph nodes in cancer of the breast. (Source:* L. H. Garland, "Rationale and Results of Simple Mastectomy Plus Radiotherapy in Primary Cancer of the Breast," American Journal of Roentgenology, Radium Therapy, and Nuclear Medicine, *Dec. 1954, p. 929.*

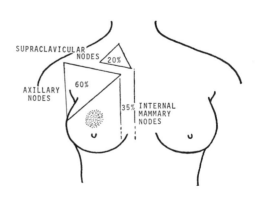

From the above considerations on the lymphatic and bloodstream spread in cancer of the breast, two dilemmas arise to confront the surgeon who is about to perform a classical radical mastectomy:

1. What is the true extent of the lymphatic involvement at the time of surgical intervention?

2. What is the status of the dissemination of the disease in the bloodstream at the moment of surgical intervention?

An answer to the second question may lead to an uncomfortable prospect indeed, for it can indicate that the cancer has become a generalized disorder beyond the scope of surgical therapy without the patient or the surgeon having been aware of it. Unfortunately, current studies on bloodstream dissemination do not offer reliable data. The surgeon has to assume that, in the absence of discernible distant metastases, which are searched for by X-rays of the chest and bones before the operation, the cancer is localized at the site of the tumor and has not spread beyond the regional lymph nodes.

The two dilemmas presenting themselves to the surgeon before breast surgery have led in the past 10 years to variations in the type of mastectomy used in the treatment of breast cancer. Briefly, surgical therapy of breast cancer can take three forms:

1. *Simple mastectomy,* consisting of the removal of the breast, but not removal of the pectoral muscles, and with variable removal of the axillary lymph nodes (depending upon the findings at the time of surgery).

2. *Classical radical mastectomy* of Halsted, the long hard procedure and the one still generally accepted in the treatment of cancer of the breast.

3. *Super-radical mastectomy,* an extended operation which, in carefully selected cases, includes not only the classical radical mastectomy but the removal of the supraclavicular nodes and of the internal mammary nodes, together with the axillary nodes.

The first-listed, simpler operation preserves the form and function of the chest wall and of the arm and reduces the possibility of lymphedema in the arm. The third, or extended operation, the super-radical mastectomy, strives for cure of the disease, not for preservation of form and function.

How can the patient and surgeon decide for minimal or maximal surgery? The decision must be made on the basis of clinical studies and their end results. What is known of the general survival from cancer of the breast treated by different surgical approaches over the past 50 years, the modern era? Let us examine the existing data.

REAL VERSUS APPARENT CURABILITY

We would, of course, like to assess and measure the absolute curability of breast cancer, but all the collected data are in terms of a 5-year survival rate as the standard of cure. The number of patients surviving breast cancer five years after treatment represents the apparent cure rate. The real cure rate, however, would be represented by the difference between the survival rate of all treated cases and what would have been the survival of these same cases had they been left untreated. The control data on untreated cases are very difficult to obtain, for doctors invariably recommend some type of treatment for breast cancer, regardless of the stage at which it presents itself, and patients rarely refuse the treatment offered. The control data on survival after untreated breast cancer comes from a rather small and biased selection of patients who, for a variety of personal reasons, have refused recommended treatment.

We have already said that patients with breast cancer coming to treatment without metastasis to the axillary lymph nodes have a much higher survival, or arrest, rate, than those coming to treatment with involvement of these nodes. Recognizing cancer early and treating it early, then, means treating it prior to metastasis to the lymph nodes. The importance of early diagnosis and early treatment cannot be overemphasized. The current techniques for early diagnosis of breast cancer, in addition to physical examination, include mammography, xerography, and thermography. To be truly meaningful and to make an impact on the disease, however, these techniques must be practiced on a mass population screening basis.

THE NATURAL HISTORY OF BREAST CANCER—
BIOLOGIC PREDETERMINISM

It must regretfully be recorded that there has been no improvement in the death rate from breast cancer in the last 60 years. Furthermore, during the past 30 years the incidence of breast cancer has not diminished, regardless of the therapeutic methods recommended to lessen its occurrence. In the chapter dealing with the statistics of cancer it was noted that if breast cancer were actually cured women treated for the disease would die at the same rate as women of the same age in the general population. A cure, in other words, would be absolute only if the patient survived and died from another cause and autopsy revealed no evidence of residual cancer. But the fact is that, even after 20 years, the primary cause of death for these women still arises from metastases from the original breast cancer.

Even if some individual patients are indubitably cured of breast cancer, we have failed to alter the mortality from this disease in the large masses of our population. The question raised for surgery is then: What should be the anatomical limits of surgical excision of cancer of the breast, in order to heighten the survival rate in large groups of the population? What are the criteria for choosing one type of surgical intervention over another? Could mere removal of the breast cancer itself yield an equal cure rate without mastectomy if the lesion were diagnosed in its formative stages?

It is by no means simple to answer the foregoing questions, for the facts, or lack of them, concerning each case are numerous and largely unknown. Let us take as an example the balance between the tumor and the host, the degree of the patient's immunological response, which we have already discussed in theory. This balance is established very early in the period when the tumor is invisible, below a size detectable by palpation. When the patient comes to the physician the behavior of her cancer has already been determined. This behavior is highly individual and depends upon the patient's biologic potential, which is expressed in the concept of *biologic predeterminism*. When assessing the results of breast cancer therapy this concept must be reckoned with, yet its expression in quantitative terms is impossible. One patient will have a slow-growing tumor, with a good chance of cure by surgical excision, for it will tend to spread slowly in size and metastasize late to the axillary lymph nodes. Another patient will have a small tumor, but it will be of virulent biologic potential; it might well still be "occult," therefore impalpable, but have already spread to the axillary lymph nodes before it makes its presence known.

Another example of what confronts the concerned surgeon before intervention is his knowledge that the larger the tumor, the greater the chances that the axillary lymph nodes will be invaded by cancer. But he also knows that 30 percent of the times when the nodes in the axilla are palpable they are *not* involved by tumor microscopically; distressingly, in another 30 percent of the cases, when the nodes cannot be felt by palpation, they *are* involved by tumor on microscopic examination.

These hard facts, and others, must be acknowledged when the surgeon weighs one method of surgery against another, when he analyzes the usefulness of each treatment. It is often beyond his power to make a truly sound and scientific decision. He must make empirical decisions, for there is at the present time no certainty about the absolute worth of any chosen surgical therapy. Absolute appraisal of spread to the regional lymph nodes requires a prior commitment on the part of the surgeon to a given surgical technique, in order to obtain the nodes for analysis. The natural history of any given breast cancer thereby becomes extremely difficult to assess.

Conflicts in real versus apparent curability of cancer of the breast by surgery, and the unfathomable depths of the variable history of the disease in each patient, have led to numerous modalities, extensions, and combinations of surgical therapies for breast cancer. In an effort to improve the end results, surgeons have at times rejected the classical radical mastectomy of Halsted in favor of the simple mastectomy of Crile. Others have felt that the surgical approach has not been radical enough and have explored the super-radical mastectomy of Urban and Wangensteen, the selected radical mastectomy of Haagensen, or the McWhirter technique. We will analyze these diverse approaches at greater length in the following subsections, but first let us return to an even more basic question.

This question is: Should lymph nodes be removed, irradiated, or left alone in the treatment of breast cancer, or, indeed, in the treatment of cancer in general? The long-awaited answer to this question is still no closer at hand. It cannot be reached if we hold fast to the teachings of our forebears, however illustrious, and if we remain unwilling to conduct controlled clinical experiments which may separate us from our comfortable but unconfirmed convictions. A powerful figure propagates a clinical doctrine and hundreds of patients are treated on the basis of a blind acceptance of current dogmas. Is it less ethical to admit that knowledge must still be gained in a clinical problem and that we still have to discover sound principles on which the therapy of cancer can be designed and evaluated?

Let us look, then, at the current apparent cure rates in the treatment of breast cancer, and analyze the results as clearly as we possibly can. Hopefully this will resolve some of the present dilemmas in the surgical treatment of breast cancer.

THE CLASSICAL RADICAL MASTECTOMY

Halsted proposed the classical radical mastectomy in 1906. By 1925, it had become apparent that the techniques developed by Halsted were unsuited to many advanced cancer cases. It became necessary to evaluate the results, first, on the basis of a clinical assessment of the cancer prior to surgical treatment, and, secondly, on the available pathologic information following the mastectomy. The clinical classification before surgery was determined by physical examination of the breast, axilla, and neck, and by radiographic examination of the chest and bones. The pathological classification after surgery was based upon the presence of lymph-node involvement and the degree of this involvement. Clearly, the radical mastectomy of Halsted is of great worth in establishing a pathological estimate of the spread of a breast cancer, since it provides the excised axillary lymph nodes to the pathologist for microscopic examination.

Obviously a clinical classification is quite different from a pathological classification. What can be seen or felt in a clinical examination does not reveal the true extent of the disease, and indeed it can be misleading, for in 30 percent of the cases when the clinician feels no axillary lymph nodes on palpation the nodes are found to be involved on pathological examination. Conversely, in another, and distressing, 30 percent of the cases wherein the clinician can palpate the lymph nodes these nodes are found to be free of cancer on pathological examination. A total of at least 50 percent chance of error is therefore incorporated in the purely clinical classification of breast cancer.

The current *clinical classification* for cancer of the breast comprises four stages, or classes (see also fig. 11-1).

1. CLASS A. The tumor is limited to the breast
            No axillary lymph nodes are palpable
2. CLASS B. The tumor is confined to the breast but mobile lymph nodes palpable in the axilla (less than 2 cm in size)
3. CLASS C. The growth extends beyond the breast, as evidenced by skin invasion or fixation of the skin to the tumor
            Tumor is fixed to the underlying muscle, or
            Axillary lymph nodes larger than 2 cm in size are present in palpation
4. CLASS D. The growth extends beyond the breast, as evidenced by fixation and matting of axillary lymph nodes
            Fixation of the tumor to the chest wall
            Metastases (shown by X-rays of the chest and bones)

The *pathological classification* comprises three stages:

1. CLASS A. The tumor is limited to the breast
            The axillary lymph nodes are not involved histologically
2. CLASS B. The tumor is present in the breast and
            The axillary lymph nodes are involved histologically
3. CLASS C. The tumor extends beyond the breast and
            The axillary lymph nodes, as evidenced by:
            Radiologic or additional pathological studies on the neck nodes and internal mammary nodes

The results of several large series of breast cancers managed by radical mastectomy are now available, and the correlation with clinical staging is apparent in the following tabulation.

Authors	Clinical Stage	Number of Patients	5-year Survivals (percent)	Total (percent)
Butcher	A	216	76	
(1963)	B	135	48	60
	C	48	48	
	D	26	11	

Authors	Clinical Stage	Number of Patients	5-year Survivals (percent)	Total (percent)
Handley &	A	77	75	
Thackeray	B	58	57	65
(1963)	C	8	25	
	D	0	0	
Haagensen &	A	344	84	
Cooley	B	138	59	72
(1963)	C	63	43	
	D	11	18	

These are the results from clinical staging of the disease. If one is to give the results on the basis of pathological staging, radical mastectomy produces the following results (in percent):

1. STAGE A.   5-year Survival   80 to 85
2. STAGE B.   5-year Survival   45 to 50
3. STAGE C.   5-year Survival   20 to 25

The differences between clinical versus pathological staging of breast cancer bring out into the open the two dilemmas facing the surgeon.

1. The true extent of lymphatic involvement is not known at the time of surgery.

2. The status of bloodstream dissemination is never known in stage 1 and stage 2 of either the clinical or pathological classification, and the biological potential of the tumor is likewise unknown. It is only later, in the postoperative course, that the discovery of metastases, and the rapidity of their appearance, clarify the assessment of these dilemmas.

Recognition of these dilemmas led, in the 1950's, to more exact studies on the lymphatic spread of breast cancer, for surgeons were, and remain, unwilling to accept the gloomy prospect that breast cancer can be, from its inception, a generalized disorder, biologically predetermined. The new studies showed that (as we have stated before) in at least 25 percent of the cases cancer of the breast spread to the lymph nodes within the chest wall, along the internal mammary chain, and less frequently to the supraclavicular nodes. The spread to the internal mammary chain is more prone to occur if the tumor of the breast is situated in the inner quadrant of the breast, but also, unfortunately, in all cases after the axillary lymph nodes have become invaded by tumor. The supraclavicular nodes are almost invariably involved after the axillary lymph nodes and the nodes of the internal mammary chain are blocked by tumor.

Certain surgeons have long maintained that, in those cases beyond the stage B of the clinical classification, a radical mastectomy is of no avail. Fixation of the tumor to the skin, the muscles, or matting of the axillary lymph nodes, denote to many surgeons that the lesion is inoperable, just as everyone agrees that radical mastectomy is not indicated if the lesion has already spread beyond the breast and the axillary lymph nodes. The uncertain nature of involvement of supraclavicular nodes and internal mammary nodes and axillary nodes with tumor led some pioneering physicians to introduce new methods in the surgical treatment of cancer of the breast in the 1950's. Unfortunately, the fundamental statistical and biological principles for conducting controlled clinical trials of alternate therapeutic methods were not clearly understood by these early pioneers, and irrefutable answers to clinical questions were and remain hard to obtain from the new treatments proposed. Nevertheless Robert McWhirter forged ahead with a new treatment which combined simple mastectomy with irradiation of the supraclavicular, axillary, and internal mammary nodes and his work did much to stimulate current concepts in the clinical treatment of breast and other cancers.

THE MCWHIRTER TECHNIQUE

McWhirter, reflecting upon the growing store of knowledge on the lymphatic spread of breast cancer, concluded in the 1950's that by the time patients come to surgery their fate has already been sealed in over half the cases by the unsuspected spread of the malignant cells beyond the limits of the surgical procedure. Why not, then, remove the breast and its tumor by simple mastectomy, and treat *all* of the regional lymph nodes—the axillary, the supraclavicular, and the internal mammary chains—by irradiation? The simple mastectomy is an innocuous procedure: it improves the quality of the patient's life by removing the anxiety associated with the malignant lump, reduces the rate of local recurrence, and prevents ulceration yet provokes no malfunction or swelling of the arm. McWhirter (1955) persuaded many British surgeons to follow his technique, for which the 5-year survival rate has been shown to compare very favorably with that of radical mastectomy, with or without postoperative irradiation. In fact, the 5-year survival rate for all of his cases treated by this method was 55 percent, equal to any other form of therapy for all cases in clinical stages 1 and 2. Notice here that the McWhirter approach does not give us any information on the status of the lymph nodes prior to the treatment by irradiation, and that the only statistical evaluation that can be made is on the basis of all cases coming with cancer of the breast for treatment in a given period of time.

The McWhirter method, then, cannot provide any information on the histological nature of the regional lymph nodes. There is no way of comparing the results of this technique in any given case with the results of the classical radical mastectomy in any given case wherein the presence or absence of axillary lymph-node involvement on a histological basis is known. It remains uncertain whether the McWhirter method is better than the classical radical mastectomy in any given patient. If the lymph nodes are uninvolved, the classical operation may indeed be better, and the irradiation of all the nodes by the McWhirter method may be unnecessary or even harmful.

The idea of McWhirter was good, but the approach, lacking in random selection of treatment alternatives, did not yield a definitive answer to the treatment dilemma, and most surgeons became willing to admit that the McWhirter treatment might be good in the advanced case but was not desirable in the clinical stage 1 carcinoma of the breast, which was still best treated by the classical radical mastectomy.

THE EXTENDED OPERATION

Three regional lymph-node chains are apt to be involved in metastatic cancer of the breast: the axillary, supraclavicular, and internal mammary. Two special circumstances predispose to internal mammary chain involvement: (1) metastases to over 50 percent of the axillary lymph nodes, and (2) a lesion in the inner quadrant of the breast.

With these facts in mind in the 1950's some surgeons proposed an extended operation for cancer of the breast, conducting first the classical radical mastectomy, but following this by the removal of the supraclavicular and internal mammary lymph nodes. The champions for extended radical mastectomy in this country were Drs. Jerome Urban and Owen Wangensteen. Over 100 operations were done and the 5-year survival rate for classes A and B of the clinical classification was identical with that for radical mastectomy. The 5-year survival rate for classes A to D was slightly better, 70 percent compared to 65 percent, but the difference is not statistically significant. Extending the scope of the operation did not demonstrate a clear-cut improvement in results, even on the basis of the 5-year survival rates as the measure of arrest of the cancer. If one cannot improve the clinical curability of cancer by extending the scope of the operation, should not one become more selective in the employment of even the classical radical mastectomy operation? Cushman Haagensen, one of America's foremost surgeons for breast cancer, directed his efforts to the solution of this question. He devised a selected radical mastectomy in an effort to better classify the cases and correlate the results of treatment with the improved classification and staging of the disease at the moment of initiation of treatment.

HAAGENSEN'S SELECTED RADICAL OPERATION

After reviewing the results from the classical radical operation, the McWhirter method, and the extended radical operation, Haagensen decided that the radical mastectomy should be applied only to selected early cases of breast cancer. He based his selection of patients for radical mastectomy on a triple biopsy technique. Before the breast surgery he performed biopsies of one of the highest axillary lymph nodes, one of the nodes of the internal mammary chain, and one of the nodes of the supraclavicular area. Only if the triple biopsy proved negative would he perform the classical radical operation.

More advanced cases with metastases to the lymph nodes would, he believed, benefit from radiotherapy. When he used this careful selection of cases, the 5-year survival rate of patients subjected to radical mastectomy reached 90 percent.

Haagensen's approach provided two useful bits of evidence:

1. The 5-year survival rate in clinical class A was 84 percent, but dropped to 59 percent in class B. Careful selection of cases on the basis of the triple biopsy enabled the surgeon to limit the radical mastectomy to patients who would have a 90 percent chance of a 5-year arrest.

2. Cases not treated by radical mastectomy were then subjected to radiotherapy, and, as evidenced by the work of Dr. Ruth Guttmann, to which we shall return, were definitely benefited by radiation therapy.

His work also reawakened interest in two highly important questions: (1) The real role of the lymph nodes in the containment of cancer, and (2) the possibility of killing the cancer in regional lymph nodes by intensive irradiation, since irradiation therapy could then be administered to patients with proven nodal metastases.

Haagensen's work raised the theoretical possibility that, if the regional lymph nodes were not involved, they need not be removed, and indeed George Crile, a few years later, adopted simple mastectomy as a possible treatment for breast cancer. His work also provided Dr. Guttmann, a radiotherapist, with the opportunity of studying the effects of radiation therapy in a group of cases with clear involvement of internal mammary or supraclavicular nodes on the basis of the triple biopsy technique. Guttmann was thereby able to show that metastatic lymph nodes could be treated successfully by irradiation therapy. The cancer at least was contained, if not arrested or "cured."

The 5-year survival rate of 90 percent in Haagensen's series of patients subjected to radical mastectomy is clearly the result of biased selection of patients and explains his favorable results. Of necessity it fails to include all patients who might have benefited from surgical therapy, and his results cannot justifiably be compared with other groups operated upon under less stringent terms in the clinical stages

A and B. Haagensen eliminated in his series some patients in clinical stages A and B who might have benefited from radical mastectomy.

SIMPLE MASTECTOMY OF CRILE

From 1960 on, Dr. George Crile attempted to answer the problem of breast cancer by varying treatment in each case; the treatment employed varied with the findings at the time of simple mastectomy. He believed that regional lymph nodes might be an important part of the immunological defense of the patient against the spread of cancer, and that, as a consequence, normal axillary lymph nodes should not be removed in the treatment of breast cancer. In a classical radical mastectomy the axillary lymph nodes are removed as a preventive measure. Crile's procedure consists of a simple mastectomy (removal of the breast and of the tumor it contains), and an opening of the axilla but not removal of the axillary lymph nodes unless they are palpably involved at the time of open exploration. Thus his cases include patients whose axillary lymph nodes have been left intact, and patients whose lymph nodes have been removed upon clinical estimation, at the operating table, of nodal involvement. The former group of patients was in turn divided into two groups: the first treated by irradiation prophylactically (preventively), and the second treated by irradiation only after the nodes had become palpable.

Crile found that the delay in removing axillary lymph nodes until involvement did not appear to promote spread of cancer from node to node; furthermore, a moderate delay in treating occult cancer in the nodes (that is, waiting until the nodes became involved before they were removed) did not seem to affect the patients' survival. Crile's postulate was, that in human breast cancer, just as in transplantable cancers of mice, the invasion of lymph nodes by tumor indicates that the patient has failed to become immune to the cancer, or that the immunity has been overriden by an excess of cancer cells. Normal lymph nodes are left undisturbed to preserve their immunological surveillance.

Among the patients who had no metastases to the axillary lymph nodes, and who were treated by simple mastectomy, the 5-year survival rate was slightly higher than that of patients undergoing radical mastectomy, 82 percent as compared to 65 percent in his own series. If the axillary lymph nodes were involved, both surgery and irradiation therapy seemed equally effective for survival. These results imply that, if there is no involvement in the lymph nodes, harm seems to be done either by removing or irradiating them. However, before this conclusion can be accepted wholeheartedly, confirming data from other groups will have to be produced.

Do uninvolved regional lymph nodes actually contribute to the immunological defenses of the patient against cancer? Should they be removed only if decidedly involved? To answer the first question a large randomized study of patients will have to be carefully evaluated before there is certainty that removal of uninvolved lymph nodes is unnecessary or even harmful. To the second question every surgeon has to find a personal and practical response every time he faces the need to operate upon a woman for breast cancer. If he is conservative and considers the morbidity of large operations, and the unavoidable sacrifice of regional tissues in a radical mastectomy, if he decides against it but later learns that he has left some occult cancer behind after the first operation, the ultimate cure of his patient may well be impossible, and his timidity may have lessened disfigurement but conceivably lost his patient's life. The value of simple mastectomy as against that of radical mastectomy remains to be established more definitely, but the time has come for undertaking random clinical trials to evaluate both types of surgical therapy.

IRRADIATION OF LYMPH NODES

During the 10 years before 1963, Dr. Ruth Guttmann, a radiotherapist working in close proximity with Dr. Haagensen, seized the unique opportunity to treat with 2 million volt irradiation a rather large number of patients whom Haagensen deemed inoperable on the basis of his triple biopsy technique. Dr. Guttmann treated these patients by irradiating the supraclavicular and infraclavicular areas, the axilla, and the internal mammary area; the breast itself was irradiated by two tangential fields. After five weeks of therapy and a total dose of 5,000 roentgens the patients experienced minimal side effects: small changes in the skin, negligible changes in blood count, insignificant lymphedema of the arm, and mild irradiation fibrosis in the lungs, evident from dry cough, some shortness of breath, and minimal changes in the lungs shown in subsequent X-rays (Guttmann, 1967).

Among these patients 45 percent had positive nodes in two of the biopsied areas. Her results provide the best clear-cut evidence that it is possible to kill cancer in lymph nodes by radiotherapy. Several patients later came to autopsy without any evidence of cancer in the area that had been irradiated. So long as the nodes are 3 cm in size (or less) they can be freed from cancer by irradiation.

On a 10-year follow-up of these patients Guttmann could claim an overall 5-year survival rate of 60 percent and a 10-year survival rate of 30 percent (table 11-1). The closest comparable series are those of Urban, who practiced extended radical mastectomy, followed by irradiation of the supraclavicular nodes (5-year survival rate of 48 percent), and of Handley, who employed radical mastectomy combined with irradiation of the internal mammary chain. Both of these series had less favorable results than the method of Guttmann.

TABLE 11–1

Survival at various intervals after treatment
for cancer of the breast by irradiation alone
(Guttmann technique)

Interval after treatment (years)	Total patients treated 1952–1963	Surviving	
		Number	Percent
4	168	106	63
5	148	89	60
6	123	64	52
7	110	48	44
8	98	34	35
9	65	20	31
10	46	14	30
10 to 14	30	7	23

In addition to a 60 percent 5-year survival rate of those patients with lymph-node metastases, Guttmann showed a clear 25 to 30 percent 5-year survival rate in inoperable, hopelessly advanced cancer of the breast, proving that irradiation with megavolt units has

an indisputable place in the management of a number of patients
with breast cancer.

ROUTINE PREOPERATIVE AND POSTOPERATIVE X-RAY THERAPY

Since Dr. Guttmann's results in radiotherapy of breast cancers were
definitely favorable, the question naturally arises: why not treat all
patients with cancer of the breast with irradiation therapy, either
preoperatively, or postoperatively, as a matter of routine? In Guttmann's series, of course, the status of involvement of the three nodal
areas was known through open biopsy. In preoperative irradiation
this status would *not* be known. In postoperative irradiation it would
be known only in the case of extended radical mastectomy, wherein
the three regional lymph nodes are excised and biopsied.

Theoretically routine preoperative irradiation has some advantages: it might seal in the tumor prior to surgery, or it might alter
the immunological nature of the tumor so that the patient would
mount a stronger immunological rejection response against the
tumor. But studies made in the 1930's and 1940's had failed to show
any alteration of the 5-year survival rate with the use of preoperative
irradiation, and more recently no solid data could be gathered in
favor of its merit (fig. 11-5). By and large most physicians frown
upon preoperative irradiation on the basis of these total experiences.

As for irradiation after radical mastectomy or extended radical
mastectomy, it too has failed to show any improvement in the 5-year
survival rate when used in a routine fashion. Indeed a recent controlled clinical study by Fisher and his colleagues (1968) suggests
that routine postoperative irradiation therapy may alter the immuno-

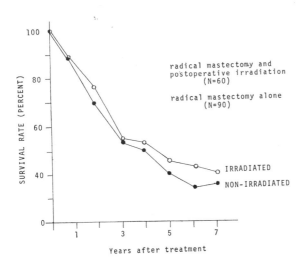

radical mastectomy and
postoperative irradiation
(N=60)

radical mastectomy alone
(N=90)

○ IRRADIATED

● NON-IRRADIATED

SURVIVAL RATE (PERCENT)

Years after treatment

FIGURE 11–5. *Comparison of
survival rates after radical
mastectomies with and
without postoperative
irradiation shows that the
difference between the two
treatments is statistically
insignificant. (Modified from
A. P. M. Forrest and P. B.
Kunkler,* Prognostic Factors
in Breast Cancer, *Williams &
Wilkins, Baltimore, 1968, p.
150.)*

logical responsiveness of the host to the extent that systemic or generalized recurrences occur somewhat more frequently than they might have if the patient had not been irradiated. This is surprising in view of the fact that Guttmann obtained such positive results in her treatment of breast cancer through radiotherapy, but it must be remembered that only in her series was the exact status of lymph-node involvement known, and patients were only irradiated if they had involvement of the lymph nodes with cancer. The ineffectiveness of postoperative irradiation therapy was demonstrated both on the continent by R. Patterson (1959), and in the United States at the Barnes Hospital (Butcher *et al.,* 1964). Recent carefully controlled clinical trial studies (Fisher *et al.,* 1968), clearly showed that prophylactic irradiation is not of value and indeed may be harmful.

Postoperative irradiation should then be reserved for patients who develop proven recurrences or metastases. The only exception to this is possibly in young women with cancer in the inner quadrant of the breast. However, most clinicians think that in young women with inner quadrant lesions it is prudent to administer X-ray therapy to the internal mammary chain at the present time. This irradiation therapy of course is given on a prophylactic basis and it can be justified in light of the McWhirter experience and of the subsequent experience by Kaee and Johanson, wherein patients with breast cancer who were treated by simple mastectomy followed by irradiation showed an overall 5-year survival rate of 65 to 70 percent in clinical Class A, and a lower 50 percent rate in clinical Class B.

In summary, neither preoperative nor postoperative X-ray therapy should be administered on a routine basis to women with cancer of the breast. Such treatment should be reserved for carefully selected cases.

ASSOCIATED ISSUES IN BREAST CANCER SURGERY

Several important issues need to be considered in the treatment of breast cancer. They center on observations previously discussed, namely, that cancer of the breast is not purely an autonomous growth but depends upon the hormonal environment of the body. As a consequence of this hormone dependency should the ovaries be removed in young women who have cancer but are still menstruating? Should pregnancy be permitted or should it be terminated? What should be done in cases of unilateral breast cancer in order to prevent cancer in the second breast at a later date? Should endocrine ablative procedures, such as adrenalectomy and hypophysectomy, be performed? Answers to these questions are not purely medical or scientific but are made delicate and crucial by the various ethical and religious attitudes of doctors and patients alike.

OOPHORECTOMY

Breast cancer tends to have a poor prognosis in young women. In addition, more than half the patients whose lymph nodes are involved carry living cancer cells in their body after a mastectomy. These facts have led to the proposal that castration (oophorectomy) should be performed in young women suffering from breast cancer, particularly if there is nodal involvement. As early as 1896, G. T. Baetson had shown that removal of the ovaries in animals with experimental cancer of the breast tends to retard the growth of the tumor. Later several clinical studies in women showed that the estrogenic stimulation of the first half of the normal menstrual cycle is associated with stimulation of the growth of the breast cancer. Logically then, castration should have a favorable influence on the prognosis of breast cancer in young women. Yet the evidence in this direction is still unconvincing. Unfortunately, oophorectomy in young women stimulates the production by the adrenals of hormones comparable to those produced by the ovaries.

The idea of castration is painful and troubling for most young women. Since oophorectomy has not been demonstrated to have a favorable influence on primary cancer of the breast, most physicians reserve it for use as a therapeutic measure when the cancer recurs. This again, of course, is for women who are not more than five years beyond the menopause. In women with recurrent breast cancer who are still menstruating or who are less than five years beyond the menopause, oophorectomy should be employed as a therapeutic measure, particularly if there has been a free interval of cancer of at least two years after the mastectomy and if the recurrence is in the soft tissues or the bones. When castration is used as a therapeutic measure the response of the patient to the operation may serve as a guide for the possible success of further endocrine ablative therapy. Most surgeons, then, use castration as a therapeutic measure rather than as a prophylactic measure in the treatment of breast cancer.

Castration can be accomplished either by irradiation or by surgery. Surgery is more expedient and certain. Castration is without question desirable in young women with recurrent disease who have had a free interval of at least two years prior to the onset of the recurrence which indicates advance of the disease, which might be altered by a prompt hormonal change.

In summary, removal of the ovaries as a preventive measure may delay appearance of recurrences but does not improve the overall survival. Oophorectomy is employed as a therapeutic measure when metastases are present in young women, so that its effect upon these metastases can be evaluated. Therapeutic castration may then serve as an indicator of the value of future endocrine ablative therapy.

CANCER OF THE BREAST DURING PREGNANCY

In every 10,000 pregnancies there are three cases of breast cancer. It is difficult to detect breast cancer in pregnant women, whose breasts undergo a natural change and enlargement with pregnancy. About 75 percent of the patients present involvement of the axillary lymph nodes at the time of diagnosis. The 5-year survival rate in a group of women whose axillary lymph nodes are invaded by cancer is 17 to 20 percent, but it can reach 65 percent if these nodes are free of cancer. This fact speaks strongly in favor of early diagnosis of breast cancer in pregnant women, or in women who have just had a child.

Should pregnancy be interrupted in the event that a cancer of the breast appears during pregnancy? Many patients and doctors alike feel that a bold course of action may be safest. In the words of Shakespeare: "Diseases desperate grown / By desperate appliance are relieved." The decision is difficult to make. A women with advanced breast cancer, who is bearing a child, may well wonder who will take care of her baby in the future. Whatever her thoughts, she is beset with conflicting and powerful emotions. Each case requires an absolutely individual answer.

No current statistics on cancer of the breast in pregnancy prove that interrupting pregnancy by itself will influence the patient's survival, or have any direct effect on the disease process. And if the cancer is totally removed, there is no evidence of added risk to the patient from her pregnancy or a future pregnancy. But since breast cancer tends to have a poor prognosis in young women, subsequent pregnancies should be viewed with a clear understanding of the guarded prognosis for the mother. Generally physicians advise a three-year interval after treatment of the primary breast cancer during which there are no recurrences. The wisest policy is to face each case anew, not only on the basis of the anticipated prognosis, but also on the religious convictions and emotional attitudes of the mother and father and their desire for children. Love and hope are strong in young people; yet they cannot transform the course of their lives and they must be made aware of the poor prognosis if, unfortunately, the young woman's breast cancer is already advanced.

When physicians feel that interruption of the pregnancy is desirable, a simple therapeutic abortion is performed in the first three months after conception. Surgical removal of the fetus by an abdominal operation is required in the second trimester of pregnancy. If the third trimester of pregnancy has been reached, abortion is ill-advised, and the pregnancy is allowed to come to term.

The breast cancer itself must be treated, usually by radical mastectomy or conventional therapy identical to that which would be employed if the patient were not pregnant.

RECURRENT BREAST CANCER

In 10 to 15 percent of mastectomy cases, when a patient survives five years, the remaining breast develops cancer. It is occasionally suspected that the tumor in the second breast is a metastasis from the first breast cancer, rather than a new primary tumor. If, at the time of removal of the first breast, a patient is known to belong to a family which has a definite history of breast cancer, or if there are palpable lumps in the second breast, or if the microscopic examination of the removed breast indicates extensive chronic cystic mastitis (a disease of the breast with cyst formation), or other abnormalities, a strong case can be made for the removal of the second breast by simple mastectomy. Yet the loss of two breasts, and one of them as a preventive measure alone, can be a traumatic experience for a woman, and the decision should be made with great care.

It is good practice for doctors to give careful follow-up examinations every few months to women who have had breast cancer. For the first five years after operation, patients should be seen at an interval of three to six months. Often clear evidence of cancer in the second breast arises between examinations; as we know, the tumor must reach a certain size before it can be detected clinically. This brings us again to the importance of early detection. Mammography is particularly important for the early diagnosis of breast cancer in women who have already had a mastectomy. By combining clinical examination with mammography, one can hopefully detect cancer in the second breast at a time when its removal offers an excellent prognosis. Indeed the most likely group of women to subject to frequent and repeated mammograms is the group which has had a carcinoma removed from one breast.

EARLY DETECTION

Routine mammography, thermography, and xerography are valuable adjuncts in the early diagnosis of breast cancer. As an example, the recent screening of 31,450 women in a New York insurance plan has proved that mammography plus clinical examination is capable of detecting breast cancer on an average of 10 months earlier than conventional methods (Hutchinson and Shapiro, 1968). Mammography is currently the best available technique and numerous recent studies show that this method can detect early carcinoma in the breast of 1 cm or less in size. Statistical results in breast cancer clearly indicate that, if the lesion is 3.5 cm in size when first discovered, the overall 5-year survival rate is only 45 to 50 percent. If the lesion is 1 cm or less in size when first discovered, only 30 percent of the cases have metastases and the overall survival rate is in excess of 80 percent. Early detection, then, remains the prime method for the successful control of breast cancer.

ENDOCRINE ABLATIVE THERAPY

Since 1945 many workers have sought to establish guides which would help doctors predict the response of a given patient to endocrine ablative therapy (removal of endocrine glands) with a high degree of accuracy. These guides, or indicators, are of a clinical and of a biochemical nature.

Among the clinical indicators, we have already mentioned the importance of the length of the free interval between the time of removal of the primary tumor and the appearance of metastatic disease. A free interval of at least three years is to be desired. To be considered also is the site of the first metastasis. If it is to skin and bones rather than to the liver and lungs, the response to adrenalectomy will be better. On the other hand, the histological character of a tumor is a poor clinical guide. So is the age of the patient. Still another clinical indicator is the prior response of the patient to the administration of hormones, or, in young women, to oophorectomy; neither response is highly reliable, the first much less than the second. In general, the likelihood of a favorable response to adrenalectomy at the present time, in patients who are carefully selected, is only 30 to 40 percent, basing the judgment for adrenalectomy on the clinical grounds discussed above.

The biochemical indicators are unfortunately no better in predicting the success of adrenalectomy. The best biochemical discriminant now known is the Bulbrook–Hayward discriminant, based on the study of the urinary steroid secretion pattern in breast cancer. A high output of etiocholanolone with respect to the 17 hydroxy corticoids indicates the likelihood of a favorable response to adrenalectomy. The initial results employed in the Bulbrook–Hayward discriminant were reasonably successful, but since 1950 it has been found less valuable than had been originally hoped. There is at the present time no good biochemical discriminant which can be utilized to select patients who will respond favorably to endocrine ablative therapy.

Only 30 to 40 percent of the patients benefit from adrenalectomy or hypophysectomy, or both, in metastatic breast cancer. Endocrine ablative procedures are not really curative, but provide the patient with an average period of comfortable results and improvement of 12 to 16 months. At the end of the 12 to 16 months of improvement, unfortunately, the cancer again progresses. Hypophysectomy is no better than adrenalectomy and the management of patients after hypophysectomy is much more difficult than following adrenalec-tomy, because hormones other than adrenal hormones may have to be replaced. The disturbance of pituitrin secretion often creates an excess of body water (diabetes insipidus, or "innocent" diabetes) which has to be controlled.

It must be recognized that different types of tumors respond to hormones in different ways and that large-scale studies are still needed for clearer knowledge about endocrine ablative therapy. The clinical and biochemical discriminants, however, can give indications that might be helpful. At the present time it is not possible to predict accurately who is likely to receive benefit from this form of treatment, and who is not, but the cases most suitable seem to be those who have had a long free interval between the initial removal of the cancer and its recurrence, and those in whom the recurrence is primarily in the soft tissues and bones rather than in the lungs and liver.

ADDITIVE THERAPY

Additive therapy with sex hormones in the treatment of ad-vanced breast cancer is, of course, the opposite of endocrine ablative therapy. As related earlier, there is no good clinical or biochemical discriminant which will enable us to predict who will respond to hormonal additive therapy. But early clinical experience has shown that women with breast cancer under 65 may manifest increased growth of the tumor under estrogen therapy. For that reason doctors do not like to use estrogens in young women. In very elderly patients, however, that is, in patients whose disease has become established in an estrogen-free environment, estrogens are quite useful in the treatment of metastases to the skin and bones.

Male sex hormones (androgens) are employed for palliation of advanced breast cancer and give favorable results in 30 to 40 percent of the cases. When 100 milligrams of androgenic hormone are given three times a week, the overall regression rate reaches 20 percent. In general the rate of response to androgens is best for lesions in the soft tissues, less so for osseous or visceral lesions. Here again a period of a free interval of at least three years between treatment of the original tumor and metastasis is almost indispensable for favorable results. The favorable results generally last six to eight months before the cancer again gains ground.

In large doses androgenic hormones produce disturbing side effects, hirsutism of the face, changes in the patient's psyche, and increase in libido. For some curious reason a small number of patients show signs of hypercalcemia (increase of the calcium level of the blood and urine) which is very distressing. These signs include nausea, vomiting, and lethargy, and if untreated may lead to coma, convulsions, and death. Hypercalcemia can be recognized early, and treated. When it is diagnosed, the administration of androgenic hormones is, of course, interrupted.

Other hormones (thyroid, cortisone, and so on) have been tried with no real success.

GENERAL CONCLUSIONS

The foregoing discussion has not been provided to belittle or detract from the value of cancer surgery, but to offer a perspective on a biological problem. Surgery answers admirably some of the questions inherent in our understanding of the nature of cancer. It can also serve as a tool in investigating a number of questions presented by cancer. Hopefully, a critical review of the accomplishments of surgery will encourage carefully designed, internationally based studies to evaluate the optimal surgical procedure at various stages of the disease. In the meantime, surgeons must employ the standard radical mastectomy for the majority of cases. They must weigh as best they can the possible morbidity of the procedure for each patient, as well as its effects upon the well-being and happiness of each patient. We have repeatedly emphasized the value of the patient's life, for existence alone cannot be equated with joy, or at least the satisfaction and comfort of living. If it can be shown that radical surgery is not advantageous, that lymph nodes need not be removed, that metastatic nodes can be sterilized by X-rays, the work of the surgeon and his results will be far more pleasurable for all in the future. This is why properly designed and controlled clinical trials, capable of answering intricate biological questions raised by cancer seem imperative. The crucial questions to be answered by surgery include:

1. What is the biological potential and growth of a given tumor?
2. How radical should the local excision of a cancer be?

3. Should the operation include in all cases the excision of lymph nodes, whether involved or not?

4. Can metastatic lymph nodes be treated as well by irradiation as by surgery?

5. What is the true role of lymph nodes in the biological immunity and the cancer-host relationship?

Some of these problems can also be explored by studying the outcome of irradiation and of chemotherapy in the treatment of cancer.

12
THE IRRADIATION
OF CANCER

*"Evil things are
neighbors to good."*
OVID

The irradiation of cancer is the treatment of the disease by X-rays or other forms of radioactivity. The object of radiation therapy is to deliver a lethal dose to the tumor with a minimum dose to the surrounding tissues and organs. X-rays affect all tissues, but fortunately cancer tissue is more susceptible than normal tissues to the damaging effects of irradiation.

The past 10 years have seen great progress in radiotherapy and great improvement in the results of this method in the treatment of cancer. This is primarily due to two developments. First, the technical equipment which is now available permits the delivery of extremely intense radiations; second, the methods of therapy currently in existence make possible even total body irradiation if desired. However, just as there are limits to the usefulness of surgery in the treatment of cancer, so, too, some factors are emerging which indicate the limits of radiotherapy in the treatment of cancer.

Our model for portraying and developing an understanding of surgical treatment of cancer has been cancer of the breast. In this chapter the models for describing cancer treatment by irradiation will be cancer of the cervix in women and lymphomas in young or middle-aged individuals. Cervical cancer is a localized disease; lymphomas are commonly generalized, requiring widespread bodily irradiation for treatment.

All radiations, natural or man-made, are absorbed by matter with transfer of energy from the radiation source to the molecules of the matter they strike. In their ordinary state molecules are electrically neutral. When radiation falls upon them the molecules split up into positive and negative ions. Ionization produces a biological change in the cells, and their metabolism is altered. This changed chemical activity not only has profound effects upon the life of the cells but may even provoke their death.

Ionizing radiations are generated in two ways—electrically and radioactively. In electrical generation electrons are accelerated to a high kinetic energy and bombard a target where part of the electron energy is converted into electromagnetic radiations, or X-rays. Before 1950 the X-ray tubes in widespread use had common characteristics and were similar in principle to those first developed. The conventional X-ray tube is a vacuum tube wherein a negative cathode is heated by an electrical current. The cathode gives off electrons which hit a positive tungsten anode, the target. The radiations produced are X-rays. Electron energies of the order of 200,000 to 300,000 electron volts are obtained with minimum problems of insulation.

X-rays are a part of the electromagnetic spectrum (as are radio waves, infrared light, visible light waves, and ultraviolet light) but their wavelengths are much shorter; gamma rays have an even shorter wavelength (see table 12–1). X-rays are invisible, and when they penetrate matter they are scattered just as light rays are scattered when they travel through air. In his quantum theory Max Planck expressed the idea that roentgen rays and all of the electromagnetic spectrum rays are small bundles of energy, or "quanta" of energy, which are called photons.

Other forms of radiation are corpuscular, that is, they are actually made up of subatomic particles: examples of these are the alpha and beta rays emitted by radioactive elements such as radium.

Since 1950 the use of high-energy radiations in radiotherapy has been greatly facilitated by new apparatus. These sources of high-energy radiations are:

1. Telecobalt units, producing energies of the order of 1.17 to 1.33 million electron volts (Mev).

2. Linear accelerators, with electron energies of 4 to 35 Mev, but generally of 4 to 5 Mev.

TABLE 12–1

Some characteristics of
common environmental radiations

Type of radiation	Relative biologic effectiveness (RBE)[a]	Approximate energy[b]	Approximate penetrating ability		
			Air	Tissue	Lead
Alpha particle	10	5.0 Mev	4 cm	0.05 mm	0
Beta particle	1–2	0.05 to 1.0 Mev	6.300 cm	0.06 4.0 mm	0.005 0.3 mm
Gamma rays (high energy)	1	1.0 Mev	400 meters	50 cm	30 mm
X-rays	1	90. Kev peak 250.0 Kev peak	120 m 240 m	15 cm 30 cm	0.3 mm 1.2 mm
Cosmic rays (secondary)	1 5–10		(Some components very high)		

SOURCE: John B. Little, "Ionizing Radiations," *New Eng, J. Med.,* Oct. 27, 1966.
 a Factor in which absorbed radiation dose in rads must be multiplied to give biologically effective dose in rem.
 b These units are Kev, thousand electron volts, and Mev, million electron volts.

3. Cyclic accelerators, such as the cyclotron and betatron, capable of going up to a billion electron volts but generally operating in an area of 4 to 35 Mev.

There are at the present time 2,000 to 3,000 telecobalt units in the world, about 300 to 400 linear accelerators, and 35 to 50 cyclotrons and betatrons.

Telecobalt units present many advantages. Their maintenance cost is low, their monitoring is simple, their handling is easy, and the conditions of treatment can be reproduced with certainty. Their main disadvantage is a penumbra, or shadow effect, requiring the use of a larger field in order to get a homogeneous dose into the tumor. This penumbra effect can be reduced to some degree by special manipulation of the telecobalt unit.

Linear accelerators accelerate electrons in a straight line along a straight vacuum tube. These electrons hit the target and produce X-rays. Cyclic accelerators accelerate electrons many times along a circular path; the electrons then hit the target and produce X-rays.

Both the linear and cyclic accelerators present two main advantages in the treatment of cancer.

1. Their high output makes possible the administration of a good depth dose with a minimal skin dose and as a consequence the treatment of deeply seated tumors is possible using only two or three external fields.

2. They can be used to generate electrons directly, a new development in radiation therapy. The machines can be designed in such a way that the electrons produced in the accelerator, instead of hitting a target and thereby producing X-rays, can be projected directly into the body of the patient where the radiation effect occurs.

Electron therapy with high-energy electrons offers a new approach to the treatment of cancer, for these electrons have a limited track dose (depth of penetration) in the tissues, the length of which is proportional to the energy. For example, the track of a 20,000,000 volt electron in the tissues is about 10 cm; the dose falls off sharply up to a certain depth, then to nothing at all at a depth greater than the maximal track length. Therefore the use of electron beams allows healthy tissues beyond the target to be spared. Of course the skin-sparing effect is much less than with high-energy photons. Electron therapy is particularly good in the treatment of surface lesions, in contrast to the high-energy X-ray therapy which is also possible with the accelerators, and which is especially suited to the treatment of deep-seated lesions. Accelerators, however, are costly machines, requiring complicated maintenance, and they are not yet as widely used as telecobalt units.

MEASURES OF RADIATION

The quantity of ionizing radiation can be measured; the unit of measure is named the *roentgen*. It is not a dosage unit. The radiation dose to a given tissue is a measure of the energy imparted to that tissue by ionizing radiation, and the unit of measure is named the *rad*. Roentgens can be converted to rads by appropriate calculations.

The dose delivered depends both upon the incident radiation and upon the nature of the absorbing medium. With X-rays and gamma rays of low energy, there is a marked difference between the dose received by soft tissues and bones, the bones receiving considerably larger doses. This difference of absorption can be avoided by using high-energy radiation.

The roentgen is simply a unit of radiation while the rad measures a physically equivalent dose in different tissues. Here a problem presents itself, for physically equivalent doses of different energies may not be biologically equivalent, that is, they may not provoke the same biological reactions in the tissues. Some other factors have to be considered, among them the distribution of the ions, the oxygen tension of the tissues, and the fractionation of the radiation dose.

PROPERTIES OF BEAMS

The dose of radiation in a given medium is influenced by (1) the absorption on the superficial tissues, and (2) the "inverse square law," which is associated with the divergence of the beam as it traverses space.

The absorption in the superficial tissues is dependent upon the energy of the radiation: a beam of 95 Kev X-rays is attenuated to half its surface intensity at a depth of 2.5 cm, whereas a beam of 4 Mev X-rays is attenuated to half its surface intensity at a depth of 14 cm.

The inverse square law states that the application is most effective when the source of radiation is close to the skin. Thus the dose from a source 10 cm from the skin is reduced due to this law by 80 percent at the depth of 10 cm, whereas the dose from a source at a distance of 100 cm is reduced only by 20 percent at the same depth. This fact demonstrates the necessity of treating deeply seated tumors by the most penetrating radiation at the greatest convenient distance, and explains the great obvious advantages of the telecobalt unit (2 to 3 Mev) and of the linear accelerator (4 to 6 Mev) over the conventional 200 Kev machines. A second advantage of the supervoltage machines is their skin-sparing effect, due to their greater penetrating power, making trauma to the deeper structures the limiting factor in their application, not the burning of the skin. A third major advantage is their bone-sparing effect. However, one limit to this advantage of the very high-energy machines, that is those above 15 to 20 Mev, is their high exit dose. This effect cancels out some of the benefits of the increased depth dose. Their principal advantage, of course, is that they can be used to produce electrons directly and therefore the production and use of X-rays can be bypassed, the electrons being the immediate therapeutic agents. This technique is currently being explored in many centers of radiotherapy.

PLANNING FOR RADIOTHERAPY

Obviously the treatment of cancer by irradiation requires careful planning: localization of the area to be treated, proper direction of the beam, choice of the proper field to avoid injury to important contiguous structures in the body, calculation of effective tumor dose and proper fractionation of the therapy, as well as an understanding of tissue tolerance and the relative biological effectiveness (RBE) of the beam employed. The object of radiation therapy is to deliver a lethal dose to the tumor while exposing the surrounding tissues and organs to a minimum dose of irradiation. To achieve this goal proper fractionation of the therapy is essential. Fractionation means the delivery of small daily doses over a long period of time. Experience has shown that fractionation of the dose increases the effect upon the tumor cells as compared to the effect upon normal tissue. In addition, the relative biological effectiveness of the radiation beam and the relative biological susceptibility of the tissue irradiated must be calculated. High-energy beams, dose for dose in rads, appear to produce smaller biological effects than beams in the kilovoltage range.

GENERAL EFFECTS OF X-RAYS

Irradiation in proper doses can eradicate cancer. In excessive doses it can produce cancer. Yet in both instances the mechanism of action must be the same. Most authorities agree that radiations produce changes in the chromosomes of the cells by "electron hits" (fig. 12–1).

FIGURE 12–1. *Schematic representation of ionizing radiation tracking through an aggregate of tissue atoms. (A) Zigzag path (scatter) followed by a radiation beam. (B) Electrons torn away at a and b produce further destruction by ionizing surrounding tissue. (Adapted from E. C. Pollard, "Biological Action of Ionizing Radiation," American Scientist, Feb. 1969, p. 209.*

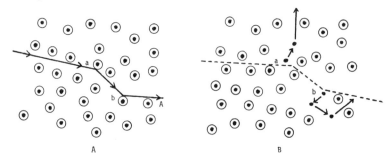

A   B

If the chromosomal damage leads to a cellular mutation which is transmissible, cancer results (fig. 12–2). If the chromosomal damage leads to the death of the cell or to the loss of cellular capacity for division and reproduction, cancer may be cured. An increasing dose of irradiation augments the number of electron hits. Such hits may have an affect upon the cytoplasm and enzymes of cells, but they are more likely to have an effect on the DNA of the nuclear chromosomes. Dr. Henry Kaplan, who has shown a lifelong interest in the mechanism of irradiation, summarizes its effects by stating: "The uniqueness of certain macromolecules in the nucleus creates a vulnerable situation in which an event which is quantitatively insignificant in radiochemical terms becomes of great importance from the standpoint of radiobiology" (see fig. 12–3).

Unfortunately, irradiation affects normal tissues as well as tumor tissues, so that the lethal dose for the tumor must be balanced against normal tissue tolerance. In large doses irradiation affects the body as a whole; the many effects of irradiation make it imperative to define the risks and the goals in irradiation therapy.

The goals of irradiation therapy may be curative or merely palliative. This will depend, of course, upon the individual situation in each patient. If the prospect of cure truly exists, irradiation is justified for curative purposes, even if it involves risks: the risks become bearable in view of an attainable goal. If the patient is incurable, irradiation can serve as a palliative measure; in such a case the treatment involves little risk and may be of inestimable value in the control of pain, ulceration, pressure effects, and similar aggravations resulting from the growth.

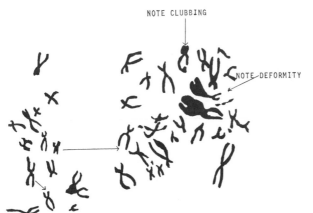

NOTE CLUBBING

NOTE DEFORMITY

NOTE FRAGMENTATION

FIGURE 12–2. *Kinds of damage done to chromosomal structures by irradiation. (Source: T. Puck, "Radiation and the Human Cell,"* Scientific American, *April 1960, p. 143.*

In order to protect the whole organism of the patient as well as the particular tissues and organs containing cancer, it is necessary to consider (1) the quality of the radiation source and its energy; (2) the total dose, its time period of delivery, and its fractionation; (3) the action of sensitizing and protective agents; and (4) the characteristics of the tissue irradiated.

Each tissue, each tumor, each individual has a different sensitivity to the same physical quantity of a given type of irradiation. The calculation of the desired radiation depth dose is obtained with the help of replicas of pressed wood, water, lucite, and the like. It is not possible at the present time to measure the dose delivered *in vivo*, and unfortunately errors may arise because the exact body contours cannot be reproduced absolutely in the replicas, and because organs and tissues are frequently displaced by disease and surgical intervention. Despite this, irradiation remains the optimal treatment for a wide variety of cancers, particularly cancer of the cervix and the lymphomas, but also some oropharyngeal cancers (mouth and pharynx), some laryngeal cancers (larynx), retinoblastomas (tumors of the retina), cancers of the central nervous system, and esophageal cancers (esophagus). Irradiation also serves as an invaluable adjunct in the total care of patients who have already had primary surgical treatment of their cancers. Radiotherapists have a notable record of achievement in the cure and containment of cancer and in the relief of suffering from cancer.

Close clinical observations during the entire course of treatment are imperative. Despite impressive developments in the administration of X-rays, most cancers are helped, not cured, by radiotherapy. Indeed we are just beginning to approach on a clinical basis the answers to two of the most important questions in the treatment of cancer by irradiation.

1. Is the intensity of the energy of the irradiation source (what we have called the quality of irradiation) of prime importance in the eradication of local lesions?

2. Should the volume of tissue irradiated include not only the primary site of the tumor but also the regional lymph nodes to which it spreads?

These questions are analogous to those confronting the surgeon, but the destructive force of irradiation is much more complex than the intervention of the surgeon's scalpel.

EFFECTIVENESS OF VARIOUS IRRADIATIONS

The relative biological effectiveness (RBE) of a radiation is the impact of this particular radiation on a tissue and is determined by the energy absorbed and the wavelength used. With soft X-rays the photoelectric effect of radiation predominates, and the maximum energy interchange takes place in the first layers of tissues. With hard X-rays an effect known as the Compton effect predominates, and the maximum energy interchange takes place in the deeper tissues. As previously noted, X-rays are scattered in matter just as light rays are scattered in air; the Compton effect is the action of these scattered rays within the tissues.

From a clinical standpoint the use of X-rays from a high-energy source such as the telecobalt unit (1.17 to 1.33 Mev) or the linear accelerator (4 to 5 Mev) results in (1) a greater penetration of the tissues with higher depth dose, (2) better beam definition and uniformity of irradiation, (3) less difference in the energy transfer between the soft tissues and bones, (4) minimal skin reaction and skin burning, and (5) much greater comfort to the patient with less effect to the patient's system as a whole.

If one exceeds 6 or 8 Mev, there is an increase of the exit dose and the favorable ratio in tissue and bone absorption disappears. In short, the use of telecobalt units and linear accelerators (supervoltage therapy) is far more comfortable to the patient, and results in much less burning of the skin than the earlier kilovolt X-ray machines (orthovoltage therapy).

SEALED RADIOACTIVE SOURCES

In certain situations it is advantageous to place a number of small sealed radioactive sources emitting gamma rays within or on a tumor rather than to bombard it from a distant source of radiation, for the highest dose is thus delivered to the tumor with a rapid falloff of the dose to the surrounding normal tissues. This technique is particularly applicable to cancer of the tongue and cancer of the cervix. In the case of cancer of the tongue this method presents the additional advantage of avoiding mutilation, of preserving function, and ultimately of keeping the patient's existence useful and comfortable. Few will choose total removal of the tongue when the eradication of cancer by radium application can be equally successful.

The most widely used radioactive material in a sealed source is radium 226. The container, in the form of needles, is easily inserted in the affected area. Other sealed sources are thin wires containing cobalt 60, gold 198, uranium 192, or small grains of gold 198 and uranium 192. Radioactive elements with a very short half-life (the time required for one half of the atoms to disintegrate), such as gold 198, can be left permanently in place: this procedure is particularly advantageous in the treatment of pleural effusions from metastatic cancer to the linings of the lungs.

ADVANTAGES OF IRRADIATION THERAPY

In recent years, cancer treatment in general has made progress through the combining of radiotherapy with surgery and chemotherapy. Care of patients is becoming more and more a group effort, with close cooperation between radiotherapists, surgeons, and chemotherapists. Such shared treatment, however, varies with the location of the cancer. For cancer of the breast, the primary lesion is best treated surgically, and the lymph nodes, particularly the internal mammary nodes, may be best treated by radiotherapy. For some pharyngeolaryngeal cancers, the primary lesion is best treated by irradiation, and surgery is more suited to the removal of the lymph-bearing area. The combination of treatments enables preservation of function with the least trauma to the area being treated.

At the present time there is a tendency to extend preoperative therapy, particularly when local recurrence in the area operated on is an important factor in operative failure. Preoperative irradiation is most worthy of consideration when there is doubt about the operability of the primary tumor, or when there is a reasonable chance that surgery cannot completely eradicate the primary tumor. Preoperative irradiation may also reduce the incidence of recurrences in the operative field from spilled cancer cells or cancer cells remaining during or after surgery. When there is a strong chance of the cancer cells being stimulated by the trauma of surgical procedure, or when the area involved with cancer may be greater than that removed by the surgical excision, X-ray therapy, either preoperatively or post-operatively, or both, may also be indicated.

Postoperative radiotherapy is often indicated after surgery when the surgeon feels that the excision of the cancer has been incomplete. Examples of areas where this is possible are the thyroid, the breast, the esophagus, and the lung. Conversely, extensive surgery may be required after unsuccessful irradiation therapy. An example of this is the use of radical pelvic exenteration in selected cases, following recurrences of cancer of the cervix after extensive irradiation.

DISADVANTAGES OF IRRADIATION THERAPY

A radiotherapist may exercise the highest competence and still be plagued on occasion with complications due to the inherent nature of ionizing radiations and the disease under treatment. In general, the complications of irradiation therapy fall into the following categories: (1) generalized radiation sickness, (2) inadvertent damage to specific organs, notably the gut or spinal cord, (3) obstructive edema of the limbs from obliteration of lymphatics, (4) alteration of the immune response of the patient to his cancer, and (5) treatment failure because of either the growth potential of the tumor or inadequate recognition of its spread during the course of therapy.

RADIATION SICKNESS

Any radiation therapy may lead to anorexia and nausea, or vomiting and diarrhea, particularly if the stomach, liver, and pancreas are included in the irradiated part of the body (fig. 12–3). Extensive radiation leads to a drop in the blood count and anemia. Symptoms can generally be controlled by antispasmodic drugs, by alteration of the dose rate and fractionation of the dose, and by administration of antibiotics. Radiation sickness is troublesome but it can be tolerated and is a small price to pay for the containment of cancer.

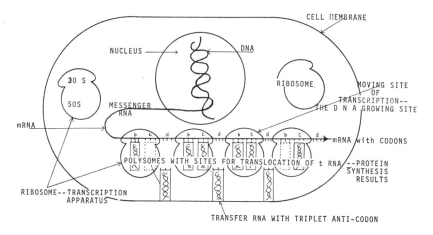

FIGURE 12–3. *Schematic diagram of larger molecular events in irradiation injury to a cell. Maximum injury occurs at DNA transcription sites. (Adapted from Pollard, "Biological Action of Ionizing Radiation," p. 225.*

INADVERTENT DAMAGE TO SPECIFIC ORGANS

The gastrointestinal tract is rarely the target of irradiation but organs such as the uterus, kidneys, bladder, and lymph nodes cannot be irradiated without also irradiating the intestines. Fortunately, the small intestine is in continual peristaltic motion, and rarely becomes involved in radiation enteritis unless it is fixed by adhesions from previous surgery. The large bowel, particularly the rectum and the sigmoid colon, is fixed, usually close to the target organ, especially in the treatment of uterine cancer, and is therefore subject to damage by radiation enteritis. Close observation of the patient makes radiation enteritis avoidable and suspension of treatment may become necessary, but the sensitivity of individuals is extremely variable and delayed radiation effects are often unpredictable. The maximum dose that can be given to the intestine is 4,500 to 5,000 rads in four to five weeks of cobalt therapy. Unfortunately, some tumors require larger doses for eradication. At present, therefore, the intestines form an insurmountable obstacle to the administration of cancericidal dosage of many tumors.

The bladder can stand radiation doses of up to 6,000 or 7,000 rads, but the kidneys cannot take doses in excess of 2,000 rads without radiation nephritis and possible renal failure. The spinal cord cannot take doses in excess of 4,000 rads without possibility of damage. Fortunately, the skilled radiotherapist with a proper treatment plan can avoid injury to these organs, yet deliver effective cancericidal doses to the majority of tumors he treats.

OBSTRUCTIVE EDEMA

In malignant disease the lymphatics draining an extremity are often choked by lymphatic disease. Treatment by irradiation may eradicate the tumor in the lymph nodes, but may produce an intense fibrosis of the lymph nodes, which again obstructs and intensifies the compression of the surrounding veins. Furthermore the primary lymph nodes are often removed in the surgical treatment of cancer, and the available channels are additionally reduced by irradiation therapy. This is particularly true in the arm following radical mastectomy, and in the pelvis and groin following radical surgical excision of cancer of the pelvis with dissection of the iliac and periaortic nodes. The combination, then, of surgical removal of the lymph-bearing area with irradiation of the secondary or residual channels oftentimes results in extensive edema of the arms and legs. This is further complicated by an increased susceptibility to infection in the part involved with edema. A vicious circle is thus unfortunately initiated, with infection leading to additional fibrosis, and fibrosis leading in turn to more obstructive edema.

Treatment of such an obstructive edema is most difficult. The best course of treatment is avoidance of infection, or vigorous use of antibiotics if infection is present, elevation of the affected part, and use of pressure dressings (elastic bandages and sleeves) to prevent additional edema. Operative procedures have been devised to relieve the edema, but by and large they are unsatisfactory.

ALTERATION OF THE IMMUNE RESPONSE

This is an extremely complex question about which relatively little is known, and concerning which much future research is imperative. Cancerous cells, altered by irradiation, may show a change in their antigenicity and may be used to stimulate an immune reaction by the host against the tumor. In this sense, then, preoperative and postoperative radiation therapy would be helpful to the host, and indeed initial therapy would not have to eradicate every last cancer cell in the patient. On the other hand, there is the question as to whether the irradiation of uninvolved lymph nodes may be harmful. This is the same question discussed in detail in chapter 11. Recently, there have been several reports in reasonably controlled clinical studies which would suggest that irradiation of uninvolved lymph nodes, particularly in cancer of the breast, might be harmful (Hollingsworth, 1969). However, the interrelationships of irradiation to immunity and the effects of irradiation on cellular antigenicity will require continued research.

GROWTH POTENTIAL AND SPREAD OF THE TUMOR

This is truly not a complication of irradiation therapy but explains the failure of irradiation in the treatment of many cancers, and the increasing frequency of complications from radiation therapy as we try to contain cancer by this method. The specific sensitivity of any given cancer cell to irradiation is not known, but in general the therapist tries to give the maximal dose. The exact area of spread of any given tumor is not known but it would appear that tumors to be cured by irradiation should be treated more widely than the local manifestation of the tumor would suggest. Irradiation failure, then, may result either because of lack of radiosensitivity of the tumor cells to irradiation, or from inadequate extent of irradiation.

LYMPHANGIOGRAPHY

Crucial to the treatment of any cancer is the mapping of the extent of the disease. The frequency with which lymph nodes are involved in each of the nodal areas is being studied by a new technique called *lymphangiography*. It consists of the introduction of a radiopaque iodinated oil into the lymphatics adjacent to the tumor, with dissemination of this oil to the regional lymph nodes. The regional lymph nodes then become radiopaque and can be visualized by subsequent X-ray examination, that is, the taking of radiograms. This technique has the following advantages.

1. It tends to clarify the extent of the disease and therefore direct the extent of irradiation required; lymphangiography thereby helps reduce irradiation failures due to inadequate extent of the irradiation field.

2. Irradiation of areas in which the chances of involvement are slight can be avoided.

3. Clear knowledge of spread of the tumor before irradiation will avoid the danger of carrying out localized intensive irradiation if the cancer is already generalized.

Lymphangiography represents considerable progress, since involvement of the lymph nodes is not clinically apparent. It enables the physician to establish whether or not the cancer is localized or generalized when treatment is initiated, and to follow the effects of irradiation on the lymph nodes.

IRRADIATION AND LYMPHORETICULAR DISEASES

Lymphomas, lymphosarcomas, and Hodgkin's disease are malignant disorders of the lymphoid tissues. They make up 3.4 percent of all malignant disorders and are equal in frequency to cancers of the ovary or rectum. The cause of these diseases is unknown, but if any human cancer is due to a virus, the lymphomas may be. The lymphosarcoma in African children described by Burkitt has been shown to contain a herpes-like virus, but there is still no proof that this is the cause of the lymphosarcoma rather than merely a passenger virus. These disorders, which can occur at any age, have two curious peaks of incidence, one in young adults 20 to 30 years of age, and another in persons in the sixth and seventh decades of life. The commonest clinical type is Hodgkin's disease, characterized by painless, progressive enlargement of superficial lymph nodes, or associated involvement of the deep mediastinal chest nodes, often with malaise, fever, and weakness. The *New York Times* has recently stated: "Many people die needlessly of Hodgkin's disease because their doctors are ignorant of the major advances in treatment made during recent years. The lack of knowledge is so widespread that even the majority of young medical students graduating from medical schools this spring will know no more as to how this disease should be handled than did their predecessors a decade ago." It is certainly true that diagnostic and therapeutic techniques introduced during the past decade, notably lymphangiography and intensive wide-field megavoltage radiotherapy, have remarkably altered the clinical course and the results of irradiation treatment of these diseases. The traditional pessimism concerning such disorders can now be abandoned, for many patients with early lesions can be cured.

The subsequent discussion will apply largely to Hodgkin's disease. The diagnosis of Hodgkin's disease requires biopsy and microscopic examination of the tissue removed. Classification of the tumor is of paramount importance and an international staging classification was worked out in 1966 (Lukes and Butler, 1966). The classification in brief terms is as follows.

Stage 1. Disease limited to one anatomic region or two contiguous anatomic regions on the same side of the diaphragm.

Stage 2. Disease in more than two anatomic regions or in two noncontiguous regions on the same side of the diaphragm.

Stage 3. Lesions on both sides of the diaphragm but not extending beyond involvement of the lymph nodes in the lower chest or upper abdomen.

Stage 4. Involvement of bone marrow, lungs, pleura, liver, bones, kidney, gastrointestinal tract.

Proper staging is crucial to any consideration of treatment in Hodgkin's disease. It is not meaningful if it is based solely on the usual history, physical examination, blood count, liver function tests, and routine X-rays of the chest, kidneys, and gastrointestinal tract. Proper staging requires the exploration of the status of the lymph nodes by lymphangiography. No diagnosis of localized Hodgkin's disease, that is, stage 1 and 2, appears secure without a negative lymphangiogram. Indeed, 50 to 90 percent of lymphangiograms on persons who, by clinical criteria are in stage 1 or 2, reveal lymph-node involvement at a distance from the primary involvement. The only contra-indications to lymphangiography include allergy to io-dized oils, severe pulmonary disease, or far-advanced abdominal lymph-node involvement on clinical examination. In these situations, special X-ray studies can be done to provide comparable informa-tion or exploratory laparotomy can be used for staging.

At the present time, radiotherapy is the only established method for curative treatment of malignant lymphomas. The involved nodes together with one set of uninvolved nodes on either side of the in-volved lymph nodes are treated. Fundamental to all attempts at cur-ative treatment of Hodgkin's disease is the assumption that the pro-cess is localized in the beginning, but then spreads to contiguous areas. Indeed recent work has demonstrated that the disease spreads from lymph node to lymph node. The use of lymphangiography is therefore essential in delineating the extent of the disease. Treatment with curative intent is indicated for all patients in stage 1, 2, or 3, unless their general condition is poor. Palliative treatment is indicated in stage 4, and consists of chemotherapy associated with palliative radiotherapy. In stage 4 cases there is seldom hope of cure because of widespread involvement of radiosensitive normal tissues.

It should again be emphasized that the primary management of Hodgkin's disease is of greatest importance, and that in young patients with stage 1 or 2 of the disease the chances of cure by appropriate widefield megavoltage therapy are good. It is imperative to dispel the commonly held notion that the disease is invariably fatal. Current favorable results stem from a better understanding of how the disease spreads from one lymph node to the next, and the identification of lymph-node involvement at early stages by lymphangiography. Certainly there can no longer be justification for a negative view of the effects of treatment of the malignant lymphomas with widespread extensive megavoltage irradiation.

Some research centers are beginning to explore the treatment of Hodgkin's disease by irradiation of essentially all the lymph-bearing areas of the body. In this regard it is important to note that as the disease progresses there is a deficit in antibody formation by the patient's body and an interruption of his immunological response. Since extensive radiation therapy itself alters antibody formation, the interrelationship between the natural history of the disease and this consequence of radiotherapy becomes quite complicated. Is it wise to irradiate the uninvolved lymph nodes excessively, thereby dulling the total immunologic responsiveness of the host to foreign antigens? Here again we are confronted with the same considerations of the lymph nodes in the containment of cancer that we discussed under surgical therapy of cancer. Continued research in this area is of extreme importance and should be carried out in a controlled manner in a few selected centers.

TREATMENT OF FEMALE GENITAL CANCERS

Cancer of the cervix is the most common female genital cancer and is exceeded only by cancer of the breast in overall frequency. Early screening has remarkably reduced the death rate from cancer of the cervix in marked contrast to the present status of treatment of carcinoma of the breast (fig. 12–4). Early and proper screening by means of the Papanicolaou technique could now eradicate invasive carcinoma of the cervix and 16,000 lives could be saved yearly in the United States. It can be detected in what is called the incipient stage, the carcinoma *in situ* stage, when it is still confined to a very restricted area of the cervix or uterus. Most of the patients present postmenopausal uterine bleeding or premenopausal irregular bleeding, and such symptoms demand full and complete investigation.

Yet the disease is still seen in its invasive stage, and the course it is going to take is closely related to the type of tumor and to the degree of invasiveness when the patient is first encountered. The disease can be readily biopsied and, most important of all, invasion of normal tissues by aberrant, disorderly, or immature cells can be easily recognized. Delay permits the cancer to enlarge and to extend to neighboring tissues and organs and to metastasize to distant foci. Here again, the primary site of spread is to the regional lymph nodes in the tissues around the uterus, the parametrial tissues.

There are two general periods during which treatment for cancer of the cervix is most effective. The most favorable period is the preinvasive stage, or the stage of carcinoma *in situ*. The second, and far more complicated period, is the invasive stage, when the cancer is

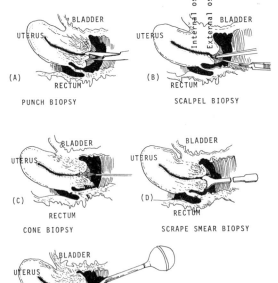

FIGURE 12–4. *Various techniques used in early diagnosis of cancer of the cervix. (Adapted from R. C. Benson, "Cancer of the Cervix,"* CA—A Cancer Journal for Clinicians, *17(4): 180.*

still small but clinically confined to the cervix. As with cancer of the breast, cancer of the cervix can be staged clinically, and the following international staging has been agreed upon.

STAGE 0. Carcinoma *in situ.*
STAGE 1. Cancer confined to the cervix.
STAGE 2a. Involving outer parametrium (a part of the uterus) and/or upper two-thirds of the vagina.
STAGE 2b. Involving outer parametrium but not fixed to the pelvic wall.
STAGE 3. Extending to the pelvic wall and/or the lower third of the vagina.
STAGE 4. Involving the bladder, rectum, or beyond the limits of the true pelvis.

This clinical staging is intended to assist in the statistical evaluation of results and to assess current treatment.

Let us now return to two fundamental questions and examine radiological treatment of carcinoma of the cervix in a manner comparable to that for surgical treatment of cancer of the breast. The two questions are as follows.

1. Are the clinical results improved by increasing the intensity of the irradiation and the depth of the dose delivered?

2. Is the current concept of treatment, namely, intracavitary radium combined with external beam therapy of the regional lymph nodes correct, or is it undesirable to irradiate the regional lymph nodes unless they are involved?

The current technique, of course, employs a high primary dose to the cervix itself, with a very homogeneous dose throughout the pelvis and to the regional lymph nodes of the parametrium and pelvis.

RESULTS OF VARIOUS TREATMENT METHODS

Fortunately, clinicians have been classifying carcinoma of the cervix for a number of years, and the results of therapy are available for various stages, 0 to 4, with both the conventional 220 kilovolt machines, cobalt teletherapy, and the more recent therapy with the linear accelerator. With the exception of stage 0, which can be treated adequately by hysterectomy, the results listed below are for those cases treated primarily by radiation therapy in one of the above stages. The results from conventional 220 kilovolt machines are as follows.

STAGE 1. 5-year survival rate between 75 and 80 percent.
STAGE 2. 5-year survival rate of 50 percent.
STAGE 3. 5-year survival rate of 25 percent.
STAGE 4. 5-year survival rate of 6 percent.

The complications from intensive radiotherapy to cancer of the cervix include bleeding from the uterus; radiation enteritis of the bowel; fistulae between the bladder and the vagina, or the rectum and vagina, or the rectum, bladder, and vagina; anemia; and, in the late cases, obstruction of the canals between the kidneys and the bladder (ureters), with resultant uremia, a toxic condition arising from the inability of the kidneys to excrete the urinary constituents from the blood.

The essential question is, can these results be improved by increasing the intensity of the radiation source? It will be profitable now to look at the recently available results of careful studies of the use of the linear accelerator in the treatment of cervical cancer (Bagshaw, 1967).

In 168 primary cases in Bagshaw's linear accelerator series, patients were treated with both radium applications in the uterus and homogeneous irradiation throughout the pelvis up to a dose of about 6,000 rads. This is very high, the usual dose being 5,000 rads; the aim was the complete destruction of the cancer in the cervix and in the regional lymph nodes. The overall 5-year survival rate for the linear accelerator group was 60 percent, while the overall 5-year survival rate of a very large group of cases nationally is only 48.5 percent. However, it should be pointed out that about 80 percent of the cases in the accelerator group were in stage 1 or 2, whereas only 62 percent of the cases in the larger national series were in stage 1 or 2. It would appear, therefore, that increasing the intensity of the dose of irradiation to 6,000 rads, with the supervoltage method of the linear accelerator, has not altered the survival rate in the treatment of cancer of the cervix.

Unfortunately, too, the linear accelerator results have demonstrated that efforts to lessen irradiation injury to the sigmoid colon and the small bowel have not been successful, despite recent attempts at shielding of the bowels. Injury to the bowels might be acceptable if the treatment meant a greater salvage of patients with advanced lesions. However, this has not been the outcome so far. An important observation from the Stanford series (Bagshaw) is that the dosage used has sterilized the carcinoma in the cervix and the regional lymph nodes of the pelvis. Nevertheless, some later deaths were the result of widespread metastases. This suggests that there are two types of cervical cancer of different biological potential: (1) a slowly growing type, occurring in young women, and less likely to be preceded by a period of carcinoma *in situ,* and (2) a rapidly growing type, often extending beyond the cervix at the time of diagnosis, tending to occur in older women, and less susceptible to cure by any method of treatment.

The treatment of cancer of the cervix by irradiation, then, is plagued by vexing questions similar to those encountered in surgery of cancer of the breast. The local lesion can be controlled by irradiation. If the pelvic nodes are involved, the cancer may be sterilized locally by intensive irradiation, but this may not in any way alter the ultimate prognosis of the disease, which may well be related to the biological potential of the tumor. If the pelvic lymph nodes are not involved, the necessity for irradiation is uncertain. In carcinoma of the breast, there is some recent evidence that irradiation of uninvolved lymph nodes may be harmful (Holloway, 1969). But we have no information on this point with regard to cancer of the cervix.

Attempts have been made to treat women with extensive stage 3 and stage 4 tumor by a combination of radiotherapy and chemotherapy. The chemotherapy consisted of large doses of a chemical agent to the cancerous area by methods of regional perfusion. Briefly, regional perfusion consists in the introduction of the agent into the blood vessels supplying the tumor. Results have been quite unsatisfactory. For example, in nine of such patients treated by the Stanford group, all had to have the chemotherapy discontinued. Seven of these patients died rather promptly, one is living but still has obvious carcinoma less than five years after treatment, and one is living with a colostomy without demonstrable gross tumor at the moment.

In selected situations, the cases with irradiation failure can be treated by radical pelvic exenteration operations. The operation, also called pelvic evisceration, requires the establishment of artificial external methods for the drainage of the urine and stool, for both the bladder and rectum are removed in the surgical procedure. The ureters are implanted into a loop of bowel and brought out to the skin in the form of a colostomy. The overall 5-year survival of patients in whom this operation is attempted, and found technically feasible, is in the order of 25 to 30 percent (Bricker, 1970). Reluctant as the surgeon may be to inflict major disability of this type upon his patients, the decision must be an individual one by the patient, for each of us values life differently. In many patients the attachment to life is such that they will accept major disability in return for even a period of relief, or, optimistically, a chance for survival of several years. The operation is not excessively difficult, but it is upsetting to patient and doctor alike.

With all the unanswered problems in the treatment of cancer of the cervix, it appears clear that solutions must follow the same line suggested for cancer questions in surgical treatment of carcinoma of the breast. But, despite the problems we have explored, it must be emphasized that prevention of cancer of the cervix is theoretically possible with present approaches, and this, of course, is feasible in the absence of a discovered cure for cancer. More emphasis should be placed on prevention, for in many parts of the country 50 percent of the women appearing for treatment of cancer of the cervix already have stage 3 or stage 4 lesions when first seen by the examining physician.

THE FUTURE OF RADIOTHERAPY

Great progress has been made in the last 20 years in radiotherapy. However, it is quite clear that the limits of success of treatment with irradiation therapy have been reached both with conventional ortho-voltage techniques and recent supervoltage techniques. Aside from the urgent necessity of standardizing these methods on an international basis, little more can be accomplished along these avenues of treatment.

Current knowledge of radiotherapy must be spread and diffused, for the relationship of present knowledge to application is indeed distressing. Current high-energy equipment is costly—approximately

$100,000 for a telecobalt unit and $150,000 for a linear accelerator. This equipment is largely unavailable in the United States, and hopelessly out of reach internationally. For the best equipment is useless, and indeed dangerous, unless operated by fully qualified radiotherapists, and here again the number of qualified personnel available —physicians, physicists, paramedical technicians, and supplementary personnel— is much too small and meager.

The future of clinical radiotherapy appears to lie in incorporating the recent advances in cellular radiobiology into clinical medicine. Three such advances are: (1) radiosensitization by oxygen, (2) differential chemical radiosensitization, and (3) synchronous cell-cycle irradiation. With these experimental approaches the cellular effects of irradiation are delivered in high concentration to the cancer tissue with a minimum impact upon normal tissues within the field of irradiation.

THE OXYGEN EFFECT

The radiosensitivity of most cells is enhanced approximately threefold in the presence of high oxygen tension (fig. 12–5). In any tumor some of the cells are living in a high oxygen atmosphere due to the local overgrowth of blood supply to the tumor, and others are severely *hypoxic* (deficient in oxygen), particularly in the areas of growth which have outstripped the blood supply. Severely hypoxic cells are extremely radioresistant, and thus tend to survive as foci for recurrent tumor growth after radiotherapy. It is possible to place patients for short periods of time in sealed chambers where the con-

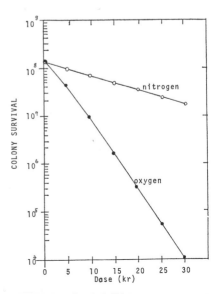

FIGURE 12–5. *Diagram showing the increasing sensitivity of cells to irradiation with increases in the supply of oxygen. (Source: Pollard, "Biological Action of Ionizing Radiation," p. 216.)*

centration of oxygen can be raised from the normal one atmosphere to three atmospheres—a change of oxygen tension in the tissues from approximately 40 to 60 mm of oxygen pressure to hopefully 1,000, or more. Irradiation is then carried out in the atmosphere high in oxygen tension. At the moment the early results indicate that the value of this technique is good in controlled animal experiments, but relatively minimal in the clinical field.

DIFFERENTIAL CHEMICAL RADIOSENSITIZATION

Certain drugs attach to cancer tissue and render the cancer tissue more susceptible to irradiation. Other drugs offer a striking radioprotective effect if they are present in cells prior to irradiation. A great deal of further research is necessary before any of these chemicals will be available for clinical use.

SYNCHRONOUS CELL-CYCLE IRRADIATION

Finally, let us mention another theoretical means of improving irradiation treatment of cancer, based on the fact that the radiosensitivity of the cell varies from one phase of its life cycle to an-

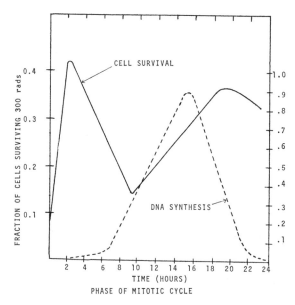

FIGURE 12–6. *Changes in radiosensitivity of cells during different stages of mitosis (cell division). (Source: Pollard, "Biological Action of Ionizing Radiation," p. 214.)*

other (fig. 12–6). After a single irradiation many cells are blocked into the premitotic phase (before division). When the cell cycle starts again a considerable proportion of the cells remain semi-synchronized and pass together through the mitotic cycle. We have described the phases of the mitotic cycle in an earlier chapter; let us remember the actual process of mitosis here designated M; it is at the stage M that most cells are most sensitive to irradiation. If, then, the tumor cells could be synchronized in their mitotic cycle, and irradiated at the crucial stage M, the effect of irradiation would be enhanced. Unfortunately, it is impossible to synchronize the mitotic phase of the tumor tissue without producing an almost identical result in normal tissues, and before this method could have usefulness one would have to know the detailed mitotic cycles of each particular tumor and the normal tissue in which the tumor is found. A vast amount of work remains to be done in these fields; so cell cycle-modulated dose fractionation, as this method is named, can have no clinical application as yet.

CONTROLLED CLINICAL TRIALS

Radiation therapy is plagued with a multitude of problems similar to those discussed under surgical approaches to cancer. Newly introduced methods are hard to evaluate from retrospective comparisons of two series of patients when the series are not entirely comparable. To achieve valid results, comparisons must be made under satisfactory statistical conditions, which means that the treatment plan should be randomized. However, randomized clinical treatments are not ethically sound if one treatment is considered to be no more effective than another at the beginning of the treatment studies. But since 50 percent of the patients with cancer are treated at some stage of their disease with radiotherapy, controlled clinical trials to establish effectiveness of treatment seem entirely justified in the light of past experiences with radiation therapy of cancer.

13

THE CHEMOTHERAPY
OF CANCER

*"A doubtful remedy
is better than none."*
LATIN PROVERB

The concept of curing cancer by the administration of a drug is beautifully simple. It is a natural outgrowth of the successful development of drugs to cure infections resulting from invasion by bacteria or parasites. In bacterial or parasitic infections, however, the drug has the specific ability to kill the offending microbe or parasite. Unfortunately this is not true for cancer. The difference between a normal cell and a cancer cell is not comparable to the difference between a bacterium and the host, and the drugs that act on cancer cells also act on normal cells in the same host. It is therefore apparent that treatment of malignant diseases which are disseminated, such as metastatic cancer, leukemia, lymphomas, or any other widespread cancer, requires an agent capable of diffusing throughout the body in uniform concentrations.

The treatment of cancer by drugs is called the chemotherapy of cancer. The outstanding shortcoming of such methods is the failure of the drugs to destroy the cancer cells specifically without simultaneously damaging the host. While normal cells, as well as cancer cells, are sensitive to the drugs used in the chemotherapy of cancer, there is a difference in the sensitivity of normal cells and cancer cells to any given drug. The crux of the problem lies in this differential sensitivity, for it is oftentimes impossible for the drug to kill the cancer cell without simultaneously damaging all of the normal cells

206

of the host. These drugs, in order to kill cancer cells, must be powerful agents, and since they are of uniform concentration throughout the body, they must have toxic effects on normal cells as well as on cancer cells. The normal cells in the body which are most susceptible to the action of these drugs reside in the bone marrow and in the gut. The administration of chemotherapeutic agents in adequate doses is therefore often complicated by depression of the bone marrow (characterized by a drop in the white corpuscles—leukopenia—and a drop in the number of platelets—thrombopenia). The damage to the intestinal tract is followed by diarrhea, anemia, suppression of the immune system of the patient, and, as a consequence of these abnormalities, an unwelcome susceptibility to infections.

Despite these problems, many cancers can be retarded in their growth by the use of chemotherapeutic agents. At the present time no drug is known to cure cancer, with the possible exception of actinomycin D and methotrexate, which are used in the treatment of *choriocarcinoma,* a cancerous growth originating in the placenta during pregnancy. The tremendous number of new drugs constantly being discovered requires careful experimentation and careful clinical screening. This is best accomplished after the basic research on the compound has been completed by controlled clinical trials on a national basis. Recognition of this fact has led our government to establish a national chemotherapy program.

Our present inability to cure cancer with drugs should not arouse undue pessimism. Many dramatic responses to these drugs have been observed and with certain drugs in certain specific cancers there is a good chance of achieving a long-term control of the disease. The accompanying tabulation lists the chemical agents available for treatment by general type (Dollinger, 1969).

Polyfunctional alkylating agents	Nitrogen mustard (Mustargen, HN2)
	Triethylenethiophosphoramide (ThioTEPA)
	Chlorambucil (Leukeran)
	Busulfan (Myleran)
	Melphalan (Alkeran)
	Cyclophosphamide (Cytoxan)

ANTIMETABOLITES

Methotrexate
9-Mercaptopurine (Purinethol)
  and 6-Thioguanine
5-Fluorouracil
Arabinosylcytosine (cytosine,
  arabinoside, CA,
  Cytarabine)

STEROID HORMONES

Androgens (testosterone,
  fluoxymestrone)
Estrogens (estradiol,
  diethylstilbestrol)
Progestational agents (6-methyl
  hydroxyprogesterone)
  (Provera), hydroxyprogesterone caporate (Delalutin)
Adrenal cortical steroids
  (prednisone,
  dexamethasone)

ANTIBIOTICS

Dactinomycin (actinomycin D,
  Cosmegen
Mithramycin*
Daunomycin*

PLANT ALKALOIDS

Vinblastine (Velban)
Vincristine (Oncovin)

MISCELLANEOUS DRUGS

Procarbazine (N methyl-
  hydrazine, Natulan)
o,p' -DDD
Quinacrine (Atabrine)

ENZYMES

1-Asparaginase*

RADIOACTIVE ISOTOPES

Radiophosphorus (32 P)
Radioiodine (131 I)
Radiogold (198 Au)

* Presently available for investigational use only
(Tabulation from "Cancer Chemotherapy," M. R. Dollinger, R. B. Golbey, and
David A. Karnofsky, *Disease-a-Month*, April 1969, p. 16.

ACTION OF CHEMOTHERAPEUTIC AGENTS

The chemical agents used in the treatment of cancer have a wide variety of biological effects on cells (fig. 13-1). They can have a direct effect upon the DNA of the cell nucleus, or they can interfere in the transfer of information from the DNA to the messenger RNA with the subsequent alteration of protein synthesis by the cell. They can act upon the mitotic process of the cell. They can interfere with the formation of hormones which are essential to the life of the cancer cell. In general, there are four major classes of drugs which are useful in blocking the synthesis of particular proteins or enzymes. These are (1) the alkylating agents, (2) the antimetabolites, (3) the steroid hormones, and (4) miscellaneous compounds with specific blocking effects.

ALKYLATING AGENTS

Alkylating agents react with some chemicals essential for the life of the cells. They act upon the DNA chain itself, producing a cross-linking of the bases of the DNA chain. This cross-linking blocks the replication of nuclear DNA during mitosis. The main alkylating agents are briefly described in the following paragraphs.

Nitrogen mustard. This drug must be given intravenously. It is used principally in treatment of lymphomas and lung cancer. It produces nausea and vomiting, but the complete course of treatment can be given in a single injection.

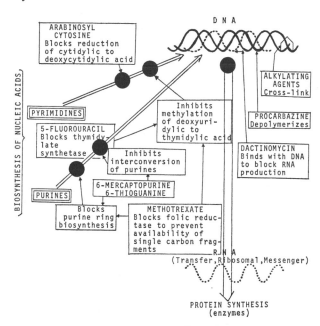

FIGURE 13–1. *Schematic diagram showing the mechanism of action of various drugs used against cancer. (Source: D. A. Karnofsky, "Mechanisms of Action of Anticancer Drugs at a Cellular Level," CA— A Cancer Journal for Clinicians, July-Aug. 1968, pp. 72–79.*

Thio-TEPA (triethylenethiophosphoramide). This is given intravenously and is used primarily in cancer of the ovaries and cancer of the breast. It can be given at weekly intervals and can be used for prolonged maintenance therapy.

Chlorambucil (Leukeran). This is the most commonly used oral alkylating agent. It is primarily used in treating chronic lymphatic leukemia, lymphomas, and breast, ovarian, and lung cancer.

Busulfan (Myleran). This is the agent of choice for chronic myelocytic leukemia, which results in destruction of marrow cells by cancer. It can be taken orally and be maintained for long periods of time.

Cyclophosphamide (Cytoxan). This drug can be taken orally or intravenously. It is particularly useful in acute leukemias of children, lymphosarcomas, ovarian cancers, and multiple myelomas. However, it has the disadvantage that it may produce baldness.

Melphalan (Alkeran). Also called sarcolysin, or phenylalanine mustard. This is effective by mouth. It is especially good in multiple myeloma, and for regional perfusion of malignant melanoma (a tumor made up of melanin-pigmented cells).

ANTIMETABOLITES

Antimetabolites inhibit the biosynthesis of nucleic acids and proteins, thereby producing cell death. The antimetabolites owe their name to the fact that their composition is close to that of cell constituents which are active in metabolism and to the fact that they block the cell's normal metabolic processes. The antimetabolites of greatest clinical usefulness are methotrexate, 6-mercaptopurine, 6-thioguanine, and 5-fluorouracil. These drugs are useful mainly in acute leukemia, chronic myelocytic leukemia, carcinoma of the digestive tract, breast cancer, and choriocarcinoma in the female.

Methotrexate. Methotrexate inhibits the synthesis of the cell's DNA by competing in the cell with folic acid (a B vitamin), which is instrumental in the sequence of chemical events leading to the formation of DNA. Methotrexate is particularly useful in the treatment of acute leukemia in children and in the treatment of the trophoblastic tumors of pregnancy, the choriocarcinomas. (A trophoblast is a tissue that supplies nutrition to the embryo and the choriocarcinomas originate in the placenta.)

6-Mercaptopurine (6 MP). This is one of the most widely used antimetabolites. Like all antimetabolites, it interferes somewhere along the chain involved in DNA synthesis. Its widest use is in acute leukemias and chronic myelocytic leukemias.

6-Thioguanine. This compound is not as useful as 6-mercaptopurine clinically, but it has the same chemical action.

5-Fluorouracil (5 FU). This is widely used in the treatment of metastatic cancer of the stomach, bowel, and breast. It is given intravenously and can be administered over prolonged periods of time, particularly if care is taken to avoid toxicity to the bone marrow and gut. It is one of the most useful chemotherapeutic agents currently available.

STEROID HORMONES

Properly administered, hormones alter the hormonal balance of the patient, and modify the growth of some cancers, notably those arising from cancer of the breast or cancer of the prostate. The mechanism of action by which the steroid hormones stimulate or inhibit cellular growth and function is not clear, but it is believed to take place within RNA prior to protein synthesis.

Adrenal steroids. Prednisone is the most widely used adrenal steroid. It is a synthetic hormone which can be taken by mouth and is useful in the treatment of leukemias in children and adults, in the treatment of lymphomas, and in the treatment of breast cancer.

Estrogens. Estrogens, the female sex hormones, are used in the treatment of metastatic cancer of the breast, or metastatic cancer of the prostrate. Diethylstilbestrol, a synthetic compound, can be taken by mouth. It may, however, cause uterine bleeding and vomiting as side effects.

Androgens. Androgens, the male sex hormones, are given for metastatic breast cancer. The synthetic compound testosterone propionate is the compound of choice. Halotestin is a similar compound, as is testonolactone. All of these can be given by mouth.

Progesterone. Progesterone, a female sex hormone, can be used in selected cases of cancer of the uterus. It is taken intramuscularly.

Thyroid hormone. Thyroid hormone is useful in initiating thyroid activity and in controlling thyroid cancer which is sensitive to both thyroid hormone and to thyrotropic-stimulating hormone from the pituitary.

MISCELLANEOUS COMPOUNDS

There are a variety of drugs which have interesting actions against cancer cells (fig. 13-2). These include the vinca alkaloids, o,p' DDD, and 1-asparaginase.

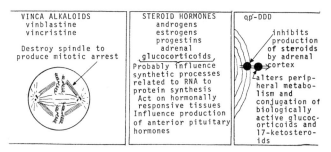

FIGURE 13–2. *The mode of action of three drugs—vinca alkaloids, steroid hormones, and o, p-DDD—used in cancer chemotherapy. (Source: Karnofsky, "Mechanisms of Action of Anticancer Drugs at a Cellular Level," p. 233.*

Vinca alkaloids. The vinca alkaloids, vincristine and vinblastine, arrest cell division. Vincristine is more active in acute leukemia; vinblastine in Hodgkin's disease. Colchicine is a comparable compound. These compounds arrest cell division and have a possible usefulness in producing cell cycle-modulated growth of the tumor during radiotherapy treatment. (Described in chapter 12.)

o, p' DDD (ortho, para prime DDD). This compound is a derivative of the insecticide DDT. It prevents excessive steroid hormone production and has been proven useful in the treatment of carcinoma of the adrenal cortex.

1-asparaginase. This is a newly discovered compound which provokes the death of cancer cells by blocking the production of a certain amino acid—1-asparagine. Normal cells appear to be unaffected by 1-asparaginase. It is most useful thus far in the treatment of acute lymphoblastic leukemias, but it is coming under investigation in a variety of neoplastic disorders.

THE PRESENT STATUS OF CANCER CHEMOTHERAPY

Cancer chemotherapy has produced results ranging from cure in a high percentage of patients with one type of cancer (trophoblastic carcinoma, or choriocarcinoma, a cancer of pregnancy originating in the trophoblast, tissue nourishing the embryo) to total failure in many forms of cancer. Cure usually refers to patients who are alive five years or more after drug administration without evidence of active or recurrent disease. Cures of this type have been produced in 70 percent of cases of choriocarcinomas. Rare cures have also been noted in some testicular tumors of childhood, in neuroblastomas, and Wilms' tumors of childhood. Some of these tumors are prone, however, to spontaneous remission.

A high degree of palliation by anticancer drugs can be produced in the acute leukemias of children, prostatic tumors, chronic lym-

Current Status of
Clinical Cancer Chemotherapy

Disease Entity	*Agents*	*Remission Rate*
Choriocarcinoma	Methotrexate, dactinomycin, velban	75 percent complete; probable cure in most responders
Burkitt lymphoma	Cyclophosphamide, methotrexate	60 percent objective; 15 percent long-term complete
Acute leukemia in children	Prednisone, vincristine, 6-mercaptopourine, methotrexate, cyclophosphamide	90 percent complete hematological; prolongation of median survival from 3 mos. (untreated) to 32 mos. combinations improve effect

Current Status of
Clinical Cancer Chemotherapy

Disease Entity	Agents	Remission Rate
Lymphomas		
Hodgkin's disease	Alkylating agents, vinca alkaloids, prednisone, procarbazine	70 percent objective with single agents; 90 percent objective, 50 percent to 90 percent complete with combinations
Lymphosarcomas and reticulum cell sarcoma	Alkylating agents, vinca alkaloids, prednisone	50 percent objective with single agent; 80 percent objective with combinations
Multiple myeloma	Melphalan, cyclophosphamide	35 percent objective
Sarcomas		
Wilms' tumor	Dactinomycin, vincristine, alkylating agents	30 to 40 percent objective; also adjuvant to surgery
Neuroblastoma and retinoblastoma in children	Cyclophosphamide, vincristine	60 percent objective; some long-term in infants
Rhabdomyosarcoma	Vincristine, dactinomycin	80 percent objective
Chronic leukemia Myelocytic	Busulfan, mercaptopurine	90 percent objective; probably no increased survival
Lymphocytic	Chlorambucil, prednisone	50 percent objective
Tumors of endocrine-influenced organs		

Current Status of
Clinical Cancer Chemotherapy

Disease Entity	Agents	Remission Rate

Breast
  Postcastration
  or postmeno-
  pause
	Androgens, fluorouracil,
	alkylating agents
		20 percent objective

Late menopause	Estrogens, androgens, fluorouracil, alkylators	30 to 40 percent objective
Ovary	Alkylating agents, fluorouracil	30 to 40 percent objective
Uterine body	Progesterone, fluorouracil, alkylating agents	40 percent objective
Prostate	Estrogens	70 percent objective
Testis	Dactinomycin, methotrexate, alkylating agents (in combination)	30 to 40 percent objective
	Mithramycin	5 percent long-term (possible cures)

FROM: James K. Luce, Gerald B. Bodey, Sr., and Emil Frei, 3rd,
The Systemic Approach in Cancer Therapy
Hospital Practice, p. 53, Oct. 1967

phatic leukemias, lymphosarcomas, Hodgkin's disease, and chronic myelocytic anemias. Palliation occurs, but is less likely, in breast cancer, testicular cancer, and ovarian cancer.

Palliation is less likely in the majority of other cancers, ranging from cancer of the lung, bowel, and stomach to cancer of the pancreas, adrenal cortex, and cervix. In this group of cancers, palliation occurs for brief duration in about 5 to 10 percent of the cases. Nevertheless, chemotherapy serves an extremely valuable role in keeping patients oriented toward proper medical therapy, and prevents the feeling of being abandoned by the physician in patients with late and hopeless cancers. Judicious employment and screening of potentially useful drugs may also prevent the spread of cancer quackery. Late and hopeless patients are particularly prone to succumb to unwarranted claims for the relief of cancer by nonphysicians, and to become prey to many types of cancer quackery. Properly based chemotherapy can serve a useful purpose in preventing improper orientation of the patient. It can also yield valuable information about a wide variety of drugs which must be subjected to clinical trial if their effectiveness is to be evaluated.

THE HAZARDS OF CHEMOTHERAPY

All chemotherapeutic agents are toxic to some degree. They are usually poisonous to the cells. Since they primarily affect DNA synthesis, they would be expected to be most toxic to the most rapidly growing cells of the body. This is, in fact, true with the primary areas of toxicity being in the bone marrow and the gastrointestinal tract. The problem is to use the drugs in a dose adequate to kill the tumor, yet not so large as to kill too many normal cells in the bone marrow and gut.

Depression of the normal content of the bone marrow is the most common toxic reaction. We have already described it as being characterized by a drop in the white count and the number of platelets of the blood. This predisposes the patient to infection and bleeding tendencies, and since these complications occur in an already debilitated patient, vigorous treatment with antibiotics, blood, and perhaps admission to a hospital may be necessary.

The gastrointestinal complications are most frequently nausea, vomiting, and diarrhea, leading ultimately to dehydration. This results from a destruction of the normal cells of the gastrointestinal tract which are rapidly turning over, or replicating, with the attendant improper absorption of food and products of digestion.

Skin rashes and loss of hair are not infrequent complications of many of these drugs. These are not serious complications, and with the increasing popularity of wigs loss of hair is not unduly distressing.

IMPROVEMENT OF CHEMOTHERAPEUTIC AGENTS

Ingenious methods for improving the effectiveness of chemotherapy have been devised. Briefly, they consist of an attempt to deliver the chemotherapeutic agent to the tumor cells in high concentration, yet diminish toxicity by reducing the dose to the body generally. These newer methods are still experimental, and the evidence concerning their usefulness is conflicting. The methods employed are (1) adjuvant chemotherapy, (2) combined chemotherapy, (3) regional infusion, and (4) regional perfusion.

Adjuvant Chemotherapy. More than a decade ago, a cooperative investigation under the auspices of the National Institutes of Health was initiated in an effort to determine the efficacy of administering drugs in conjunction with "curative cancer surgery of the breast." The hope was that the initial surgery would eradicate the bulk of the tumor, and since tumor cells were also present in the blood in a fair number of patients undergoing early cancer surgery, chemotherapy immediately after the operation would be employed to destroy the disseminated tumor cells and thereby prevent recurrences. Because of its effectiveness in palliation of mammary cancer thio-TEPA was chosen for evaluation. The drug 5-FU (fluorouracil) has also been evaluated in comparison with thio-TEPA. Twenty-three major American institutions adopted a common protocol, and the results of their investigation were reported by Fisher *et al.* (1968). Eight hundred and twenty-six patients were followed, and there were adequate numbers of patients in the premenopausal age group, the postmenopausal age group, and in control groups for both premenopausal and postmenopausal patients. The analysis could be conducted for patients whose lymph nodes were uninvolved as well as for patients whose lymph nodes were involved. All patients had the standard radical mastectomy as an initial treatment, and since in a radical mastectomy the axillary lymph nodes are dissected the degree of their involvement could be ascertained.

This study demonstrated that in all categories neither thio-TEPA nor 5-FU administered at the time or shortly after surgery, in a maximum dose compatible with the patient's safety, reduced either the recurrence of the tumor or enhanced the 5-year survival rate. The present therapeutic results obtained in adjuvant chemotherapy have been unsuccessful, but they have provided information which may be of value in future studies of this type. The study has helped to define the general principles of clinical research studies, for it involved the cooperation of a large number of institutions, with pooling of patient data. It also indicated that cells are drug sensitive during only part of their cycle of division (mitotic cycle), and that the percent reduction of neoplastic cells for a given treatment is constant, regardless of the number of cells present, and that host immunological factors may be important and altered by drug therapy. The theory of adjuvant chemotherapy is sound, but in practice it has not altered the results of any cancer to date.

Combined Therapy in Malignant Disease. The hope that use of radiotherapy together with a chemotherapeutic agent might do more for a patient with cancer than radiotherapy alone has not been substantiated. It was hoped that chemotherapy would enhance the radiation effect, that the joint action of these methods would produce an effect greater than the mathematical sum of the two component treatments. Most of the initial studies unfortunately were uncontrolled, but recent controlled studies have shown that placebos are as effective as chemotherapeutic agents in combined therapy. Until some very useful clinical benefit from combined therapy can be expected, we should probably employ just one method of treatment at a time, and indeed it has been demonstrated that patients under combined therapy have far more infections, with considerably greater toxicity, with less dose of radiation than they would have had otherwise. Furthermore, the individual response to combined therapy is more variable than it is to radiotherapy alone, and it would seem far more fruitful to pursue other meaningful approaches to the treatment of cancer than trials of this type.

Regional Infusion. Recent interest has centered on the possibility of improving the results of cancer chemotherapy by continuous intra-arterial infusion techniques. It is now technically simple, in many arteries of the body, to insert a small polyethylene catheter through a needle puncture in the skin, or by an insignificant local operation, under anesthesia, to expose the artery. The chemotherapeutic agent can then be infused directly into the arterial supply of the tumor. This, of course, provides a very high concentration of the drug to the tumor, for instead of being diluted by the total volume of the patient's blood it is merely diluted by the regional

Combined Therapy for Advanced Breast Cancer
1. Surgery first
2. Irradiation next, then
3. Treatment of metastatic breast cancer

A. Premenopausal Patients

Oophorectomy

Response   Failure

Androgens   Chemotherapy (see D)

Response   Failure

Hypophysectomy   Chemotherapy

or adrenalectomy

Chemotherapy

B. Patients One to Five Years Postmenopausal

Androgens

Response   Failure

Estrogens   Corticosteroids or Chemotherapy

Response   Failure

Hypophysectomy   Corticosteroids

or adrenalectomy

Response   Failure

Chemotherapy

C. Patients Five-Plus Years Postmenopausal

Androgens or estrogens

Response   Failure

Use other agent

Response   Failure

Corticosteroids   Chemotherapy

D. Chemotherapy
1. 5-Fluorouracil, 12 mg/kg x 5 days q 3½ to 4 weeks; after one or two courses, 12 mg/kg may be used once weekly
2. Cyclophosphamide, 100 to 150 mg daily p.o. for 21 to 24 days each month
3. Methotrexate, 1.25 t.o.d. p.o. until evidence of toxicity appears; repeat when toxicity clears
4. Vinblastine, 0.1 mg/kg daily x 2 or 3 days; then in 2 to 3 weeks 0.1 mg/kg weekly
5. Investigational programs

FROM: Robert W. Talley, Chemotherapy of Solid Tumors, Postgraduate Medicine, 48:182–189, Nov. 1970 volume flowing to the tumor area. To further protect the body from generalized toxicity, it is possible to give the patient some protective agents. Regional infusion has particular usefulness in inoperable cancers of the head and neck, where the catheter can be inserted into the external carotid artery by simple means. The technique is somewhat less useful in inoperable cancer of the pelvis and liver, where the catheter can be inserted directly either into the hypogastric artery nourishing the pelvis, or the hepatic artery supplying the liver. Long-term cannulation of these vessels is possible with small polyethylene catheters, so that the cancer cells can be exposed over a long period of time to the chemotherapeutic agent. However, since one is dealing with patients with advanced cancers, the results from this form of therapy are unpredictable, and in general mediocre. Arterial infusion therapy may also present some complications, such as inadequate catheter placement, leakage of the infused drug, hemorrhage, and drug toxicity. Tumor regression has been noted in about 20 percent of the patients, varying from a few months to a year or two. On the whole, this method of therapy, although difficult and disappointing is theoretically valuable.

Regional Perfusion. In an effort to increase the amount of drug that can be brought to a part of the body and reduce the amount of drug that spills over into the entire body, initiating toxicity, the method of regional perfusion, or isolation perfusion, has been developed. This technique works best in an extremity, particularly the lower extremity, and is primarily applicable to a disease known as malignant melanoma of the extremities. It has also been tried in the treatment of pelvic cancers, and in the treatment of liver metastases, but in these situations the technique of regional perfusion is extremely complicated, and the proportion of spillover into the body is quite large so that toxicity cannot be avoided.

In the treatment of malignant melanoma of the extremities the femoral artery and the femoral vein are first isolated. A tourniquet is then placed above the site of the incision in these two blood vessels. Blood is taken out of the femoral vein, and run through a pump oxygenator to control its temperature, its pH, and its oxygen content. The blood is then pumped back into the femoral artery, while the chemotherapeutic agent which is to accomplish the tumoricidal effects is added slowly over a period of about an hour. The tourniquet effectively isolates the limb from the rest of the body, so that the spillover of the drug into the body is limited. The drug acts usually within one or two circulations through the extremity, for the drug is utilized and destroyed within the extremity in a minute or so. Rather large doses of the drug can be given to the tumor, with minimal dosage getting into the general circulation. In isolated perfusions of an extremity the average spillover into the general circulation, during the course of an hour perfusion, is only 10 to 15 percent. In isolated perfusion of the pelvic organs and liver, the spillover may be as high as 75 percent in the same period of time. It is possible to irradiate an extremity while it is undergoing a regional perfusion. It is also possible to buttress the effects of the drug by juggling the temperature, pH, and oxygen content of the blood flowing through the extremity. The regional perfusion technique is not without complications. Approximately 20 percent of the patients will have complications with healing of the perfusion incision; about 10 to 15 percent will have severe or persistent edema of the extremity, and the most serious complication is depression of the bone marrow from spillover of the drug in about 10 percent of the cases. Occasionally arterial thrombosis (formation of a blood clot in the artery) results from the cannulations, and the leg may become gangrenous, requiring amputation. Fortunately, this complication is quite rare.

Finally, it should be noted that the technique has largely proved unsatisfactory with the exception of isolation perfusion of the extremity in cases of malignant melanoma. The future of regional chemotherapy, whether by regional perfusion or regional infusion, is still uncertain.

THE DEFECT OF CANCER CHEMOTHERAPY

The fundamental defect of all cancer chemotherapy is that no drug is specifically oriented to destroying cancer cells without producing comparable effects on normal cells. The differential effect of the drug is related, therefore, to the growth potential of the tumor against that of normal tissue. The lack of specificity of the drug for the cancer cell, and the growth potential of the cancer cell, make this at best an uncertain method of therapy. It might be compared to the difficulty of controlling an expanding colony of mice by shooting them with a smaller number of bullets than the number of mice. No matter how we calculate the firing system, one could see that inevitably, if even two mice capable of mating remained, doubling of the population would resume. This analogy corresponds to the growth of cells generally, and to the molecules of DNA concerned in cell proliferation. With chemotherapy, we have no sure shot, but we have a differential shot in which we have to consider normal cells as well as cancer cells. It is clear that we can never eliminate the last cancer cell by using antimetabolites.

The aim of chemotherapy, however, is not simply to eliminate the last cancer cell, but to do so without reducing to dangerous or lethal levels other necessary cell populations in the patient. Fortunately, we have working with us factors within the host which govern the growth potential of the tumor cell, and by bringing about a reduction in the number of cancer cells, combined with increased host resistance, hopefully chemotherapy will enable us to achieve better results in the containment of cancer.

14
THE IMMUNOLOGY
OF CANCER

"To seek to discover new truths,
new methods, new procedures;
to forge new and unknown weapons,
to battle with disease,
to stay the hand of death."
RUDOLPH MATAS

Because of its intractability, cancer is surrounded by mystery and ritualism in medical as well as popular circles. Clinical thinking about cancer has been deeply influenced by two curious dogmas. The first of these holds that malignant tumors are purely autonomous growths, not subject to the usual restraints governing normal tissues. The second dogma maintains that cure can be achieved only by the complete eradication of every last living cancer cell in the host, either by surgery, irradiation, or chemical means.

Since we are unable to cure many cancers these dogmas offer a simple explanation for our helplessness. But they are contradicted in part by what clinicians have long observed, that is, that the body has natural defenses against cancer. Many physicians have observed a patient with far-advanced, inoperable cancer, who, contrary to expectations, remained well for long periods of time, and, indeed, who came to autopsy without evidence of cancer. Whether they are complete or not, unexpected regressions of cancer do occur. Everson and Cole (1967) have gathered together 176 cases of spontaneous regressions in cancer, each impressively documented. The majority of these regressions occurred in such cancers as neuroblastoma, adrenal and renal tumors of children, and in pigmented melanomas.

Clinical and experimental evidence has been extensively cited to demonstrate that cancer cells may lie dormant for long periods of time in the host before they are aroused and suddenly grow without control. Here again natural defenses of the body against tumors appear evident, and, indeed, there are so many carcinogenic chemicals in our environment because of carelessness or abuse, the wonder is that the incidence of cancer is not far greater.

The human body possesses beautiful and natural mechanisms for its own protection and defense. These mechanisms have been designed by nature to reject foreign substances and foreign proteins in the body, or any substance or cell in the body which is not recognized as "self." The process of immunological defense against foreign tissue has been called "immunological surveillance" (fig. 14-1). It explains, not only the regressions of certain cancers, and the vagaries in dormancy of cancer cells, but also the variability in the course of a similar tumor in different patients. The cancer cell is a changed cell, different from the normal cell from which it originates. It can be regarded as "nonself" by the organism. In fact, immunologists today think that a cancer cell produces a cancer-specific antigen, thereby adding another biochemical difference between the normal cell, a cancer cell, and the tissue of origin from which the cancer arose.

FIGURE 14–1. *Graphic representation of immunological surveillance. Genetic identity is essential for a successful homograft. A foreign antigen in the donor results in rejection by the recipient.*

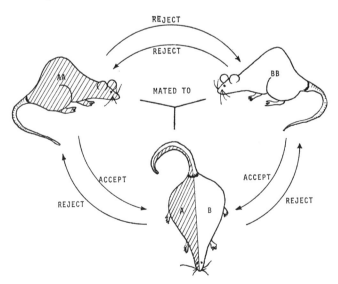

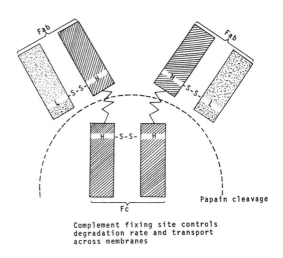

FIGURE 14–2. *Diagram showing the mechanisms and responses of a humoral antibody. Note (1) pairing of heavy (H) and light (L) chains; (2) binding of antibody to antigen at positions Fab; (3) fixing of complement by antibody at position Fc; (4) dividing of antibody into three parts at the Papain cleavage; and (5) control of degradation rate at the Fc fragment. (Adapted from* Transplant, *Medical Communications, Inc., 1969, p. 31.*

Immunological surveillance operates through two major mechanisms or responses: (1) a humoral response, or (2) a cellular response. A humoral response consists in the production of free-circulating (or humoral) antibodies against the foreign antigens of the cancer cells (fig. 14-2). The cellular response, or action of cell-bound antibodies, consists in the ability of certain specific cells to produce and bind antibodies to the surface of the cell membrane, and thereby endow the cell with the ability to destroy foreign cancer antigens (fig. 14-3).

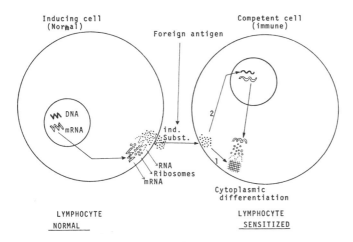

FIGURE 14–3. *Schematic representation of the process of production of a cellular antibody through sensitization of a lymphocyte. (Adapted from E. Wolff, "Embryonic Differentiation,"* Cell Differentiation and Morphogenesis, *North-Holland, Amsterdam, 1966, p. 16.)*

In theory the "nonself" cancer cells can be looked upon as a graft of foreign cells or tissue in the host, and cancer can thus be compared with the grafting or transplantation of tissue from one individual to another. The study of the rejection or acceptance of transplanted tissues in animals and man has afforded tremendous understanding of the problems of immunological tolerance and immunological surveillance. Genetically identical or inbred strains of animals are available for experimental studies in tissue and organ transplantation. Three major types of tissue transplantation are of particular interest to us. They are:

1. Syngenic grafting or the transplantation of tissues between genetically identical animals (see fig. 14-1).

2. Allogenic grafting (or homografting), the transplantation of tissues between genetically different animals, but of the same species.

3. Zenogenic grafting, the transplantation of tissues between animals of different species, that is, from mouse to rat, or from rabbit to dog, or from monkey to man.

Under controlled experimental conditions it has become possible to relate tissue transplantation and cancer transplantation between genetically known strains of animals, and to examine the progression of tumors under controlled conditions of tissue compatibility, as well as the changes induced in these tumors by immune reactions of the host under genetically controlled experiments.

METHODS OF STUDY OF TUMOR IMMUNITY

Around the turn of the century evidence of spontaneous rodent tumors was collected. These tumors could occasionally be transplanted by grafting from one animal to another, and indeed some of the transplanted tumor lines still exist under the names of Ehrlich carcinoma, Jensen sarcoma, Walker carcinoma, and others. With the data provided by these well-established experimental tumor lines, immunological thinking concerning the transplantation of cancer has passed through three successive stages.

The first stage extended from 1900 to 1930. During this time it was felt on the basis of uncontrolled transplantation experiments that an immunity against cancer could readily be produced. The second stage extended from 1930 to 1950, and during this period genetically identical strains of animals became available, so that the characteristics of transplanting normal tissue as well as cancer tissue could be studied, and it was observed that the same degree of transplantation acceptance or rejection applied to both normal and cancerous tissues. The third stage covers the period from 1950 to the present. Refined immunological techniques are now beginning to indicate that cancer-specific antigens and cancer-specific antibodies do exist and that immunological potential might ultimately be exploited in the clinical treatment of cancer. The pertinent lessons from each of these stages bear upon our understanding of cancer immunology.

As early as 1906, Ehrlich found that tumor transplants often failed to take when introduced in mice which had already received a transplant from the same or a similar tumor. He also discovered that an animal harboring a growing tumor would not accept additional transplants of this same tumor, although the original tumor continued to grow. Obviously the animals were in some kind of immunized state and he termed this immunity "concomitant immunity." Obviously, too, the degree of immunity in question was sufficient to reject the transplants of tumor, but not the originally established tumors. Hopes ran high that the cancer problem could be solved through immune mechanisms. During this period, however, Ehrlich and other investigators interested in cancer immunology were unable to work with genetically identical or inbred strains of animals. Indeed, genetically identical strains of animals were not available for experimental studies in transplantation until the late 1920's. At that time it became clear that the rejection of many of the transplanted tumors was the result, not of any specific cancer immunity, but of the normal rejection process which attends grafting between any tissue in nonidentical strains of animals. Allogenic strains of animals reject homografts of either normal or cancerous tissue to an equal degree, and what Ehrlich and others had been observing was the homograft rejection phenomenon, not cancer-specific immunity.

Studies of tumor transplants were subsequently made in the late 1920's in mice that were genetically identical (syngenic animals), in animals that were genetically different but still mice (allogenic animals), and in animals of different species (zenogenic animals), and it became clear that cancer tissue and normal tissue grafted under genetically controlled conditions followed the same acceptance and rejection response regardless of whether the tissues were normal or malignant.

The second period in our understanding of cancer immunity and tissue transplantation immunity followed with a precise analysis of transplants of both normal and neoplastic tissues in brilliantly conducted experiments by Snell, Gorer, Medawar, and Mitchison. These investigators used syngenic, allogenic, and zenogenic animals. Of a number of conclusions reached, two are of particular interest to the immunology of cancer.

1. Grafts of either normal or cancerous tissue between genetically different animals (homografts, or allografts) stimulate an immune response in the recipients because of the genetic diversity of the grafted material.

2. Rejection of transplanted tissue, either normal or malignant, does not occur in genetically identical donor and recipient animals (see fig. 14–1).

The investigations proved that the acceptance or rejection of transplanted tumors was due, not to tumor immunity, but to the inability of any foreign tissue to grow in a genetically deviant host. In other words, the same laws applied to the transplantation of tumors as to that of normal tissues. A homograft liberates into the host an antigen against which an antibody is produced, resulting in the phenomenon previously mentioned, immunological surveillance. Immunological surveillance is primarily cellular in origin, and the cell-bound antibodies are produced by the lymphocytes of the host (white blood corpuscles arising in the lymph glands and lymph nodes). These cell-bound antibodies enter the bloodstream, remain bound to the lymphocytes, reach the homograft, and destroy it in a matter of a few days. Although the lymphocytes are the key cells in this process, humoral or free-circulating antibodies also share in the rejection phenomena to a lesser degree, and subsequent studies have demonstrated that the source of these humoral antibodies are the plasma cells of the host, not the lymphocytes (fig. 14–4).

This third period in our understanding of cancer immunity has resulted in a far richer and better comprehension of the process. Since

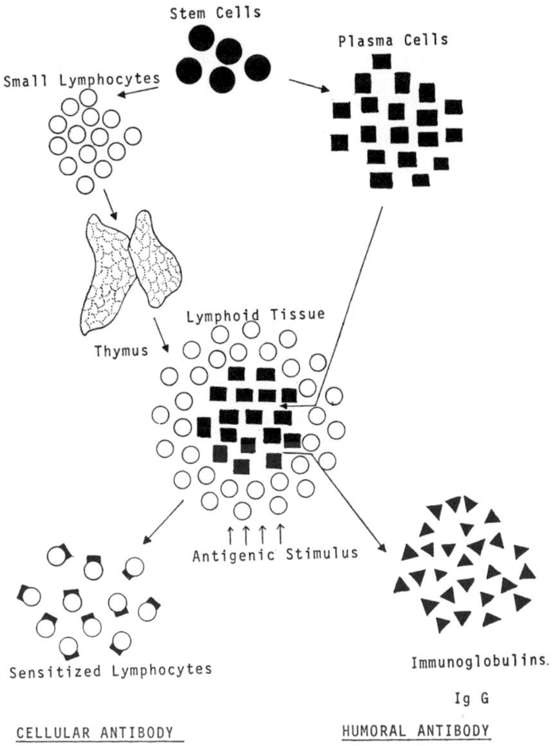

Stem Cells

Plasma Cells

Small Lymphocytes

Thymus

Lymphoid Tissue

Antigenic Stimulus

Sensitized Lymphocytes

Immunoglobulins.

Ig G

CELLULAR ANTIBODY

HUMORAL ANTIBODY

FIGURE 14–4. *Origins and interrelationships of cellular and humoral antibodies. (Adapted from Robert Good, "Immunologic Reconstitution,"* Hospital Practice, *April 1969, p. 43.)*

1960, a recrudescence of interest in tumor immunology has occurred and this time experiments have concentrated, not on large compact tissue grafts, but on the introduction of small numbers of individual neoplastic cells which can be counted and measured in the injection dose. By measuring the rejection of a few cancer cells, whose number can be verified, it has been established that tumor resistance can indeed be engendered, and that specific immunity to tumor antigens exists in a genetically identical host (syngenic host). Indeed two major types of cancer antigens can now be characterized:

1. The antigens originating in virus-induced tumors.
2. The antigens originating in chemically induced tumors.

We shall return in more detail to both the viral and chemical tumors later in this chapter, and we shall see the important differences in the antigenicities of virally versus chemically induced tumors, and how these differences have relevance to the application of tumor immunology in man.

CURRENT EXPERIMENTS IN TUMOR IMMUNOLOGY

In the 1960's scientists proved that the response of the host organism to neoplastic cells involves an antigen-antibody reaction. The body has a tendency to reject neoplastic cells just as it rejects any foreign antigens, tissues, or other substances. In the formation of a malignant tumor, the cells undergo transformation—they acquire a new tumor-specific antigen against which the body marshals its antibody response (fig. 14–5). At this point it must be emphasized that, although it has been widely confirmed that many cancer cells possess many tumor-specific antigens, these antigens must be compared to "weak" transplantation antigens, and do not evoke strong immunological responses.

We have said that both free-circulating antibodies (humoral antibodies), and cell-bound antibodies (cellular antibodies) are involved in fighting cancer antigens, but, just as in the general area of transplantation immunity, the primary reactions are mediated by the cell-bound antibodies, which remain attached to the lymphocyte cells, until they reach the foreign antigen, the so-called "target-tissue." We have also mentioned that cell-bound antibodies are produced by the lymphocytes of the lymph nodes; details of the action of the lymphocytes are not entirely known, but are currently being intensively studied in experimental animals and in the test tube. Study of the

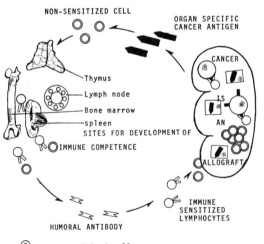

FIGURE 14–5. *Diagram showing the tumor-specific antigenic activity of a cancer cell and consequent antibody response. (Adapted from* Transplant, Medical Communications, Inc., *1969, p. 32.)*

NON-SENSITIZED CELL

ORGAN SPECIFIC CANCER ANTIGEN

Thymus
Lymph node
Bone marrow
spleen
SITES FOR DEVELOPMENT OF
IMMUNE COMPETENCE

CANCER

IS

AN

ALLOGRAFT

IMMUNE SENSITIZED LYMPHOCYTES

HUMORAL ANTIBODY

◎ non-sensitized cell
○━ graft leukocyte antigens
○≈ sensitized cell
≿≾ antibody
▬ organ-specific antigens, CANCER SPECIFIC ANTIGENS

response of man's own lymphocytes to spontaneous tumors in the cancer patient would be most helpful, but is particularly difficult. It would involve a type of human experimentation which we are only beginning to contemplate. Needless to say, this kind of experimentation would be acceptable in very special cases only. We must therefore direct our efforts at understanding the immunology of cancer with the help of either tissue culture techniques (studying man's tissues in the explanted form), or with the help of experimental cancer in inbred strains of animals.

A clear and interesting difference exists between the immunology of chemically induced tumors and that of virally induced tumors. This difference will be discussed in the following subsections.

IMMUNOLOGY OF CHEMICALLY INDUCED TUMORS

Both tumors induced by chemicals and those induced by viruses produce antigens. But, whereas each "chemical" tumor possesses its own individually distinct antigen, all "viral" tumors induced by a given virus possess the same antigen.

If the same chemical agent, say methylcholanthrene, is used to induce multiple tumors in the same animal, each tumor has a specific antigenicity: not only do the antigens vary with each tumor but the vigor of the immunological response varies in degree. The reason for the unique antigenicity of chemically induced tumors is still unknown.

FIGURE 14–6. *Chart demonstrating active immunization against tumor-specific antigens. No tumors were produced in immunized animals after transplantation. The rate of tumor production among untreated syngenic animals was 100 percent. (Adapted from E. J. Ambrose and F. J. C. Roe (eds.),* The Biology of Cancer, *Van Nostrand, 1966, p. 97.*

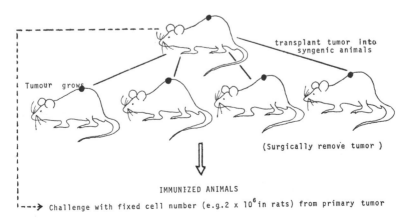

transplant tumor into syngenic animals

Tumour grows

(Surgically remove tumor)

IMMUNIZED ANIMALS

---→ Challenge with fixed cell number (e.g.2×10^6 in rats) from primary tumor

Active immunization against the tumor-specific antigens of chemically induced tumors is depicted in figure 14–6. Active immunization is the immunization effected by the formation of antibodies by each organism's own cells. Notice that this active immunity has been demonstrated in the identical host-bearing animal, or in animals of identical genetic constitution.

IMMUNOLOGY OF VIRALLY INDUCED TUMORS

The vast majority of tumors produced by viruses produce antigens which are identical for all tumors produced by a particular virus, whether it be a DNA or an RNA virus (fig. 14–7). As noted in chapter 5 the virus material becomes incorporated in the genome of the cancer cell, giving rise to genetic change in the cell which is specific for the virus, and hereditable and transmissible. Wherever the given virus makes its invasion and whatever the tumor it generates, the antigen is identical: for example, a sarcoma induced by a polyoma virus shares the same antigen with a carcinoma induced by the same virus in another animal.

Active immunity against viral antigens can be obtained, and the viral specific antibody against specific virus protects against the syn-

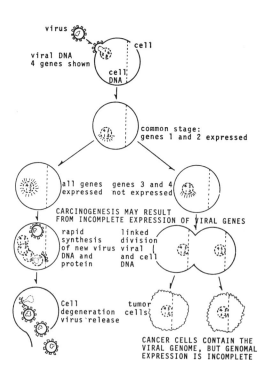

FIGURE 14–7. *Scheme showing the possible sequence of events following the infection of cells by small DNA-containing tumor viruses such as polyoma virus. Viral cancers have antigen common to the virus, can be transplanted to allogenic hosts, and incorporate virus in the host genome. (Adapted from M. Stoker, "Viral Carcinogenesis,"* Endeavour, *1966, 25: 119.)*

genic transplantation of all tumors induced by this particular virus.

Sometimes animals affected by a "viral" tumor, instead of showing an immunity reaction to the tumor, are totally unresponsive to the virus. In other words, instead of rejecting the foreign virus, they are tolerant. It is not because the tumor lacks the specific antigen that tolerance occurs, but because the animal has become tolerant of the virus as a direct result of the vertical transmission of the virus from mother to offspring. The virus then lives in a state of immunological tolerance in the host, and induces the cancer change, free of an immune response from the host. Through vertical transmission from mother to offspring the virus gains access to the future host at a time when it is immunologically immature, unresponsive, and thereby tolerant.

IMMUNOLOGICAL FACTORS FAVORING TUMOR GROWTH

Cancer often escapes the remarkable defense mechanisms of the body. Instead of checking and fighting the growth of a tumor, the body may demonstrate mechanisms through which it actually favors the growth of the tumor. Let us examine a few of these known "avoidance mechanisms." One of them is due to the loss of tumor-specific antigens. A second is related to the possibility of immuno-selection, and a third to the phenomenon of immunological tolerance.

LOSS OF TUMOR-SPECIFIC ANTIGEN

Sometimes, in experimental tumors, an antigen may disappear. Such is the case with mammary carcinoma in inbred strains of mice; it would appear that vertical passage of the tumor from mother to offspring would result in the loss of tumor-specific antigen. Similar antigenic deletion may at times appear in tumors that have been growing in the same individual for a long period of time. This phenomenon is simply explained by the concept of immuno-selection.

IMMUNO-SELECTION

Immuno-selection holds that the number and density of antigens vary on the surfaces of the cells. The cells with the largest number of antigens would provoke the formation of large numbers of antibodies, and thereby be destroyed. The more weakly antigenic cells would survive and grow, and the tumor as a whole would have escaped immunological surveillance. The weakly antigenic cells are believed to lack both the antigen for the recognition of "self," and the antigen controlling growth.

We do not know that this phenomenon is true for primary tumors in man but it is postulated from experimental animal tumors of the lymphoma and mammary groups.

IMMUNOLOGICAL TOLERANCE

Another avoidance mechanism is the system of immunological tolerance described in chapter 5. Let us remember that, during the early stages of embryological development, before the time of maturation of an organism's immunological system, it is totally unable to reject any foreign tissue. All antigens are tolerated in a state of immunological immaturity. If this were not so the female egg and the male sperm could never possibly unite; they are foreign to each other (genetically different) but tolerant of each other. In maturing, the organism shifts from tolerance to rejection of foreign substances and the antigens then provoke an immunological response of rejection through the formation of antibodies. The time of maturation of the immune system varies from animal to animal. In rats and mice the immunological system does not completely mature until the day of birth. In man the immunological system matures several months prior to birth, that is, during fetal, or embryonic, life.

Immunological tolerance is a major reason for the growth of antigenic tumors in animals when the animal is invaded by the cancer-producing agent before it has developed its immune system, as when "viral" cancers are transmitted vertically through the mother's milk. Tolerance in theory could be abolished by the introduction of antibodies into the host, or by the addition of sensitized lymphocytes, also called immunologically competent cells. Antibodies, or lymphocytes, would then take over the work of immune rejection. The sensitized lymphocytes would abrogate the state of tolerance which existed prior to their introduction into the animal.

Perhaps the most important avoidance mechanism is the unspectacular phenomenon of "sneaking through." It occurs when the growth intensity of the tumor exceeds the capacity of the host for resistance. The tumor's growth is unhampered, and, curiously, this happens in both the implantation of small or large numbers of tumor cells. It is believed that small numbers of cells grow relatively undisturbed until the tumor reaches a size rendering it capable of antigenic stimulation. This situation could be altered by a prior injection of antigenic tumor cells, or of a vaccine from the tumor itself, in an amount proper to produce immunity. On the other hand, large quantities of tumor cells seem to be capable of overwhelming the host's resistance with their excessive amount of antigen. In either situation "sneaking through" occurs.

Immunological surveillance and avoidance mechanisms are still incompletely understood. It is not known whether all or some of these theoretical systems, the formulation of which is due to experiments on animals or in the test tube, are applicable to man, and to cancer in man. They have as yet brought no clinical benefit for treatment of human cancer, but could, in the long run, provide new approaches to the therapy of cancer.

IMMUNO-SUPPRESSION AGENTS

Chemicals which interfere with the organism's natural defenses against foreign antigens suppress the normal immune response. This effect is termed "immuno-suppression" and recent evidence suggests that it has a bearing on the appearance and growth of cancer. Many drugs which are used in the treatment of cancer are capable of immuno-suppressive effects, and many of the immuno-suppressive agents used in conjunction with organ transplantation are chemically very close to chemical carcinogens. Successful organ transplantation requires the prolonged and continuous use of immuno-suppressive agents to insure that the patient does not reject the transplant.

In the 1960's, a very powerful immuno-suppressive agent was developed in the form of an antilymphocyte serum. This has recently been purified and is now used as antilymphocyte globulin (fig. 14–8). This antilymphocyte globulin could be of help in testing the hypothesis that spontaneous malignant tumors are common but rarely result in true cancers because of the body's normal surveillance mechanisms. Our testing question would be: Have human tumors

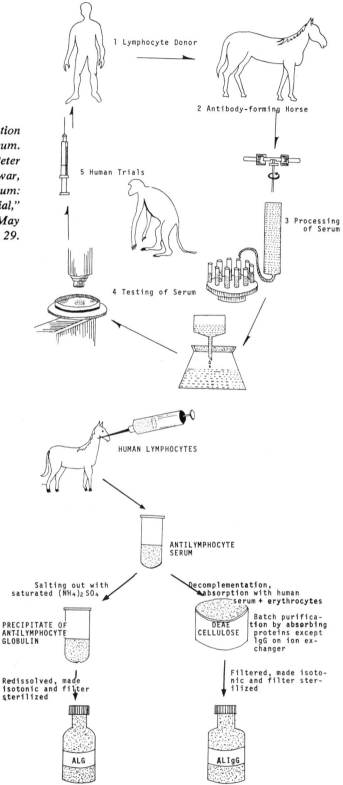

FIGURE 14–8. *Preparation of antilymphocyte serum. (Adapted from Peter Medawar, "Antilymphocyte Serum: Properties and Potential,"* Hospital Practice, *May 1969, p. 29.*

1 Lymphocyte Donor

2 Antibody-forming Horse

3 Processing of Serum

4 Testing of Serum

5 Human Trials

HUMAN LYMPHOCYTES

ANTILYMPHOCYTE SERUM

Salting out with saturated $(NH_4)_2SO_4$

Decomplementation, absorption with human serum + erythrocytes

PRECIPITATE OF ANTILYMPHOCYTE GLOBULIN

DEAE CELLULOSE

Batch purification by absorbing proteins except IgG on ion exchanger

Redissolved, made isotonic and filter sterilized

Filtered, made isotonic and filter sterilized

ALG

ALIgG

emerged under the influence of immuno-suppressive drugs? In other words, has the use of a potent immuno-suppressive drug like anti-lymphocyte globulin been instrumental in the development of some cancers?

There are three reported cases in which kidney transplants carrying malignant donor cells produced tumors which grew and metastasized in the recipient. The patient had received the standard immuno-suppressive therapy employed in all transplantation procedures. In one case the tumor was rejected, together with the transplanted kidney, after interruption of the immuno-suppressive therapy. Another renal transplant was then successful, and tumor regrowth did not occur, even under the influence of subsequent immuno-suppression. In other words, the original transplanted tumor cells had unrestrained growth under the influence of the immuno-suppressive agent, but their antigens were foreign to those of the recipient. When the immuno-suppression was stopped, spontaneous rejection of the transplanted kidney, as well as the transplanted tumor, occurred. Other reports indicate that patients receiving heavy dosages of anti-lymphocyte globulin developed lymphomas and lymphosarcomas. Indeed, if the general incidence of cancer is two per 10,000, current statistical evidence suggests that the patient receiving large doses of antilymphocyte globulin will develop cancer with a frequency of five per 1,000, a tremendous increase in the incidence of spontaneous cancer due to the abrogation of normal immune responses of lymphocytes, which are the prime host cells involved in immunological surveillance.

At the present time there are still too few cases on which to base a specific answer to our question with accuracy, but concern is indicated. It may well be that patients receiving prolonged immuno-suppressive therapy are far more vulnerable to spontaneous cancers than the normal population. Evidence indicating this is beginning to accumulate.

POSSIBLE OUTCOMES OF IMMUNOLOGY

The ultimate goal of all cancer research is of course the treatment and cure of cancer in man. Theoretically, immunology could bring to the .

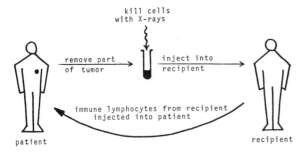

kill cells
with X-rays

remove part
of tumor →

inject into
recipient →

immune lymphocytes from recipient
injected into patient

patient

recipient

FIGURE 14–9. *Schematic diagram showing production of heterologous antilymphocyte antibody. (Adapted from* Transplant, Medical Communications, Inc., 1969, p. 44.)

cancer problem solutions of both preventive and curative type, in the form of vaccines and antisera (fig. 14–9). The vaccines would provide an active immunization against cancer; the antisera would provide a passive rejection of the cancer once it occurred and became established.

It is clear that an immunological approach to cancer therapy would be far simpler for virally induced tumors than for chemically induced tumors, since the former have specific antigens common to all cancers induced by the same virus. But, at the present time, we have no proof that any cancer, with the possible exception of the Burkitt lymphoma of East and South Africa, is viral in origin. A virus has been identified in the Burkitt lymphoma, but it may be a passenger virus, and not the true cause of the cancer. The EB virus, which is found in Burkitt lymphoma, is also found in patients who have had infectious mononucleosis, thereby suggesting it is a passenger virus, not the true etiological virus.

If viral cancers are proved to exist in man, vaccination against cancer will be a useful procedure. All cancers produced by a single virus could be prevented by the injection of the attenuated virus as a univalent vaccine. A polyvalent vaccine could be used to protect against diverse viruses producing different tumors. Some problems would present themselves, for example, that of tolerance and vertical transmission—vaccination might be useless where viruses are transmitted from mother to offspring.

Tumors induced by chemicals could not be prevented by vaccination. They are of so many different antigenic origins, and the diversity of antigens is so different for each "chemical" tumor in any given host, that the task of vaccination against each individual tumor would seem almost hopeless. Perhaps polyvalent vaccines would be useful, but the likelihood of containing cancers of chemical origin by a polyvalent vaccine is far less possible than that of treating and preventing viral cancer by the use of attenuated viral vaccines.

As a preventive form of action against cancer, the entire field of immunization remains to be investigated. As a form of therapy for established tumors, active immunization has also been tried. Unfortunately, it has been found wanting. Many attempts have been made at increasing the resistance of humans to existing tumors by active immunization, but thus far they have been disappointing.

Curiously, vaccines which are not specific for cancer have been shown to enhance immunity against cancer in animals. The administration of pertussis vaccine (vaccine against whooping cough), or of BCG vaccine (a substance similar to the coat of tubercle bacilli), reinforces the host's own immune response. It must be remembered that extreme caution is essential in injecting hazardous agents in debilitated patients, whose immune response is already weakened or altogether suppressed by the invasion of cancer. However, BCG has recently been tried in man and has been found helpful in producing an active immunity against melanoma cells in patients with metastatic melanoma. The entire field of agents that might enhance the normal immunological response must be further investigated.

Striking regressions in tumors borne by animals have been obtained by the injection of sensitized or "immuno-competent" lymphocytes, accompanied by whole body irradiation (fig. 14–10). Similar attempts have been made in man and are possibly achieving success in the treatment of leukemia. Yet efforts at reducing tumor growth should employ more conventional and well-recognized methods— immunotherapy with sensitized lymphocytes being used as an ad-

FIGURE 14–10. *Possible method of stimulating a patient's immune reaction to tumors by injection of irradiated cells with altered antigenicity into recipient followed by injection of immune lymphocytes into patient.* (*Adapted from J. A. V. Butler,* Gene Control in the Living Cell, *Basic Books, Inc., p. 136.*)

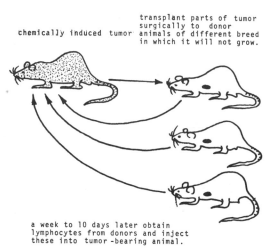

transplant parts of tumor surgically to donor animals of different breed in which it will not grow.

chemically induced tumor

a week to 10 days later obtain lymphocytes from donors and inject these into tumor -bearing animal.

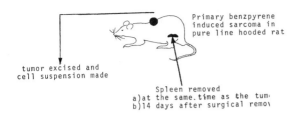

Primary benzpyrene
induced sarcoma in
pure line hooded rat

tumor excised and
cell suspension made

Spleen removed
a) at the same time as the tum
b) 14 days after surgical remo

FIGURE 14–11. *Chart showing the experimental use of immunologically competent lymphocytes to induce cancer regression. (Adapted from Ambrose and Roe,* Biology of Cancer, *p. 117.)*

juvant for the treatment of selected cases and in an experimental fashion (fig. 14–11).

Finally, antisera have been developed between patients afflicted with cancer. They are directed specifically to a given tumor and their use has given some hope of benefit in the treatment of melanoma (a skin cancer), but no conclusive evidence exists that the use of antisera, transferred passively from one patient to another, will destroy or eradicate an existing cancer, even though it might attenuate its vigorous growth. The passive transfer of sera containing antibodies against cancer from one patient to another with a similar cancer is nevertheless worthy of investigation. The following tabulation shows the potential applications of immune therapy to cancer.

Active Immunization by Vaccines
    1. Prevention. Viral Tumors: Univalent Vaccine
                    Chemical Tumors: Polyvalent Vaccine
    2. Therapy.   (a) Cancer-cell reducing methods
                        Surgery
                        X-rays
                        Chemotherapy
                (b) Immunologic Stimulation
                        BCG
                        Injection of irradiated cells
                        Interferons: viral resistance
                (c) Experimental
                        Cell fusion
                        Cell hybridization
                        Foreign marrow grafts
Passive Rejection (Antisera)
Humoral (Human or heterologous antisera)
                (a) Univalent Serum
                (b) Polyvalent Serum
    Cellular (Antisera)
                (a) Syngenic cultured lymphocytes
                (b) Homogenic cultured lymphocytes: Graft versus host reaction may also ensue

The new and wide knowledge born out of immunological studies has led to enthusiastic clinical experimentation, yet has failed to provide meaningful forms of treatment. However, our reaction should not be one of discouragement, for it was only a few years ago that the idea that immunology could contribute to the treatment of cancer seemed as absurd as Jenner's hope of preventing smallpox by vaccination in the 1700's. Yet the ideas and potentialities are identical, if indeed cancers have a demonstrable chemical or viral origin.

If the hopes are modest, they are real. Immune reactions against cancer exist, both in man and in animals, and host resistance to cancer can no longer be dismissed. Even a guarded optimist can now envision the immunotherapy of cancer as, initially, an adjunct to the usual methods for reducing the number of tumor cells, and, ultimately, as a true curative procedure. Further research will bring new advances in these directions. New techniques will be developed for the study of human cancer cells in the test tube, so that the antibody reaction of an individual's own lymphocytes can be studied. His own defenses against cancer could then be assessed. New techniques will be developed, too, for the isolation and identification of viruses, based on the hope that many human cancers will prove to be viral in origin.

PROSPECTS FOR IMMUNOTHERAPY

For the present we must adhere to the three accepted methods for fighting cancer—surgery, irradiation, and chemotherapy. But, for many cancers, these three accepted forms of therapy ultimately fail. Sympathy for the cancer victim demands optimism for emerging and potential forms of therapy. Prolongation of the cancer patient's life alone is an inadequate goal. Improvement in the quality of life must also be achieved. The important consideration is always the individual, and the quality of his life. In the therapy of cancer, fresh ideas must be explored, particularly if they are founded on sound scientific premises. The key to cancer control lies in understanding the body defense mechanisms, and in stimulating its rejection factors. Immunotherapy might not even have to be the primary form of treatment. It might well be that its prime value will be as a supplement to conventional means of therapy, and that the major portions of the cancer will be eradicated by surgery or irradiation, and immunotherapy will be called upon to rid the body of only the few remaining malignant cells that give rise to late metastases or recurrences. What are some of the current experiments by which researchers are attempting to bolster immunological defenses against cancer?

Cell-free cancer tissue homogenates are being injected into terminal or inoperable cancer patients in several institutions. In about 20 percent of the cases treatment of this type has either halted tumor growth, reduced the size of the tumor, or eliminated the tumor entirely for periods of up to two years. Sera from these patients have demonstrated an increased cytotoxic activity against their own tumor cells.

Refined immunological techniques have also recently demonstrated that the lymphocytes of patients with malignant melanoma can be stimulated when cultured in the test tube by extracts of their own tumor. Extracts from a melanoma tumor contain a mitogenic material in the tumor fluid, which has the structure of a beta globulin, and antisera can be developed against this material which seems to be fairly identical for all types of human melanoma. It would appear, then, that malignant melanomas share a tumor-specific antigen which is identical for many melanomas, even though it is immunologically weak. The lymphocytes can be specifically sensitized against this antigen, and the immunological response can thereby be strengthened, hopefully making this form of therapy available for the treatment of metastatic melanoma. Other workers have recently shown that BCG stimulates the immune response of the host, and between these various methods of provoking immunological responsiveness, immunotherapy looms as a potential adjunct in the treatment of malignant melanoma. Similar antigens have recently been found in human tumors of the Wilms' type (carcinoma of the kidney, the lung, and the colon). We are just beginning to gather reliable information that tumor-specific antigens occur in at least several kinds of human cancer. Thus it becomes reasonable to postulate that immunologic phenomena will have increasing relevance to clinical medicine as further clarification and study of antigenic material develop.

Viruses have also recently been used in the clinical treatment of cancer. In the treatment of cancer, injection with viruses may have the following beneficial effects: (1) Direct destruction of the cancer cells by multiplication of the virus, if the virus homes in the cancer cell; (2) immunological cytolysis (dissolution of cells) by both cell-mediated and humoral responses to "budding" viruses which incorporate the cell membrane into their coat, and confer virus-antigen determinants on the surface of infected cells, and (3) interference with the production of interferons by viruses.

In using viruses as cytolytic agents (that is, agents causing the destruction of cells), the ideal situation would be to have the virus attach itself to the tumor cell but not to the normal cell of the host. Antibodies could then be injected against the virus, thereby destroying both the virus and the attached tumor cell. Some cells have now been shown to have specific receptors for certain viruses. This type of therapy would be particularly advantageous in diseases such as leukemia, where the malignant cells are in the circulation, and attachment of the virus to such cells would make them readily accessible to antibodies against the virus, which could be either humoral or cell-bound in origin.

Viruses can be also used to stimulate the immunologic response of even a weakened host. As an example, the injection of a newly isolated, nonpathogenic (NP) virus into terminal cancer patients has resulted in extensive destruction of cancer cells in all sites throughout the body. The viruses apparently replicate in the cancer cells, to form a haptene complex with cellular antigens. (A haptene is a partial antigen, which can produce its antibody only if united to some other substance.) The haptene is recognized by the body as foreign and stimulates the host's defensive response against its own malignant cells. A similar mechanism operates with other viruses, notably the type 3 Rheo viruses in the malignant leukemias and lymphomas of mice. Unfortunately the successes of immunotherapy are impressive but they are never complete or permanent. The remissions thus far have lasted only a matter of months. Yet the therapeutic possibilities are exciting enough to make this an important new area of clinical research, despite the minimal dangers of injecting viruses into patients.

Immunological cytolysis occurs with many viruses which "bud off" from the cell membrane. The lipoviruses, or viruses with lipoprotein coat (a lipoprotein is a compound of protein with a lipid, or fat), have a particular knack of attaching to cells and producing "buds" on the cell membrane. These "buds" change the antigenicity of the cell surface and make the cell antigenic in the original host. The immune responses engendered by these "budding" viruses may be humoral or cell-mediated. In this way, even passenger viruses would be helpful in producing immunological cytolysis, if they localized to cancer cells. This fact of treating the host with a harmless virus of the "budding" type may be entirely comparable to the use of lymphoreticular stimulants, such as BCG. The lymphoreticular stimulants or the "budding" viruses enhance the capacity of the host to produce antibodies against the infected cells.

Another new promising approach to cancer therapy uses poly I:C, an anti-viral interferon inducer. Poly I:C is a combination of polyriboinosinic and polyribocytidylic acids. Viruses produce interferons, which interfere with the growth of the oncogenic virus, or the transformed cell. The level of interferons in patients can be increased by the intravenous injection of poly I:C, and this substance then affects the interaction between the host and the virus, raising the body's sluggish defenses against cancer.

The most exciting and promising aspect of all this recent work is the potential for stimulation of both the humoral and cell-mediated immunity against neoplastic cells by viruses, lymphoreticular stimulants, cytolytic agents, and interferons. These reactions seem particularly valuable against minimal quantities of malignant cells. The future therapy of cancer may then involve the eradication of the bulk of the tumor by conventional means, combined with the destruction of the last few remaining tumor cells by immunological reactions, stimulated within the host by new agents enhancing immunological surveillance. Immunological mechanisms must in the future, however, be probed more directly in the cancer patient, rather than in a foreign or atypical host. The quality of life for the hopeless cancer patient will not be impaired by these important new avenues of clinical research.

PART FOUR

PSYCHO-SOCIAL PROBLEMS

BY DENISE SCOTT

15
SMOKING AND CANCER

A cigarette is the
perfect type of a perfect pleasure.
It is exquisite, and it leaves one
unsatisfied. What more can you want?
OSCAR WILDE

An Arab legend gives the following account of the origin of tobacco. As the Prophet was walking in the country he found a snake dying from cold on the ground. In his compassion he raised the snake to his chest and tried to revive him, but the animal's only reaction was one of anger, for, said he: "Thy race persecutes mine and I have sworn to Allah that I shall seek revenge." The Prophet said: "How canst thou be so ungrateful?" and the snake answered that gratefulness did not exist upon earth. He then bit the Prophet, who immediately sucked the venom from his wound and spat it on the ground. At that very place grew a plant, which, the story says, combines the compassion of the Prophet and the venom of the serpent. That plant is tobacco. As the legend demonstrates, even in remote times the double-edged nature of the plant was known.

Today, in the modern USA, a little girl watches television. She sees and hears a grim warning from the American Cancer Society: smoking may cause cancer—beware. Immediately afterward she sees a magazine ad praising a well-known brand of cigarettes. She exclaims: "Daddy, that doesn't make sense." She cannot reconcile the two conflicting and almost simultaneous versions of the same fact. She does not understand that two entirely different motives underlie the two communications. She is confused.

If you are her father what should you be thinking at that moment? Let us suppose you are lighting a cigarette. You relax in your chair and inhale the warm smoke. You exhale, see the smoke spread in the air, or you watch it curl from the cigarette that you hold between your fingers. Do you enjoy the cigarette? Do you feel that smoking relaxes you? Do you like the taste of tobacco? Do you dislike the habit and wish you could put an end to it? Do you think the act of smoking is ridiculous, but is your decision to stop smoking for to-morrow?

As you enjoy (or do not enjoy) your cigarette, you reflect upon what you have heard and read for years: smoking is dangerous, smoking is the cause of lung cancer, of cancer of the larynx, of the mouth, of the lips. Your cigarette is incriminated in lung cancer, but pipe smokers are not immune to cancer; they may develop cancer of the lips, whereas cigar smokers may become the victims of cancer of the tongue. Perhaps you think that the hot little object which rests on the ashtray so innocently is not innocent after all. You may know that in the gracefully curling smoke, invisible, poisonous substances are contained: nicotine, arsenic, hydrocarbons, and hydrogen cy-anide. You may be aware that your cigarette is the center of power-ful chemical transformations, increased by its heat, that tars can be extracted from the elegant smoke which you contemplate idly and that they are deadly if painted on the skin of mice. (But you are a man, not a mouse!)

Your cigarette has a filter that is supposed to protect you from the harmful effects of tobacco smoke. Nevertheless, you have just read that it may be worse to smoke filtered cigarettes than unfiltered cigar-ettes if (and you are tempted, aren't you) you smoke them to the very end.

These thoughts do not bother you very much. Many smokers never develop cancer—your grandfather smoked until he died, in his eighties, and he was the healthiest person you ever knew—and what about Winston Churchill, the classical example of the heavy smoker?

Is cigarette smoking hazardous? Many authorities say yes, but some say that the hazard has not been proven by any means other than statistical evidence: as the amount of smoking throughout the world increases, the number of detected lung cancers increases too.

It has been estimated that in 1900, among a million living persons, nine developed lung cancer; in 1953, the comparable figure was 342. However, statistics are only circumstantial evidence. The crime is not proven beyond any doubt, the advocates of smoking say. It has been proven beyond reasonable doubt, say its opponents. Other culprits have been implicated, but do they exonerate cigarette smoking? It is true that the average citizen of the world lives to become older, and that consequently the number of detected lung cancers is greater. It is true that the possibilities and techniques of diagnosis and detection have greatly improved and may account partly for the larger number of lung cancers revealed. It is true that air pollution is much worse than it was several decades ago. It is true that X-rays are utilized more and more widely and they are known to be capable of inducing cancer. It is true that some cultural habits seem to have a relation to lung cancer. One instance is the fact that many Mexican women cook over a kitchen stove without any chimney and inhale a great deal of smoke; they present twice as many cases of lung cancer as Caucasian women who do not cook in similar surroundings.

Do these facts, and others, make the case against cigarette smoking any weaker?

Dr. Harry S. N. Greene, a smoker and a cancer researcher, Chairman of the Department of Pathology at Yale University, has written (Northrup, 1957): "The evidences from both approaches, statistical and experimental, do not appear sufficiently significant to me to warrant forsaking the pleasure of smoking." Dr. Alton Ochsner, a nonsmoker and a renowned surgeon who has operated on many patients with lung cancers, has said (1954): "Cigarettes cause cancer. . . . Indeed in view of research by the American Cancer Society, the National Cancer Institute, the National Institutes of Health, and scores of independent scientists throughout the world, it is appalling that anyone could doubt the shocking link between smoking and a dozen major health problems."

When equally learned and experienced men present us with opposite conclusions founded on the same facts, what are we to believe? Perhaps the smoking scientist is prejudiced in favor of his pleasure, but perhaps the nonsmoking scientist is prejudiced against a pleasure which he does not appreciate, and therefore has a tendency to condemn? Perhaps the optimist dismisses the idea of danger too easily, but perhaps the pessimist contemplates it too willingly? It would be easier to come to agreement if clinical and experimental evidences were more readily available. Obviously human experiments are out of the question. What about experiments on animals? Drs. Wynder, Graham, and Croninger (1957) discovered that tars obtained from a "smoking-machine" and applied to the skin of shaved mice can produce death if the concentration of tar is strong, and cancerous tumors if it is less potent. In two years, 44 percent of the mice presented cancers. However, the opponents of the theory linking cigarettes and cancer object that the pure strains of mice used for the experiments are extremely susceptible to cancer. They argue that the mice can develop cancers after contact with many irritants, some of them as mild as sugar water, olive oil, and tomatoes. Their conclusion, in the words of Dr. Kanematsu Sugiura: "It suggests only that there is something wrong with these animals" (Northrup, 1957). Yet in Dr. Ochsner's words (1954), after such experimentation, "the presence of a carcinogen in cigarette *smoke* was categorically proven."

In another type of experiment, Dr. Essenberg of the Chicago Medical School could produce lung cancer in mice by making smokers of the mice—placing them in glass chambers into which cigarettes were "inhaled" at the rate of one cigarette per hour. Again it was objected that the strains of mice were abnormally receptive to cancer and that the results of the experiments were not applicable to man.

To smoke or not to smoke? What do you, the smoker, think? How does the evidence look to you? If you are a woman, you may have heard that lung cancer is more frequent among men than among women, and this knowledge may entrench your smoking habit more deeply. Women smoke more and more every year without the increase in lung cancer following in proportion. According to Rosenblatt and Lisa (1967): "With so many millions of persons of both sexes smoking cigarettes regularly, parity in lung cancer mortality would have been reached a long time ago if tobacco was a main factor." They added that women seem to be biologically resistant to lung cancer and that a large number of the cancers diagnosed as primary lung cancers in women are actually due to metatases from cancers of the breast and of the genital organs.

It is not easy for the lay person to establish a valid opinion. We cannot but be impressed with the efforts of our government in the fight against cancer, and against lung cancer in particular. Before President Nixon's proposed $300 million program to fight cancer, President Johnson had launched the Acute Leukemia Task Force, the Breast Cancer Task Force, and the Lung Cancer Task Force. The director of the Lung Cancer Task Force, Dr. Kenneth Endicott, has attracted the public's attention anew to the increasing spread of lung cancer. A 1967 report by the U.S. Public Health Service presenting the findings of approximately 2,000 research studies concluded that "it is no longer a question of whether or not cigarettes cause disease . . . but how much disease they cause, and how much of it can be averted by cessation or reduction of cigarette smoking."

Lung cancer is not the only cancer to be associated with smoking. If women are relatively spared by lung cancer, they are not by cancer of the larynx. Warren H. Gardner (1966) says that 70 percent of the women included in his study of laryngectomized women had been smoking until the time of surgery, and that one woman, who had started smoking at age eleven, had been smoking four packs of cigarettes a day for 35 years. The numerous problems, both physical and psychological, which laryngectomized patients have to face are as real for women as they are for men. Such patients have to learn to speak again, using the esophagus in place of the missing larynx; they have to live with a small opening in their throats for the rest of their lives. Obviously they have to readjust their personal and professional lives.

Should everyone abstain from smoking? Is it possible to reduce the dangers of cigarette smoking? Is there such a thing as a safe cigarette? Can any amount of advice stop anyone from the habit? Who smokes? And why do we smoke? Is there a typical cigarette smoker, or are there several types of cigarette smokers? Is a rational approach successful in the fight against smoking?

Despite the absence of absolute evidence in studies to date, it is reasonable to assume that there is a strong probability that lung cancer is associated with the habit of smoking cigarettes. Some opposition has been shown to this opinion by serious researchers, but prudence (not panic) obliges us to consider the reality of a possible danger when we smoke. Even without positive assurance it would be sensible to decide that the risks are too great to be ignored. The next, and logical, step, would then be to stop smoking, or to smoke so little that the odds against one's health would be considerably diminished. But at this point one encounters a number of difficulties. If we were totally rational, the decision would be simple: smoking is in all probability dangerous, therefore we must not smoke. If we were able to say, like Sir Robert Aytoun in his Sonnet on Tobacco:

> "It's all one thing—both tend into a scope—
> To live upon Tobacco and on Hope
> The one's but smoke, the other but wind"

things would be rather simple. But are we? Most people's attitude toward smoking is, to say the least, ambiguous. They would agree with Charles Lamb, who admitted:

> "For I hate, but love, thee so,
> That, whichever thing I show,
> The plain truth will seem to be
> A constrain'd hyperbole,
> And the passion to proceed
> More from a mistress than a seed."

Lamb's attitude would be best described as addiction: when the seed, the tobacco leaf, instead of serving our pleasure, becomes a mistress and enslaves us, the salvation is far from our reach. Even though we may hate our cigarette, we love it, with a love which perhaps brings little pleasure, yet which we are not free to renounce.

Apparently some people have no difficulty in stopping smoking and in holding fast to their life of abstinence. They are able to make their own decisions and to live in accordance with that determination. For a great many others any rational exhortation to give up smoking is ineffective, or, if they can be brought to agree on the dangers of smoking, they cannot carry through the decision to abandon their habit without a long and difficult struggle.

Why? Psychologists have studied the personality of smokers and have found that various personality traits are associated with smoking. Moderate smoking, like moderate drinking, may be viewed as part of our culture, therefore somewhat acceptable, while excessive smoking (more than 25 cigarettes a day) indicates to some researchers that factors other than cultural ones are at play. They relate heavy smoking to all other types of exaggerated behavior and continue: "Heavy cigarette smoking . . . is overly determined and represents an extension of a socially accepted practice in the service of underlying frustrated needs" (Jacobs *et al.*, 1965). Smoking is, among other things, an oral activity. The researchers quoted above have established a relationship between heavy smoking and oral frustration experienced in childhood through a cold, domineering, and controlling mother. Other psychologists have linked cigarette smoking to other personality traits as well. There are so many motives impelling people to smoke that it would be idle to try to identify them all. But perhaps a story, the "true story" of a smoker, might clarify some of these motives.

The young girl was thirteen. Her mother smoked moderately, her father not at all, and they had little concern with the dangers of cigarette smoking. When their daughter asked for a cigarette they allowed her to have it, assuming that it was better to give permission than to risk the possibility of her smoking behind their backs. They felt that it was possible to control the amount of smoking she would do. So the girl smoked one or two cigarettes on Sunday in her mother's company and with her father indulgently looking on. She was not tempted to smoke more, since she did not particularly enjoy it. When the school year was over and she left with her family for a vacation by the sea things changed considerably. She began to smoke more and she also began to enjoy hiding while smoking. She and her friends liked to walk far away from her parents, find a lonely place on the rocks near the sea, and talk for hours in the hot sun, their feet playing with the wet sand or splashing in the water, their hands occupied with a cigarette. The feelings of independence, separateness, and sophistication that they experienced were profoundly enjoyable. They had contrived a situation in which what was not actually forbidden appeared to be so. It was a great joy to indulge in an adult activity without the sanction of the adults. It was as if the sensation of feeling "grown up" could not have been entirely genuine or authentic if it had been approved by the young people's parents. Since it is true that the processses of physical and mental growth happen largely in the secret recesses of body and mind, it is possible that our young girl could not have experienced her growing up in a psychological sense without putting herself in a situation of secrecy. Under the eyes of an adult things do not happen, they are only permitted. The girl's autonomy, her sense of identity, her power of decision, were expressed in an unvoiced phrase: "I am going to smoke a cigarette."

A few years later the girl stopped smoking. The change was easy. Her smoking experience had been mostly of a symbolic nature and had not developed into a habit. It is probable she stopped smoking because she had found other and better ways of asserting herself.

Some psychologists say that it is possible we smoke because we are rebellious, not merely during the normally rebellious adolescent stage, but throughout life, from a tender age through adulthood (Stewart and Livson, 1966). It is not impossible that this could apply to the girl in our story, for years later, in her twenties, she resumed smoking. This was after an early and unsuccessful marriage which ended in a divorce, after several attempts at work which she found difficult to accept and from which she escaped, and during a hard try at a demanding job. She felt unable to respond positively to the demands of her life, she felt angry and resentful, and found solace in smoking. Later, when she found the energy to return to life and to work, she felt that the tensions inherent in her life were eased by smoking, too. Both her social and her professional life were more comfortable when she had a cigarette. In fact, discussions between psychologists and young women students who smoked uncovered the same motivation: after the experiencing of sophistication, of independence, and maturity, a time would come when smoking would offer these young women a relief from their tensions: smoking had become a crutch in their student and social life (Maussner, 1966). At that time the young women began to find pleasure in inhaling cigarette smoke. This was also true of our friend. She inhaled, and she finally learned to enjoy smoking. But eventually the habit left her: she fell in love and married, and discovered that smoking held no more attraction for her. She was relaxed and happy, and needed no crutch. At the time she had become mature and had children, she never smoked at all. But later, after a serious illness during which she had been close to death, and during the marked depression which followed, she felt the need of "something" to keep herself going, and resumed the habit. Cigarette smoking did not actually relieve her anxiety. On the contrary, when she inhaled the smoke from her first cigarette in the morning, she felt a bodily distress and a dizziness which matched her mental anguish. When she reached some degree of relief from her emotional difficulties (but from sources other than smoking) she decided that smoking was too hazardous a game, and she gave up the habit.

As everyone knows, it is usually difficult to stop smoking. It was not a terrible effort for the woman of our story to quit the habit. Why? She may have belonged to a group of persons for whom mastery over their own life is more important than they perhaps know. In a self-testing kit developed by Daniel Horn, and published by the U.S. Department of Health, Education, and Welfare, she might have scored 9 or above on the mastery, or self-control, section of the testing, and she might have read: "You are bothered by the knowledge that you cannot control your desire to smoke. You are not your own master. Awareness of this challenge to your self-control may make you want to quit." But whatever the reason, she was lucky. It is, more often than not, very difficult to stop oneself from smoking.

Fortunately the difficulties of long-term psychotherapy can be dispensed with. Numerous techniques are available to those who decide that they will stop smoking. Group psychotherapy, hypnotherapy, lobeline drug therapy, and librium drug therapy were all used by Drs. Van Buren O. Hammett and Harold Graff in a recent Philadelphia project (1966): a total of 62 percent of the persons treated stopped smoking successfully, while only 11 percent achieved success in a control group which was given no therapy at all. The following comment from both therapists and patients is worthy of note. All agreed that a powerful adjuvant in the treatment was the support that therapists gave their patients; it clearly appeared to be much more difficult to break the habit with the help of drugs alone and without the element of human interest and participation from the therapist.

Obviously, in order to stop smoking, it is useful to know to which smoking style, or pattern, one belongs. Breaking the habit will itself assume a pattern dependent upon the smoking habit. Silvan Thomkins of the Center for Research in Cognition and Affect, City University of New York, is the author of a classification of smoking behavior, which includes the following patterns (1969).

Habitual Smoking—in this case the smoking has become automatic.

Positive Affect Smoking—here smoking is actually pleasurable.

Negative Affect Smoking—a psychologically soothing type of smoking.

Addictive Smoking—without a cigarette the smoker is really suffering.

The "Positive Affect" smoker, for example, is somewhat of a hedonist, who uses smoking as a pleasure, and may therefore learn to substitute another pleasure for that of smoking. One such pleasure is a deep-breathing exercise with holding of the breath—a yoga exercise which not only gives a pleasurable sensation in the chest but is also very relaxing.

In the fight against smoking, one segment of the population has attracted much attention: teenagers, who are the eventual smokers, and who are subjected to personal and social pressures to smoke. They often have difficulty in resisting these pressures. In 1958 and 1959, Dr. Horn, of the American Cancer Society, conducted an experiment in the Portland High Schools, dividing the teenagers into six experimental groups and one control group. Each group was exposed to a different approach. One group was given "sermons" on smoking, to no avail. The members of another group were instructed to warn their families about the dangers of smoking, in the hope that this tactic would influence their own view on the subject. The results were poor. Another group was presented with what was called the "contemporary" approach, pointing to the cost of smoking, while still another was given the "remote" approach, touching upon the relationship of cigarette smoking to lung cancer. This rational presentation of the problem was the most successful. Finally, a "both-sided" approach was used which permitted a small amount of smoking, accepting the fact of social and personal pleasure derived from smoking. The most rewarding tactics were the "remote" approach for the boys, and both the "remote" and "contemporary" approach for the girls. This seems to indicate that young people, when given the possibility of a rational choice, are quite able to take responsibility for their own decisions. The best, the most effective way of convincing young people not to smoke is, quite understandably, not exhortations, admonitions, or any paternalistic or authoritarian advice, but an honest presentation of the facts, leaving the conclusions and decisions to them. Nevertheless, if respected and influential figures (doctors, teachers) would set better examples the teenage smoking habit might be better resisted (Lieberman, 1969).

It is not unusual for a teenager, or even a younger child, to reproach his parents for smoking in an attempt to impart his newly found knowledge to an unwilling father or mother. He may well be astonished by the weakness of those adults who have had such a strong propensity to advise and counsel him.

Perhaps the little girl who was previously described as being puzzled by the conflicting presentations of the pleasures and dangers of smoking, will one day turn to her father when she will have learned and understood more about the problem, and ask him seriously:: "Daddy, why do you smoke? Don't you know that it is not good for you?" Perhaps her father will begin to think along new lines and he may even give her the satisfaction of seeing him stop smoking, or smoke less. Perhaps he will give himself the joy of learning from his own child.

16
PSYCHOLOGICAL PROBLEMS

*"Men are less sensitive to good
than to ill."*
LIVY

A man suffering from cancer said, again and again: "I want to go home, but there is no home." This strange saying had not come to his mind when he was told about his illness, or even shortly before, but had been his for many years, more years than he could remember. He admitted that the utterance was an old habit, a kind of compulsive motto. He had not chosen the phrase; rather, the phrase had "chosen" him, had "come to him" repeatedly, in times of stress or despondency perhaps, but also at any time at all. When did it first happen? He could not remember. But it was a long, long time ago, a time now engulfed in the depths of his past.

It is difficult to understand the man's words. He *had* a home he could go to. He had a loving wife and fine children. He loved his family. He was not unsuccessful. He had friends who liked him. He was intelligent, well-educated, had many interests in life. He did not seem unhappy or disturbed, and his reaction at discovering that he had cancer had not been unduly strong. Nevertheless there was for him no home. All beauty, all meaning belonged "elsewhere." A veil separated him from everything which he had liked and enjoyed before. What had formerly been possible, a fulfilling life, was now somehow "wrong," out of focus. His old motto possessed him with full force, and he expressed the feeling of being aware of an uncanny other self at the heart of his personality.

His recurrent, puzzling phrase, "I want to go home, but there is

258

no home," *is* troubling. What does it mean? Can one disregard it as nonsensical? Is it perhaps a line from a song or a poem he had heard many times in the past, and forgotten? But, if so, why had he retained it so faithfully, why had he repeated it so compulsively, why had he been so impressed with these simple words?

The fact that our emotional life has some influence over physical health or lack of it is now universally accepted. The vast field of psychosomatic medicine is relatively recent, in terms of systematic research and practical discoveries, but otherwise it is as old as medicine itself. The great Galen, who practiced medicine in Rome in the second century A.D., observed that cancer attacked women of a melancholic temperament more frequently than those who showed a tendency to be sanguine.

A long time has elapsed since then, and many hypotheses have been offered on the subject of the relationship of emotional factors to the onset of cancer in men and women. Although all researchers agree that more probing is desirable, evidence is beginning to accumulate that there is often a definite relationship between an emotional loss or trauma, and the onset of cancer. (We shall see later what types of loss, and at what periods of life.) A relationship, it must be emphasized, does not justify a concept of causation, however. As Dr. Roy Grinker says (1966): "We have, I hope, abandoned the convenient but restricted and artificial two-foci correlations linking single factors in causality of disease processes. Hence we need no longer argue whether a disease is *caused* by heredity, constitution, disordered chemistry or physiology, infection, trauma, or repressed pathogenic emotions. We are no longer concerned with either-or single-factor polarities but currently attempt to map out the widest possible ranges of conditions, all of which in some way and at some time, seem to be implicated in a dynamic chain of causes and effects."

To return to the cancer patient whose declaration was so persistent: it is very interesting to discover in some researchers' studies about the psychophysiological aspects of cancer, that other people suffering from one form or other of the illness also have recurrent comments, which can be linked to this man's. Certainly a saying such as "If the rock drops on the egg—poor egg. If the egg drops on the rock—poor egg" has the same desperate coloration as "I want to go

home, but there is no home." Another patient says: "It's as if all my
life I've been climbing a very steep mountain. It's very hard work.
Every now and then there are ledges I can rest on for a while and
maybe enjoy myself a little, but I've got to keep climbing, and the
mountain has no top" (LeShan, 1966).

This last patient (a woman) seems to have a more direct, a more
personal awareness that something disturbs her, has disturbed her all
her life. But it has been found that, in most cases, there is no conscious realization of any inner trouble. With the help of certain psychotherapeutic techniques, however, the cancer patients studied
came to confront a profound unhappiness, a real despair, which had
been part of themselves for very long, and to recognize it as, indeed,
the very stuff their lives were made of. Somehow there had always
been, nested in them, the conviction that they "could not make it,"
that they were doomed to a mysterious failure, no matter how hard
they tried.

> "It's everything we would have liked to do and did not do,
> Which wanted to speak and did not find the appropriate words . . ."
> JULES SUPERVIELLE

They had felt separated from the rest of the universe, singled out
for a drastic isolation. To them the following words from Jean
Anouilh's *La Sauvage* would have expressed vividly their acute sense
of separateness: "Now that I am in despair I have escaped you. I have
entered a kingdom where you could not follow me to make me yours
again."

It must be emphasized that this isolation, this despair, are not
consciously felt by most patients. On the surface their lives, up to
a certain time (which will be examined later) had been satisfying.
But it must also be emphasized that a subtle undercurrent of unhappiness, of inadequacy, a sense of not belonging, had always been
dimly perceived.

The phrases from the saying of cancer patients given above are
but a few of those reported. Dr. LeShan's study, however, involved
450 adult cancer patients (and 150 controls) over a period of 12
years and the pattern which emerged from their emotional life-history

appeared in 72 percent of the cancer patients and in 10 percent of the controls.

This pattern has three main periods. The first period appears in the patient's childhood. At that time the patient suffers some parental loss, or some other trauma, which thwarts his capacity to experience positive emotional relationships. He feels abandoned—left out—and as a consequence he retreats into himself, he gives up. What he has suffered is not violent enough for him to show any overt symptoms. On the contrary, as the years pass, he demonstrates an ability to adapt quite well to life and to the people around him, at least on the surface. He retains from his childhood the typical attitude that if something goes wrong, *he* is guilty, and not the world, or others. He shows little or no anger, little or no aggression. And in this fashion he reaches the time of young adulthood.

He is now verging on the second period, which is characterized by some positive event (perhaps love, perhaps marriage, perhaps an interesting job), and this event is going to obscure his reduced capacity for deep involvement. For an indefinite time (from as little as one year to as many as 40) he is going to live by this new and more confident type of relationship or involvement, to deepen it, to come to trust it and enjoy it. However well-covered by his seeming happiness, though, the undercurrent of despair is still present. And it shows. It may show subtly all through the years as in the repetitive phrases which we have quoted, or it may show much more definitely at the onset of the third period, when something happens which upsets a satisfactory course of life, such as the loss of the meaningful relationship or involvement which had sustained him for years. He may show a perseverant attempt at keeping life as it has been, or he may collapse; he may be seized by a sense of the futility of life so great that he may be totally overpowered by it. While it is true that practically everyone, at some time or other, ponders the futility of life, it is usually only an intellectual experience, perhaps tinged with emotion. But our man has quite another and much more intense realization of the meaning of such futility: we see here the gap which separates an ordinary understanding of a truth, and an existential, vital experience of the same truth.

Aldous Huxley once wrote: "Those who live with unpleasant

memories become neurotic, and those who live with pleasant ones become somnambulistic." In the cancer patients studied it is as if both pleasant and unpleasant memories had existed simultaneously —the pleasant ones being predominant (reflected in long stretches of satisfied living), the unpleasant ones brought to light by a shock or significant event which preceded the appearance of cancer (but always present, like an almost imperceptible musical theme).

The third, and last, of the three periods of life described by LeShan precedes the first clinical symptoms of cancer, and its length may be from eight months to eight years. While it is obvious that many people who never have developed cancer and may never show any signs of the disease often encounter similar feelings of despair, we must note that statistical data indicate clearly that these feelings appear much more often in the cancer patients than in the control groups.

Dr. Grinker has an interesting comment about the correlation between emotional factors and the appearance of cancer. He argues that, since the presence of cancer may exist undetected for months and years before any clear manifestation, and since the traumas or losses mentioned appear in the patients from eight months to eight years before the onset of the illness, it is possible that "the organism may be aware at lower levels of the presence of a destructive lesion long before it is indicated to the clinician that the patient has a malignant disease." This comment raises the problem of earlier possible detection by a systematic study of patients presenting psychological symptoms. In other words, would it be possible to hasten a diagnosis or to be alerted to the possibility of cancer, by paying more attention to typical emotional states much before any actual evidence is readable? Psychiatrists and psychologists could collaborate more closely with clinicians in the study of so vital a problem, but at the present time few physicians who treat cancer patients and the depressions triggered by the discovery of their illness are thoroughly acquainted with the bulk of psychiatric work on the subject of cancer. Not only do many researchers believe that some psychological factors influence the onset of cancer, but they also believe that for every cancer patient there are several times of serious stress: These may be at the moment of discovery, and at various times after the discovery, during treatment. Before we turn our attention to these moments of stress for the cancer patient, let us see how emotional factors may influence tumor growth.

What mechanisms, in our studies, respond to psychological stress? In what manner? What is the mysterious link between psyche and soma? Where do our "minds" and our bodies meet? How can the loss of or the separation from a loved person have any impact on leukemia and lymphoma, for instance? How can a separation have any influence in the appearance of breast cancer? Or why has it been observed that a feeling of hopelessness is present in a number of women who develop uterine cervical cancer? Why do some lung cancer patients show a definite difficulty in externalizing their emotions? (Annals of N. Y. Acad. Sci., 1966).

While no answer has been offered as to why a certain type of trauma or psychological attitude influences a certain type of cancer, a general conception of the relationship between patients' emotional lives and their illnesses can be stated in the following manner: as we know, our emotions have their origin in our brain, more specifically in the hypothalamus, which is situated in the lower portion of the brain, and which controls the function of a small but most important endocrine gland, the pituitary, or hypophysis. This small gland at the base of our brain produces many hormones and is the director of all other endocrine glands (called endocrines because they discharge their substances within the body itself, through the bloodstream). The pituitary, then, is the great controller of all our endocrine secretions. The ovaries, the testes, the adrenals, the thyroid, to cite only some of the endocrine glands, would not do their duty without the supervision of the pituitary. If, for instance, the pituitary did not manufacture a hormone like gonadotropin, the sex glands would not develop and in turn would not produce their own hormones, necessary to differentiate us as men and women.

Our emotions travel all the way from the central nervous system, from the hypothalamus, through the open passages of our endocrines (the pituitary being the first central station) to the very cells of each of our organs, and as they travel, they induce changes in hormonal production and function. The precise mechanism of these changes is not known, but to the researchers its evidence is clear.

It is also clear that some cancerous tumors are definitely related to hormonal dysfunction. Examples are prostatic cancers among men, and uterine, breast, and ovarian cancers in women. Ablation of the ovaries or administration of male hormones produce an amelioration of certain cases of uterine and breast cancer, while administration of female hormones may be beneficial to patients with prostatic cancer. We can understand now why our emotions, which are the bases of many changes in our body and the root of other psychosomatic illnesses, also have their responsibility in the induction of cancer: the hormonal troubles they provoke may lead, in certain circumstances, to the dreaded illness, cancer.

When a patient learns that he has cancer he has to face new and often very strong emotions. Everything is metamorphosed by the news. This is true even when matters are still uncertain, as for instance when surgical exploration is going to be the only way to determine the nature of a tumor. This very doubt carries within itself a powerful threat. Not knowing is perhaps just as difficult as knowing, for the human mind has a propensity to dwell on possibilities inordinately. Nothing is transparent any more, the continuity of our life is attacked. If we can admit that we are vulnerable, if we accept the thought that we have indeed limitations in dealing with unexpected and threatening facts, we shall be better equipped to come to terms with these facts. Without the admission of fear, courage is make-believe. Not bravado, or even equanimity, which are almost always façades, not genuine positions, are needed now, but the simple admission that things are going to be difficult for a while, and that we would welcome help.

The threats are many, the most formidable being perhaps the threat to our expectations and our future. The ultimate threat to our sense of indestructibility is indeed a shattering experience. It should not be surprising, then, that many people delay consulting a physician when they suspect they might have cancer, or that they find all sorts of excuses for not doing so, or that they "forget" to keep an appointment with a doctor if they have made one. It should not be surprising either that a number of cancer patients reject the news, with all the clever unconscious techniques that they have at their disposal and that they muster for their own defense. It is a familiar paradox that we may know something and at the same time not know it, for it is typical of the human mind to refuse a knowledge which hurts. It has been found that neither age, nor sex, marital status, or ethnic origin have any influence on the degree of awareness of cancer, but that there is a "positive correlation between level of awareness and education" (Moses and Cividali, 1966). If formal education can inhibit our tendency to block unwelcome knowledge, part of the answer to fear may lie in better public education about cancer—about the chances of cure and arrest of the disease, its warning signals, and the advances made in research and in the understanding of cancer in recent years.

Physicians ask themselves questions like: "What do we tell our patients?" "Is it wise, kind, or beneficial to the treatment of their illness, to tell them the truth?" "Is truth an absolute which must be acknowledged and accepted by all, regardless of the circumstances and the consequences?" These questions immediately lead to others, such as: "What kind of person is this patient?" "What does the news mean to him as a unique individual?" "How can I best communicate with him?" and also "What kind of a person am I?" "What are my own reactions to cancer?" There are no pat answers to any of these questions. They present dilemmas which must be resolved every time anew, and the more intelligent and sensitive a doctor, the more searching his thoughts on the subject. Most doctors do not tell their patients that they have cancer. In a study of Philadelphia physicians' attitudes to such disclosures, it was found that 57 percent of them do not usually tell, 28 percent usually tell, 12 percent never tell, and 3 percent always tell. (Fitts and Radvin, 1953). In another more recent study, it was shown that 88 percent of the doctors questioned do not tell their patients that they have cancer, in contrast to 12 percent who do (Oken, 1961).

What is the meaning of such a prevalent attitude, particularly in view of a parallel finding that most patients say that they *want* to know whether they have cancer? One possible explanation is that doctors may very well be aware that people say one thing and desire another. Their experience with patients may have taught them that prudence in such matters is the best possible course. Yet there is a school of thought, not prevalent in this country, which advocates telling the truth no matter what. Interestingly enough, it is a belief which exists predominantly in Scandinavian countries, where (says Dr. Morton Bard, who has lectured in medical schools and hospitals in Denmark, Iceland, Finland, Norway, and Sweden) "independence and self-reliance are highly valued characteristics," and where "the patient is usually self-reliant and stoical, apparently content in the knowledge that he will be well-cared for." It is significant to note that Minnesota, with a population largely Scandinavian in origin, is the state where the telling of the truth to cancer patients is most advocated.

Conflicting attitudes concerning what to tell cancer patients can only be resolved by looking at the problem from the patient's point of view rather than the doctor's. A clear awareness of the patient's philosophy of life is indispensable to the physician before he decides what to say about the nature of the illness. But the physician must also look at himself and become aware of his own reactions to cancer. As a professional his attitude may be of one kind, but as a man he may have another. Fortunately many doctors are aware of their personal attitude toward cancer, and they know that this attitude influences their manner of approaching and communicating with their cancer patients, both at the moment of telling them about their illness and also during treatment.

The principal treatment for cancer remains surgery, either accompanied with irradiation or without it. Surgery is traumatic, but the trauma is perhaps less physical than psychological. In surgery our physical integrity has been attacked, we have been cut open, we have been turned into objects. Our wholeness has been interfered with, and this is a shocking experience. It has even been noted that there is such a phenomenon as "postoperative psychosis," a type of panic reaction experienced after surgery by some patients. This occurs rarely, says Dr. R. C. Mastrovito (1966) and it can be treated with adequate medication, and with reassurance. This reassurance is indispensable to the patient who has shown an acute reaction to surgery or to anesthesia, or to both. "Reassurance should be given that there is no question of mental weakness or potential psychosis and that the patient will in all probability never undergo this experience again."

There are milder reactions to surgery. While anxiety is a fairly common reaction before surgical intervention, depression is most common after cancer surgery. Anxiety can be alleviated by adequate preparation of the patient, including a frank and sympathetic discussion of what he is to expect. When depression occurs, antidepressants may be given to the patient until he is able to view his situation in a quieter frame of mind. In some cases it will be advisable for the patient to seek advice and treatment from a psychiatrist thoroughly acquainted with the problems of cancer patients.

A type of psychotherapy not yet widespread, but of possible benefit, is hypnotherapy. Paul Sacerdote, of the Montefiore Hospital in New York, believes that "hypnosis properly used is a *psychotherapeutic* means 'par excellence' and especially effective when the problem is more specifically a 'psychosomatic' one." He adds—and this comment might be of special interest to those who regard hypnosis with suspicion—that a misunderstanding about this method of therapy "involves the identification of hypnosis with certain modalities of induction. In reality formal induction is not always necessary nor desirable; not only do many patients at one time or another act or react to direct or indirect hypnotic suggestions, but also they are often capable of gaining insight, where to the uninitiated onlooker no hypnosis appears to have taken place."

We have said that some people react to cancer, and therefore to the possibility of cancer treatment, with a denial of the reality of the illness. An interesting suggestion has been offered for the approach to these cases by Dr. S. L. Foder, from the Department of Psychiatry at Mount Sinai Hospital in New York. He thinks that LSD might be a useful means of breakthrough since "if anything produces a phenomenal discharge of all kinds of tensions, physical, chemical, psychological, it would be LSD." LSD has already been used in the treatment of some psychiatric patients (not cancer patients), and seems to speed up therapy, although perhaps provoking reactions of an intensity seldom seen in more orthodox approaches.

Finally, there is an important point to be considered in the psychological relationship that doctors have with terminal cancer patients. It has been found that some doctors (Sacerdote, 1966) and also nurses (LeShan, 1966) are reluctant to get personally involved with dying cancer patients. LeShan reports that he made an experiment in a New York hospital, the results of which appear shocking. "On a cancer floor, I had the chief of service rate all the patients as to how close they were to death. Then I sat by the nurses' call board with a stop watch and a notebook. I simply took down the time that it took from when a light went on showing a patient had called until the nurse got into his room. There was a direct and rather high correlation—the closer the patient was to death, the longer it took the nurse to get into his room, after the bell had been rung. This is, I think, a real problem. And much research in this field will be blocked until we can understand and perhaps do something about it."

The nurses were quite unaware of their reaction to dying patients, and shocked at the discovery. There must be ways to re-educate all of us to the presence of death in our midst. In our culture death is a subject which is almost taboo. Yet death is with us, and it should belong *to us* as we belong to it. As Rilke writes in his poem *Finale*:

> Death is great.
> Laughing
> We are his.
> When we feel at the heart of life
> He dares to weep
> In us.

We must learn to face the awesomeness of death, for our own sake and for the sake of others who depend upon us and upon our care in their last moments. Believers and unbelievers, atheists, agnostics, all have reasons, however different, not to be robbed of the meaning of their death and of our participation in their death. Many unfinished tasks, of a practical or nonpractical nature, may call them. Facing the inevitable may prove to be the most important time of their lives. In the words of Bertrand Russell (1903): "In the spectacle of death .... there is a sacredness, an overpowering awe, a feeling of vastness, the depth, the inexhaustible mystery of existence, in which, as by some strange marriage of pain, the sufferer is bound to the world by bonds of sorrow. In these moments of insight, we lose all eagerness of temporary desire, all struggling and striving for petty ends, all care for the little trivial things that, to a superficial view, make up the common life of day by day."

It can be affirmed that even an illness like cancer can be an experience of positive value in a life. Many cancer patients do not have to face death from their illness, and in their experience, there can be much to be thankful for. There is always a great deal to be discovered in a new experience, however disagreeable. In illness there is a weakening of the ego, which can be a revealing experience, and may even bring some degree of enjoyment. Other people become all-important because we are in need of them. They present us with the image of a life which we must reconquer. Objects become more perceptible. A patch of sun, a design on a wall, water running from a faucet, drops of rain bouncing on a window sill—when do we have time to visualize such things in a simple, but profoundly enjoyable way? When do we ever experience awakening in its fullness? Not when we have to rush from bed to shower to breakfast and to work, not when the telephone is ringing and the children are calling. In illness, in forced dependence and idleness, we can know a paradoxical freedom, unlike anything else we have encountered before. When we awaken there are no demands on our time. We emerge from unconsciousness; a delicate life dances, flickers, dies again. We return to life, immobile, drowsy, surprised—simple birth, fragile anticipation—a pleasure of the mind worth the humiliation of being sick.

Whatever their state, the sick are entitled to understanding and to help from those who participate in their care. We have seen how impossible it is to separate some patients' cancer from their whole life, from their psychological make-up, from their childhood no less than from their adult life. Clinicians, psychiatrists, psychologists, researchers of many disciplines, can unite for a better understanding of cancer, and for the best total care of their patients.

17
CANCER QUACKERY

"A quack's words are heard,
but no one trusts himself to him
when he is sick."
CATO

Unfortunately, the words of Cato, the Stoic philosopher, do not apply to many of those suffering from cancer. All too often instead they seek the advice and help of unqualified or unprincipled therapists. At the present time, cancer is cured in only a third of the cases. The fear of the illness, and of a possibly fatal outcome, leads people to look for remedies other than the orthodox and recognized treatments. The latter, people may feel, do not offer certainty of recovery. In their search for miracle cures, patients suffering from cancer are encouraged by sensational reports in the daily press, in magazines, books, by some radio and television programs, and by the testimonials of cancer patients who believe they have been helped by new or unproved methods, often sponsored by famous persons.

If someone suspects that he has cancer or if he has been treated less than successfully, he has the choice of consulting reputable physicians, or of abandoning himself to the hands of unqualified therapists. He may travel far and wide in search of new, unproved treatments: to Switzerland, where an organization utilizes mistletoe therapy (fir tree mistletoe for males, apple tree mistletoe for females); to Lyons, France, where a chemist has developed a method of ether inhalations; to Mexico, where, among other techniques, he will be able to try Chinese acupuncture; to Germany, New Zealand, Canada, India, England, Italy, or Uruguay; and within the United States he will find numerous organizations which will present him with various methods which are of no objective value in the diagnosis and treatment of cancer. No country has a monopoly on unproved, and therefore unsafe, methods for the cure of cancer.

Tear extract? Ox bile? Llama placenta? Lemon juice enemas? Clam extract? Diamond carbon compound? These substances and many others have been or are currently being offered for the treatment of cancer. Hundreds of methods, in the United States and abroad, have been labelled unproved by the American Cancer Society. The American Cancer Society publishes at regular intervals detailed compilations of *Unproven Methods of Cancer Treatment.* It also publishes an idex of its file material on *New or Unproven Methods of Treatment of Cancer,* the pages of which seem to increase with the years. These methods vary in their approach. They may involve diets, machines, biological products (compounded from cancer tissue for instance), drugs; all are ineffective and sometimes positively harmful in the treatment of cancer.

Not all men who advocate untested methods for cancer treatment are quacks. Some of them are doctors and scientists who otherwise excel in their professions and who, out of concern for the victims of cancer, experiment with new drugs and remedies. Yet, until these drugs and remedies are thoroughly investigated they cannot be trusted. Many agencies throughout the U.S. and indeed in many other countries carry on such investigations and report on their findings in a wide variety of scientific journals and other publications.

These investigating agencies include the National Cancer Institute, the American Medical Association, the Federal Food and Drug Administration, the U.S. Public Health Service, and certain independent agencies. They all have strict standards of investigation. These include examination of clinical evidence presented by the treatment proponent (as the examination of biopsy slides and of X-ray pictures); analysis of the new drug; experiments in animals; tests for consistency (through treatment of a large number of patients); and reviews of the results of the autopsies of patients who have died after having received the new remedy or treatment.

No honest and serious researcher can have any objection to scientific investigation of his methods. But there are so many new, still unproved treatments for cancer that it is not possible to investigate them all; a choice must be made of which treatments merit investigation; others have to be abandoned, at least for the present.

Some proponents of untested cancer therapies are laymen who, although well intentioned, lack the capacity to evaluate their discoveries scientifically. They err mainly through ignorance. Other people are motivated by the desire for financial gain or ego gratification; they are the unscrupulous quacks.

Anyone may practice quackery. In his play "Doctor Knock," Jules Romains describes a hilarious quack, relatively harmless, but totally without scruples, who is making fast money out of uneducated French country people, and whose motto is: "Every man in good health is a sick man who ignores illness"; but when professional and nonprofessional men apply therapies which endanger the lives of cancer patients, our reaction is one of horror. Everyone should therefore be aware that there are at the present time only three methods unequivocally recognized for the treatment of cancer: surgery, irradiation therapy, and chemotherapy (the use of certain drugs definitely beneficial to cancer patients).

Among the hundreds of unproved cancer treatments, let us consider three. One, a diet, the "grape diet." A second, involving a machine called the "orgone machine." A third, a drug treatment, was made famous by a long and sensational trial reported in the press throughout the country, the Krebiozen treatment. These three methods are ineffective in treating cancer and may serve as models of what should be avoided by cancer patients if they want (and obviously they do) all the power and knowledge of science on the side of their recovery.

The "grape cure," which is supposed to be very old, was revived in 1925 by Johanna Brandt, Ph.N., N.D. (Philosopher of Naturotherapy and Doctor of Naturotherapy). The treatment utilizes grapes and unsweetened grape juice. The fruit is first taken without the addition of any other food. After a few weeks other fruits and sour milk are included in the diet. Then a raw food diet is introduced, including salads, nuts, honey, olive oil, and milk products. Sometimes the patient takes one cooked meal a day, at which time he does not drink anything or eat any raw food. Grapes are used, not only as a food, but also at times as poultices on external cancer, and juice is taken in gargles and enemas. At both the Federal and State levels (California), action has been taken against the advocating of the "grape cure," which the American Cancer Society has found to be "of no objective benefit for the treatment of cancer in human beings."

The "Orgone machine," or "Orgone-Energy-Accumulator," was introduced by Wilhelm Reich, M.D., in the 1940's. It consisted of a tall box, called the "Shooter box," in which the patient was placed. "Orgone-energy" was then concentrated on the site of the cancer to be treated. Bedridden patients were treated with the help of an "Orgone-blanket"; an "Orgone-cone" was used for head treatments. Dr. Reich claimed that his machine captured "cosmic orgone energy," and that this energy, relea ed on the sites of various cancers, was effective in the cure of the disease. Under the sponsorship of the Federal Food and Drug Administration, doctors and physicists tested the "Orgone-machine," and found that it was without value in the treatment of cancer. Moreover, the "orgone-energy" was undetectable. Federal action was taken against Dr. Reich and his device was barred from public use.

Krebiozen was another instance of a worthless cancer treatment. Yet the claims for Krebiozen attracted countless patients. The new drug, a serum supposedly obtained from inoculated horses, was brought into this country by a Yugoslavian doctor, Stevan Durovic, who interested an American physician, Dr. Andrew C. Ivy of the University of Illinois, in his product. When Krebiozen was analyzed by the FDA, some ampules were found to contain creatine, which was discovered to be of no value in the treatment of cancer. Some of the ampules contained mineral oil alone. In 1963, the National Cancer Institute concluded its testing of Krebiozen and stated that it was a worthless drug. In 1966 Drs. Durovic and Ivy were acquitted in a jury trial from the charges brought against them by the FDA. Their acquittal, however, could not affect the scientific findings of the FDA and the National Cancer Institute; Krebiozen was banned from interstate commerce.

The Krebiozen story is well-known. It has received wide coverage in the press and much publicity. It should serve as a warning that many other worthless cancer treatments are being practiced today and will be practiced in the future. The reasons why cancer patients, frightened and sometimes desperate, turn to unsafe practices, are understandable. Nevertheless, it must be repeated that the utmost caution is necessary.

Some doctors who are not permitted to pursue their cancer treatments in the U.S. find a refuge and the possibility of a lucrative practice in Mexico, where the laws governing the practice of medicine are not as stringent as in this country. One author tells the moving story of a desperate mother whose little boy was dying of leukemia, and who went to Tijuana in the hope of saving her child (Smith, 1968). In February 1965, the child received his first treatment there ("Blood-cleansing" and "antitoxin" shots, with "cellular-therapy"— the injection of dried cells obtained from freshly killed animals). Six months later, in August, despite the repeated treatments, the little boy's condition was much worse. The physician in charge finally decided against further treatments and sent the child back to an American hospital. Very soon the little boy died—of leukemia.

It would be possible to argue that a number of the unorthodox therapies for cancer are not positively harmful, on the grounds that they seldom utilize dangerous drugs or remedies; or that they encourage hope in patients; or that they keep active in the patients the desire and love for life. Such arguments are specious. Countless cancer patients are distracted from the roads to safe and proven methods of cancer cure by the lure of miracles. Even if they did not die as a direct consequence of unacceptable methods, they would be deprived of the benefits from proven treatments, and from the discoveries which are being made and which will be made in the future by researchers who accept the severe but safe standards of all true scientific work. Cancer quackery can never be condoned or countenanced on the basis of promises that in the end prove to be false.

18
DEATH AND CANCER

"The beauty of failure
is the only lasting beauty.
Who does not understand failure
is lost."
JEAN COCTEAU

In the world of medicine where all efforts are dedicated to success—the overcoming of illness, the restoration of the sick to a healthy life—the admission of failure may seem absurd. Failure? An insult, almost, to doctors and patients alike. Even if it is at times accepted as unavoidable, failure is always acknowledged as unfortunate. But if one examines the meaning of failure more closely one may come to quite different conclusions.

Where there is failure there has also been effort. Without effort failure would make no sense. Effort leads to success and to failure, and indeed many successes are failures in disguise. They do not leave the successful man with a feeling of fullness, of completeness, but with a feeling of emptiness and sometimes of fear. Success, to be complete, must satisfy the beholder. Paradoxically, failure may, and at times does, satisfy the person who has failed, because it brings with itself the realization of the attempt, a particular quality of fulfillment.

We fail only because and after we have tried. We reach the destination of failure not because we are inert or powerless, but for just the opposite reasons. It is often because we have looked in all directions and tried all avenues available to us. We are not powerless: our power finds limits within and without. After many a failure, the best of us, and the best in each of us, rises again. But there comes a time when we have to confront the ultimate failure, our death and the death of others. If we know how to transform this apparent failure into an accomplishment, we shall have defeated death itself, at least to the limits of our individual capacities. How does one defeat death? How does one prove stronger than annihilation?

Perhaps if we understand what death really is we shall also find the answer to our other question, how to defeat death: for understanding alters our point of view and therefore allows attitudes which were unknown to us, or appeared impossible. Although we may see death as a clear termination of life, a definite break with living, an irreversible event which happens once and only once, it may be denied to be that simple. For one does not actually die once, never to return again. Like life, death is a continuing process, as the process of aging and dying of our body cells demonstrates. From the time of birth one grows into death at a slow but steady pace: this growing into death encompasses psychological and spiritual as well as physical changes. The physical changes, viewed as the natural process of growth, are not necessarily painful. The discovery of one's separateness from others, of pain, of sickness, even of joy and happiness are often incommunicable and increase our sense of being alone. The fear of being alone contains the germ of our death, the ultimate separation.

Some people go through the changes and small deaths of their lives with a completely natural acceptance. Few or no questions are asked. People like these are steeped in life and its vicissitudes so thoroughly that, like healthy children, they remain largely untouched. They have an innocence which protects them all through their years and the suffering common to all does not find them rebellious.

A woman who was told by her doctor that her cancer was probably incurable reacted in a way which exemplifies this fundamental trust in life, and the acceptance of the end of life. She said that it was all very interesting, that she was looking forward to this new experience, that since it was unavoidable she was determined to enjoy it in the sense of embarking on an unknown and therefore fascinating voyage. She would welcome drugs or sedatives only when the pain became too difficult to bear, and she hoped she would be conscious of all that lay ahead of her, including her own death. This woman was not trying to impress her doctor, she was not pretending to be superior to fate, for she actually maintained her attitude quite naturally until her death. There was an innate grandeur in her faith in herself which carried her through the ordeal exactly as she had foreseen.

Not everyone is capable of instinctive faith in all the processes of life, including death. The extreme neurotic attitude toward life and death, which we all share at times, confuses death and life, takes one for the other, and searches for death where it is not, and for life where it is not either. Fear dominates, not the natural fear of frightful realities, but a fear detached from actual happenings, free-floating and always ready to invade the psychic life. For the neurotic "what is called death . . . mainly because it is dark and unknown, is a new life trying to break into consciousness; what he calls life because it is familiar is but a dying pattern he tries to keep alive" (Hillman, 1964). He clings to the past, to habitual reactions, out of fear of what has never been experienced. The small deaths of his universe do not find him ready and accepting, but fill him with apprehension and resistance. Facing real death may thus prove extremely difficult for him and his confusion may be extreme. He may desire death, he may feel an impulse to suicide: but this is entirely different from the true facing of death: he runs to death out of his need for annihilation, out of his fears, whereas, for facing the death which comes to him, at its own time and place, he would need presence of mind and body; it is a conscious confrontation which is required of him, and of which he is incapable, for his very need is to flee and disappear.

Midway between the attitude of total acceptance and that of total refusal lies the attitude of the ordinary man, who is neither completely at ease with life and death, nor entirely in rebellion. The ordinary man oscillates between yes and no, and he will do the same if he is faced with death from an incurable illness. This ordinary man is depicted to perfection by Pirandello in his play, *The Man With The Flower in His Mouth*. The man has an epithelioma: "Death passed my way. It planted this flower in my mouth and said to me: 'Keep it, friend, I'll be back in eight or ten months'." An ordinary man (in the play he does not even have a name, he is just "the man"), the sick hero oscillates between cheerful sarcasm, amused acceptance, and terror. He struggles for peace through his imagination. "I never let my imagination rest, even for a moment. I use it to cling continually to the lives of others. . . . If you only knew how well it works! I see somebody's house and I live in it. I feel a part of it. . . ." But later he says: "In fact I do it because I want to share everyone else's troubles, be able to judge life as silly and vain. If you can make yourself feel that way, then it won't matter if you have to come to the end of it." He has now oscillated to the no. But the yes comes back to him. He remembers the sensuous joys of life: "These wonderful apricots are in season now. . . . How do you eat them? With the skin on, don't you? You break them in half, you squeeze them in your fingers slowly. . . . Like a pair of juicy lips. . . . Ah, delicious!" Then he returns to resentful rage: "We all feel this terrible thirst for life, though we have no idea what it consists of. But it's there, there, like an ache in our throats that can never be satisfied. . . . Life, by God, the mere thought of losing it—especially when you know it's a matter of days. . . . ."

The ordinary man's death, which is the death that most of us will encounter, is described at length by Thomas Bell (1961). His book is the record of his last year. Bell, a not very successful writer as he admits himself, has a malignant tumor near his liver and his pancreas. He knows that he will die. After an exploratory operation his surgeon has decided that the excision of the tumor is impossible. The X-ray treatments Bell receives are ineffectual, the drugs he takes have no power. What is his reaction? He is sometimes frightened and discouraged, disgusted at the sight of his body invaded by the tumor, sad for himself and his wife, puzzled by the mystery of fate, but above all courageous and dignified. His book opens with the words: "I said to myself: "I'll make a journal of it, a book; put down all these thoughts and fears as they come and so get rid of them. Once they're written out in words they won't be confined inside my skull, making trouble." Not everyone is a writer, but everyone may decide to face his own thoughts and fears. All through the book one witnesses the author's love of life, which both sustains and saddens him. ("My curiosity is insatiable, my pleasure in reading undiminished. . . . I like, as I always have, privacy and solitude, they are as necessary to me as air. . . . My appetite is excellent and my pleasure in food has never been greater.")

According to Weisman and Hackett (1961) when we are near

death a new world opens up to our perception. While "the fear of dying is the sense of impending dissolution or disintegration of all familiar ways of thought and action," while "the world normally at one with our perceptions suddenly becomes alien, disjointed, and runs along without us," while "few patients save the truly predilected, approach death without despair," it is also "frequently clear that in the terminal phase the sharp antithesis of living and dying gradually become modulated into a dampened harmonic line," and that "for the majority of dying patients, it is likely that there is neither complete acceptance nor total repudiation of the imminence of death."

The fear and rebellion experienced at the coming of one's own death is admittedly stronger in young people who have not yet lived full lives, whose hopes, expectations, and responsibilities are threatened beyond their endurance, whose sense of an unjust fate cannot easily be dismissed. Fortunately "during the decades from fifteen to forty years, there is a relatively low . . . toll of deaths, largely due to fatal accidents and a few cancers" (Hinton, 1967). However, for the young, there is no comfort in statistics. One's life is unique and precious. To younger people the sense of failure from an imminent death cannot be anything but acute. Yet there must be some way to prove stronger than one's fate. When Cocteau writes that the "beauty of failure is the only lasting beauty" doesn't he offer us the solution? In other words everything eventually deserts us, and at a time that we have not chosen; but the power to face our bankruptcy remains our privilege: in so doing we penetrate it and master it, we transmute it through imagination, understanding, and the will to stay in control. The beauty and grandeur of such mastery is exemplified at its most sublime in the death of Christ, in the death of Socrates.

Failure, the success in reverse, can be the success of the ordinary men, who, like Bell and many others, feel "a kind of despairing, dragged-by-the-hand unwillingness," and also, "for no obvious reason . . . smile in the darkness." It is not easy to "smile in the darkness" if one has no previous experience of what that darkness is. In Francis Bacon's words "Man fears death as the child fears the dark," and truly the child in us will always fear the dark until he has gone through it once and for all, willingly and thoroughly. What is this darkness? Is it not the unknown in us, the unresolved, the intricacies and mysteries of an inner life not totally adult, and does not this darkness take its most vivid and its most valid symbol in death, the last question, the perfect unknown? But the exploration of our night can bring strength and a peaceful acceptance of life and of death. In the effort at understanding oneself and one's fears, the frightening bugbear, death, appears in a much gentler light. Death may remain the image of all the unattainables. However, these unattainables, these unreachables, these failures, can become a simple question mark, troubling, but incapable of destroying one any longer.

Hope, "the thing with feathers," in Emily Dickinson's words, almost always "perches in the soul," regardless of our nearness to death, regardless of the mortal quality of our illness, regardless of how small a material hope we harbor. For hope is a quality of being, rather than a rational expectation. And in that sense hope can and must be implanted in the person who is fatally ill.

The quantity and the quality of care that a dying patient receives are powerful adjuvants to the growth of hope, of openness to whatever future may be his. This case is dependent upon the kind of persons physicians are—or nurses, psychiatrists, social workers, family, and friends—all of those who are in contact with the patient in the terminal stage of his illness. Certain qualities are demanded. A profound sense of right judgments. A subtle and supple mind. No preconceived or unchangeable opinions. A willingness to meet the patients on their own terms. No moralistic or religious zeal on the part of the "believing" doctor, nurse, or relative. No skepticism or hardened professional "scientism" from the unbelievers. The first thing to remember about dying patients is that it is *their* death.

Some patients do not want to know of their impending death. Many studies indicate that this wish is rare. Yet in the words of Dr. Paul R. Rhoads "honesty should often be tempered with optimistic uncertainty" (Ross, 1965). He illustrates the necessity of this attitude: two patients present the same type of cancer at the same time: both have a retroperitoneal lymphosarcoma of about the same size in the same site; they receive the same X-ray treatment. One dies within three months, the other lives an active life for nine years. The future is unpredictable, even in some apparently desperate cases, and optimism and hope can be maintained in many instances, perhaps even when they do not seem warranted by the facts known to the physician, or by his experience.

Dr. Alvarez writes (1965): "I doubt if a physician who has examined an old man and found an inoperable cancer of the prostate gland need always tell about it. Especially when the man has high blood pressure and heart disease or has had some minor strokes, it may be that he will die of one of these before the cancer kills him, and then it may be best to let him live in mental peace."

A reasonable and perceptive openness to the improbable does not mean dishonesty. However, when patients indicate that they desire to know that they may die in the near future, there is little doubt that they must be told the truth. It is a great comfort to some people to be given the time and opportunity to put their affairs in order, to arrange material details with their families, to explore their thoughts, to deepen and enjoy their relationships. Yet even in those who wish to confront their own death, fears still exist, and they should be encouraged to speak freely about themselves, and about everything and anything that troubles them. "Many a dying man," writes Dr. Alvarez (1952), "would like to discuss the problems that are in his mind, but he would like to do this dispassionately, much as if it were someone else whose troubles were being talked about."

Dr. John Hinton has explored many aspects of the act of dying, many attitudes toward death, and a number of ways to make the end of a life more peaceful and more comfortable, mentally and physically (Hinton, 1967). He points out that if a patient receives all the relief from pain to which he is entitled, with the help of drugs and surgery (surgery in such instances is purely palliative and entirely justified on this basis as it allows the sick person to live his remaining days in less discomfort), he will be offered the first and indispensable condition for a painless and peaceful death.

"A painless, peaceful death," are the words used in the dictionary to define euthanasia, which is at other times vividly described as "mercy-killing." In August, 1967, a young man killed his mother who was dying of leukemia. "She reportedly had begged him to kill her, and even as he was arrested, his mother's sister embraced him saying, 'God bless you' " (Kinsolving, 1967). One can easily understand the pity that husbands, wives, children, parents feel for a loved person who is going to die, who is suffering without much hope, or without any hope at all. One can understand the pity that the doctor feels for a patient to whom he can no longer offer anything but a "painless, peaceful death." But one cannot help but be overwhelmed with the immense problems and responsibilities that euthanasia would present, even to those who have no religious convictions against the taking of a life and even to those who would never kill in any other circumstance. For if euthanasia were to be considered acceptable in cases of terminal cancer, why should it not be acceptable as well in other painful illnesses which are not leading to death? In an editorial in *The Lancet* (Anon., 1961), we read that "in his recent study, Exton-Smith found that unrelievable enduring pain and misery is worst not, as the public suppose, among patients dying of cancer whose pain, if present, he found controllable and relatively short, but in the victims of locomotor disorders not essentially lethal. If 'euthanasia' is granted to the first class, can it be long denied to the second?"

Euthanasia is a "painless, peaceful death," and also "a means of producing it." Must this means be of necessity killing? Rarely can an easy and happy death be produced by killing, for, despite the hope of relief that the promise of death does bring, death by killing carries violence within itself. What if the patient who desired to die reconsidered at the last minute and nobody but himself was aware of his reconsideration? If euthanasia were ever to be legalized, would not the anguish of making such a decision add an insufferable weight to the already difficult task of facing an involuntary death? The task, by adding a new stress to the stress already existing, would make the act of deciding almost impossible.

But there are alternatives to the stark conception of euthanasia as "mercy-killing." A painless, peaceful death can be given to people in the terminal stage of cancer. In a letter to the editor of *The Lancet* (1961), Cicely Saunders writes: "We are now always able to control pain in terminal cancer . . . and only very rarely indeed do we have to make (patients) continually asleep in doing so." And in a later editorial in the same medical journal (1961) one reads: "If euthanasia . . . were put on a par with, say, safe childbirth; if the known means to make death comfortable were applied by individual and collective effort with intelligence and energy, could not all but a few deaths be made at least easy?"

An important consideration is, is it desirable to prolong life when death is very near? A number of means to prolong life artificially do not add to the quality of life of a very sick person. According to one observer, J. W. Reid (1964), perhaps "the patient . . . lies in bed surrounded by standards from which dangle bottles of various solutions with tubing running to arms fixed to boards projecting on either side of the bed as though he were nailed to a cross. A nurse stands at one side, and the intern on the other side is injecting a new drug that has successfully prolonged life in a small series (of patients) for a few weeks and (the clincher) as long as a year in one authenticated case! The wife stands uncertainly in the doorway wanting to be with her husband in these last hours but diffident about pushing her way through the busy traffic around the bed." The author goes on to say: "Is not all this activity to keep alive a dying man more often merely an educated cruelty?"

His opinion is echoed by many physicians. The prolongation of life often does more harm than good in the pursuit of a peaceful death. The quality of a human life, which at that stage is synonymous with physical comfort and mental peace, must be the only consideration.

Together with the problem of prolonging or not prolonging life, doctors face that of the free use of powerful drugs to relieve pain as completely as possible. Heroin and morphine are addictive drugs, but what is the importance of addiction at a stage of life when death is so near? The answer seems obvious. However, Dr. John Hinton expresses the opinion that "there is too much error on the side of caution." He believes that "given in adequate and frequent enough doses to begin with, so that the patient is confident that the pain is controllable, the need to increase the dose of morphia or heroin and the undue dependence of the patient on the drug do not often constitute a great problem in dying patients" (Hinton, 1967). This inducement of confidence in the patient seems extremely important, for if he knows from the very beginning that his physical pain will be controlled, his fear of future suffering will be greatly alleviated. The anticipation of pain is as difficult to bear as the pain itself, and more frightening. The certainty that one's doctor is able to control both of these by his skill in the handling of the drugs available, is deeply comforting to the dying patient. Such practices can result in true euthanasia, a means to a painless, peaceful death.

Finally, mental suffering often accompanies physical pain in terminal cancer. Sometimes psychiatric intervention is indispensable, perhaps more often than is the common practice. Its object is, as expressed by Weisman and Hackett (1961), "to help the dying patient preserve his identity and dignity as a unique individual, despite the disease, or, in some cases, because of it." They introduce the concept of "appropriate death." It is "an aspect of euthanasia—death without suffering—for patients whose death is imminent . . . the conventional concept of euthanasia as the hastening of the death of the incurably ill patients is the antithesis of the appropriate attitude towards death which psychiatric intervention advocates. In conventional euthanasia the patient's personality is ignored; in the proposal of therapeutic dissociation of the patient from the disease, the personality in its unique dignity is enhanced." Nonpsychiatrists express similar ideas when, like Dr. Cicely Saunders, they say (1961): "We try, and we believe very often with success, to enable our patients to remain themselves throughout their illness, to find their own key to the situation and to use it. They make of it (consciously or unconsciously) not just a long defeat of living but a positive achievement of dying."

All religions and most philosophies have recognized death as a challenge, as a beginning. In the words of Plato, "Those who tackle philosophy aright are simply and solely practicing dying, practicing death, all the time, but nobody sees it." One does not have to be religious, or a philosopher, to confront death in a manly way. One has only to be human, to realize that the acceptance of everything which is our lot is under the control of our intellect and of our sensibility. Everything which happens to us is ours if we make it so. It is within our power of understanding. This is where hope enters. It is when one may hear what W. H. Auden calls the "imaginary song":

> You, alone, o imaginary song
> Are unable to say an existence is wrong.

Our existence before death is worth living to the fullest. All of us, within limits, can measure up to the last "failure." Jean Cocteau says that who does not understand failure is lost: he is lost to the hope and to the deepening of experience that failure offers. In the elation of success, when we ride the crest of the wave, our sense of power blinds us. Success is intoxicating, and the intoxication is authentic, as are all our experiences. But success is not the whole. In the hollow of the wave, in failure and in the approach of death, we can experience a humble power, and the knowledge of peace. Physicians and families care best for the dying patient by helping to make death an inevitable but positive experience, from which none of us is spared.

CANCER--1977

"First dire chimeras conquest was enjoined
A mingled monster of no mortal kind
Behind the lion's mane and head
A goat's body and dragon's fiery tail was spread."
BELLEROPHON'S TASK

Five years ago the United States declared open war on cancer. Hopes ran high that rapid and brilliant research accomplishments in molecular biology, virology, and immunology would reveal the true nature of the underlying cellular defect. Mass screening programs of high-risk segments of the population with novel clinical, radiological, biochemical, and physical techniques would detect silent cancers early enough to permit simple cures. Expanded horizons in standard therapy, employing appropriate combinations of surgery, irradiation, chemotherapy, and immunotherapy in a multi-modality attack would optimistically eradicate existing cancers in the majority of patients. The National Cancer Act was passed, elevating the National Cancer Institute (NCI) to a separate and privileged status within the National Institutes of Health, and creating a three-member President's Cancer Panel, which provided direct access to the White House for support of cancer programs. Truly vast sums of money were poured into cancer research at all levels. The NCI, with an expanded budget of 700 million dollars yearly, joined with the American Cancer Society to establish cancer screening clinics for the early detection of breast cancer throughout the land, and controlled clinical trials were supported on a regional basis to bring the fruits of research to the people through the use of new drugs, diagnostic techniques, surgical and radiological skills, and other therapies.

In spite of the war on cancer, the facts and figures of the National Cancer Institute and the American Cancer Society for 1976 stated that 675,000 new cases of cancer were expected in 1976 and that only one-third of these cancer victims would be alive in 5 years. Cancer still occurs at any age, killing more children between the ages of 3 to 14 than any other disease. One in four people now living will eventually have cancer. In the 70's it is estimated there will be 6.5 million new cancer cases, 3.5 million cancer deaths, and more than 10 million people under medical care for cancer in the United States. One of every six deaths from all causes in the U.S. is from cancer, and this year at least 370,000 will die of the disease. Cancer remains the second leading cause of death in America, exceeded only by deaths from cardiovascular disease.

Misgivings and concern about the effectiveness of the war on cancer, in spite of vast sums of government money, is currently leading to a review and examination of public policy in the areas of biomedical and behavioral research. The Senate has formed a Health Subcommittee which has started off its probing into biomedical research by questioning the concept that pouring vast sums of federal money into basic research on fundamental problems, like cancer, will best serve the public interest and need. Questions are being raised about the relative merits of basic versus applied research, and whether scientists are being responsive to social obligations by struggling with the acquisition of new and fundamental knowledge. Might they more properly be directing their efforts toward a more practical solution of current problems by disseminating the fruits of existing knowledge? The implication is that the public is not getting its money's worth from research unless the scientist's mission is prevention, diagnosis, and treatment of disease through judicious employment of advanced existing skill and technology in the conquest of a specific illness, like cancer.

The problem of scientific freedom and responsibility is not new, but the cost of basic scientific research is mounting rapidly at a time when mass communications are unfolding unbelievable vistas of a glorious life freed from hunger, poverty, and illness by applied science. The truth of the argument rests on a balanced judgment of history, for the pendulum of science swings between the acquisition of new knowledge and its judicious application. Scientific freedom is necessary for the advancement of knowledge from which society may benefit; the application of science to enlarge our intellectual, cultural, and social realities and horizons emerges from our understanding of life and its interrelationship to the total universe. Science and technology, basic and applied, have become inseparably entwined in the core of our existence and salvation, much like the double-helical strands of DNA, the essence of the origin of life, its replication, and its genetic specificity.

Nowhere are the problems of scientific freedom and social responsibility more complex and striking than in the current status of cancer research and treatment. We have not solved the cancer problem at either the level of scientific understanding or applied technology, but the last 5 years have witnessed rapid strides in our basic knowledge of the origin of genes for cancer and the cellular alterations that lead to tumorigenicity, invasiveness, cell destruction, and metastases. Practical control, prevention, and cure of cancer have not been achieved, but new approaches are emerging for early diagnosis and improved treatment. New scientific knowledge bears on cancer, but more importantly its application is capable of releasing immense new forces into our environment which may well shape the future history of man and our species.

BIOLOGICAL PROGRESS IN CANCER: 1972–1977

THE CENTRAL DOGMA OF MOLECULAR BIOLOGY UP TO 1972

We must begin by trying to understand the origin and nature of life. A presumptuous approach is to briefly review what by 1970 came to be called the "central dogma of molecular biology." Life succeeds in creating order from randomness in an infinite variety of forms which are biologically unique, yet each unique form has the ability to utilize energy and replicate itself through genetic information. Plants take the energy of the sun and with it mould orchids to algae from carbon dioxide, water, and a few nutrients. Animals take plants or other animals, break them down into appropriate miniscule particles through digestion, and from these reconstruct and reproduce themselves as ants to elephants, biologically unique as individuals, but replicative as an identifiable species—ontogeny and phylogeny. All forms of life evolve from primitive chemical elements uniting to form simple gases which mix, fuse, and join with emerging compounds and water to form a primordial stew out of which life originates, changes in response to its environment, and procreates. The extraordinary organization of living things, the ability to replicate and pass on hereditable information, and the opportunity to evolve to meet changing fortunes has finally come to be understood in terms of two classes of molecules—the nucleic acids and the proteins.

The principal nucleic acid in all living things is desoxyribonucleic acid—DNA. This ubiquitous DNA is composed of a 5 carbon sugar, phosphate groups, and only 4 possible organic bases: adenine (A); thymine (T); guanine (G); and cytosine (C) (fig. 1). One of the organic bases joins with the deoxyribose sugar and a phosphate group to form a nucleotide. A strand of DNA is then a chain of nucleotides, each consisting of a deoxyribose sugar and a phosphate group, and one of four organic bases: A, T, G, or C. DNA was proven to be a double-stranded molecule. The sugars and phosphates constitute the backbone of the strand, and the paired bases, linked by hydrogen bonds, connect the two strands. In any DNA chain the number of A molecules equals the number of T molecules, and the number of G molecules equals the number of C molecules.

Brilliant studies by innumerable erudite scientists in the 1950's and 1960's led to the realization that the sequence of organic bases coded for, or specified construction of, a specific amino acid, the building blocks of protein. There are only 20 amino acids essential for life, and in order for them to be coded for by only 4 possible organic bases, A,T,C, or G, the sequence of any 3 of these bases would be required to code for one amino acid. The nucleus of the cell was known to contain large amounts of DNA; the cytoplasm of the cell was found capable of synthetizing protein on its ribosomes. Resulting from 25 to 30 years of high-level research on the nature and structure of DNA, in 1963 Watson and Crick formulated the Watson-Crick hypothesis (Watson, 1965). This hypothesis rapidly

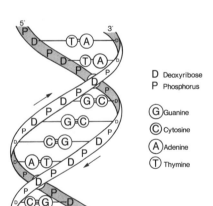

D Deoxyribose
P Phosphorus

G Guanine
C Cytosine
A Adenine
T Thymine

FIGURE 1. *DNA is a double helix. The strands consist of a desoxyribose sugar and a phosphate group. They are bound together by 4 bases. Guanine invariably binds to cytosine and adenine invariably binds to thymine.*

became the central dogma of molecular biology. The double helix was the name applied to the double spiral stairway-like structure of DNA (fig. 2). The sugar and phosphate groups made up the backbone of each spiral, and the purine and pyrimidine bases, A, T, C, and G, made up the central core with an A invariably being bound to a T and a G invariably being bound to a C by hydrogen bonding. The sequence of any 3 bases would code for a specific amino acid.

Inherent in the separation of the chain into 2 component strands was the possibility that a portion of the single strand might act as a messenger to be carried into the cytoplasm, serving as a template for the synthesis of specific amino acids and proteins—the so-called messenger RNA or mRNA. The single strand carrying the complete sequence of A, T, G, and C in a linear tape could also code for its identical reproduction, since A only binds to T and G to C in the double strand, thereby accounting for the transmission of genetic or inherited information. The chromosomes of a cell transmit the hereditary material; they are composed of genes in variable numbers, the genes are double-stranded DNA which can code both for the transmission of genetic material from cell to cell and for the production of specific proteins through activated bits of a single-strand passing into the cytoplasm as messenger RNA, mRNA.

The central dogma of molecular biology until 1970 was that genetic information is transferred from DNA to RNA to protein. The curious ability of a small piece of Rous sarcoma virus, a very small bit of ribonucleic acid, a RNA virus, to convert a normal chicken cell into a cancer cell was unexplained (see chapter 6, page 75).

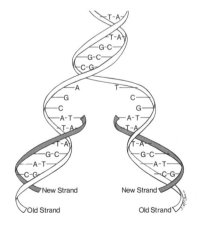

FIGURE 2. *In DNA replication, each strand separates into a single messenger strand—mRNA—and a second non-replicating strand. The mRNA strand serves as a template for the exact reproduction of the original DNA helix.*

VIROLOGY, MOLECULAR BIOLOGY, AND CANCER

With over 30 years of intense and brilliant research required to understand the overall structure and function of DNA, efforts now turned to an in-depth analysis of genes by working with the simplest of living organisms: bacteria and viruses, which have only a few genes and replicate rapidly. A single gene codes for a single protein with a single specific function. Not all genes in a chromosome are active at any one time. Some of the bacteria have specific enzyme or protein functions which can be isolated and studied to look into problems of gene activation. Particles of genetic material can be separately isolated from bacteria for genetic manipulation. Currently the most attractive of these are extra-chromosomal structures called plasmids. These plasmids made it possible to study genetic engineering and recombinations of DNA in living cells. Viruses have equally great attraction for the experimental biologist, for they can be either of the DNA or RNA type, and both types can induce cancer in normal cells under properly controlled conditions. Some of the RNA viruses are so small they contain only 5 proteins, that is 5 genes, and the entire sequence of purine and pyrimidine bases (A,T,G,C) for each gene could be worked out. (Three bases code for an amino acid; 30 to 50 amino acids make up a single protein. Therefore, the total sequential base composition for some small DNA viruses would only be 600 to 1000 bases). The RNA viruses have the unique ability to convert a normal cell to a cancer cell in defiance of the central dogma of molecular biology. Both DNA and RNA viruses can induce cancer. Viruses, then, can be used to map out the essential differences between cancer cells and their normal counterparts and to elucidate new mechanisms for the transmission of hereditable material.

Ellerman and Bang (1908) and Peyton Rous (1911) opened the field of mammalian tumor virology, but in the absence of inbred strains of animals and appropriate laboratory technology the field lay dormant until the great awakenings of mid-century. Obviously, it is impossible in this brief account to pay tribute to the many brilliant concepts and experiments of all contributors to this burgeoning field of knowledge. Some of the crucial work has been reviewed earlier in prior chapters, but I would now like to look at the works of Gross, Rubin, Dulbecco, Baltimore, Spiegelman, and Temin, all of whom have won either the Laster Awards for medical research in American medicine or the Nobel Prize for science during the past 10 years. As yet no one has proved that any human cancer is due to a virus, but the relationships of viruses to cancer make us realize "how economical, elegant, and intelligent are the accidents of evolution that have been maintained by selection. A virologist is among the luckiest of biologists because he can see into his chosen pet down to the details of all of its molecules. The virologist sees how an extreme parasite functions using just the most fundamental aspects of biological behavior" (Baltimore, 1976).

Mouse mammary cancer, an experimental cancer of proven viral origin in C3H mice, was demonstrated by Bittner (1936) to be transmitted through the milk from mother to offspring. Gross then suspected that tumor-inducing viruses were transmitted from one generation to the next by "*vertical transmission,*" that is by a latent viral gene going from mother to offspring as part of the normal hereditable material, in contrast to "*horizontal transmission*" of contagious pathogenic agents, such as those causing measles, scarlet fever, or chickenpox. He developed two inbred strains of mice, C58 and Ak, that had a 90% spontaneous incidence of mouse leukemia, which he suspected was due to a virus. He tried to transmit mouse leukemia into other strains of mice either through mother's milk or through cell-free filtrates of embryonic extracts of the C58 or Ak embryos. Convinced as he was that mouse leukemia was due to a virus, he could never prove it by classic methods of viral transmission. He even obtained C3H mice from Bittner, but could not produce leukemia in these mice by any method: foster-nursing experiments; injection of cell-free filtrates of embryonic C58 or Ak mice; or even by direct injection of these C3H mice with cell-free filtrates of leukemic spleens or leukemic tumors or leukemic mice.

These frustrating failures to transmit mouse leukemia consumed his life from 1940 to 1949. In 1949 Gross attended a lecture on the *immunological unresponsiveness* of newborn animals less than 48 hours of age. He immediately repeated his viral transmission experiments on immunologically tolerant newborn mice. He proved the vertical transmission of mouse leukemia virus for newborn mice and rats, and the ability to pass the virus between newborn mice and rats. He next took C3H and C57 black mice, normally free of spontaneous leukemia, and induced leukemia in these mice by repeated total body X-ray irradiation in amounts sufficient to suppress normal immune responses. Extracts from mice in whom radiation leukemia was induced were rendered cell free, and these cell-free extracts were able to induce leukemia in newborn mice. Radiation-induced leukemia was, therefore, caused by a virus.

Curiously, some of the mice inoculated with leukemia virus did not develop leukemia alone but also developed bilateral parotid gland carcinomas and other salivary gland tumors. Gross quickly demonstrated that in addition to the mouse leukemia virus these animals had a second smaller heat-and ether-resistant virus, which he designated the "parotid-tumor virus." This "parotid-tumor virus" was later proved to be the polyoma virus so named by Eddy and Stewart who isolated it in tissue cultures. The polyoma virus, isolated in 1958, has been shown to be a small DNA virus about 40 mu in diameter. It is present in many mice without causing tumors, but can be activated by propagation in tissue culture or by blind passage in newborn mice. The polyoma virus was joined a few years later by the discovery of another papovirus, the SV 40 virus. Both of these viruses were so small that their molecular biology could ultimately be worked out by emerging technology, and laid the foundation for Dulbecco and his brilliant collaborators to study the molecular basis of cancer induction by oncogenic DNA viruses.

Rubin, a gentle philosopher in search of truth and a lifelong opponent of scientific dogma, elected to study cancer induction in the early 1940's, at a time when DNA was known to carry genetic information, but RNA was just beginning to be understood as a translator for converting DNA messages into protein. He returned to the Rous sarcoma virus, a RNA virus known to produce cancer in chicken fibroblasts grown in tissue culture. Quantitation of the relationships of RSV to cancer were studied by measuring the discrete foci of altered chicken embryo cells infected with Rous sarcoma virus in tissue culture. The relationship of other RNA viruses, the so-called Rous associated viruses (RAV viruses), to RSV and cancer induction could also be studied. Rubin concluded that the RNA of RSV virus became integrated into the DNA of the cell and thereby coded for cancer and that RNA viruses which coded for cancer were incomplete viruses. These RNA viruses became part of the DNA of the cell, coded for cancer, but they could not replicate themselves in the cell unless help for replication was obtained from Rous-associated viruses. Viral replication killed the cell; incomplete assimilation of the RNA into DNA coded for cancer. The flow of information from RNA to DNA defied the central dogma of molecular biology.

From the concept that RNA viruses inducing cancer were incomplete viruses emerged the luminous and scholarly research by Baltimore and Temin clarifying the interactions of RNA viruses on cells in the induction of cancer. Rubin won the Lasker award of American medicine; Dulbecco—his teacher, Temin—his student, and Baltimore won the 1976 Nobel prize in medicine; and the relationships of DNA viruses, RNA viruses, polymerases, and proviruses to cancer are at the forefront of current research. Before we review the conclusions of these great researchers on the origins of cancer, we should introduce the exciting work of Spiegelman on the test tube synthesis of viral nucleic acid and the development and use of molecular hydridization techniques in molecular analysis.

Spiegelman started with the premise that RNA viruses must carry out their life cycle in cells that use DNA as genetic material but in which RNA can serve as a genetic messenger. Either the DNA of the host cell contained a molecular sequence of A,T,G,C homologous to the viral RNA or such a sequence was introduced into the cell from the viral RNA by a reversal of transcription. By either explanation, sequences of A,T,C,G complementary to the viral RNA must ultimately exist in the DNA of the cell. Spiegelman first showed, using MS–2–RNA bacteriophage, that there were no detectable sequences in the RNA complementary to the viral RNA either before or after infection. In 1962 he postulated that RNA viruses generate RNA copies from RNA by a new type of replicase, a RNA-dependent RNA polymerase, and made the further intuitive guess that this replicase would be specific for its own template, and not copy any RNA molecule of sequence other than the template. He proved the specificity of replicases in 1963 by identifying the replicase for MS–2 bacteriophage in *Eschericia coli* and another replicase, the Qb replicase, which was specific for another unrelated RNA virus known as Qb virus. Qb replicase proved to be extremely stable and easily isolated as a free enzyme. With it Spiegelman was able to synthesize RNA in a test tube and show that the enzyme could not distinguish between authentic viral RNA and its synthetic counterpart. All the genetic information required to produce a virus had been faithfully copied in the test tube synthesis of the viral RNA, and subsequent experiments proved this synthetic RNA to be equally infectious, ug to ug in weight, to the authentic virus.

Qb virus and Qb replicase proved to be a particularly fortuitous choice, for Qb virus has a wildtype which grows at any temperature and a temperature-sensitive mutant which can be easily identified, for it can not grow at 41 C. Qb replicase, very stable and not temperature-dependent, reproduces both types of Qb virus. The viral RNA was shown to be the instructive agent for replication; in controlled synthetic experiments the product was mutant if the initiating template was mutant, and the product was wildtype if the initiating template was wildtype. RNA could be synthesized in a test tube, and with the Qb replicase system RNA was the instructive agent for self-replication.

Strangely, the Qb replicase system is still the only one in which indefinite molecular replication of RNA in a test tube can be achieved, another example of serendipitous choice of experimental design. The system has been used for detailed study of nucleic acid synthesis, and has shown that erplication is not only conplementary but involves plus and minus strands. The sequence of the nucleotides of plus and minus strands over 218 nucleotides in length has been worked out, and the strands are essentially mirror-images of each other, with the intrastrand anti-parallel complements binding into secondary and tertiary structures with two- and three-dimensional consequences. The secondary and teritary structures permit phenotypic evolution from both greater length and complexity of the molecules. Replication from plus and minus strands also offers an evolutionary advantage, for a desirable sequence present in one complement will be inserted into the other with appropriate secondary and tertiary stems and loops in the total molecule.

By the mid-1950's it was generally accepted that the flow of genetic information went from DNA to messenger RNA to protein. In 1958 Speigelman and his associates were among the first to provide evidence that there is a specific enzyme in cells whose function is to use DNA as a template to make complementary RNA copies, a DNA-directed RNA polymerase, ultimately named transcriptase. Using electrophoresis and velocity centrifugation in sucrose gradients they developed techniques for separating RNA's. They demonstrated that E. Coli infected with T bacteriophage produced a new RNA species which could be physically separated from the normal RNA found in uninfected cells. The next step was to prove that this new RNA was a complementary transcript of the viral DNA. Knowing that the two DNA strands were held together by hydrogen bonds between the complementary bases, Spiegelman reasoned that the same thing might occur between a DNA strand and its complementary RNA strand. Double isotopic labelling of the

DNA strand and RNA's was carried out, and under appropriate conditions hydrogen bonding between the two was permitted. With high-speed centrifugation techniques they demonstrated that molecular hybridization did indeed occur, and identified the T2 specific RNA as complementary to the T2 DNA. This proved that the RNA newly synthesized after viral infection specifically hybridized to the viral DNA and not to the DNA of the host.

Molecular hybridization as a technique for identifying complementary molecular bases soon became simplified by filter-paper techniques, and quantitative assay for DNA-RNA hybrids with DNA immobilized on a membrane soon followed. The RNA-DNA hybridization technique was used to clarify major issues of the day in molecular biology, particularly after it was demonstrated that "competitive hybridization" could be used to distinguish one RNA molecule from another, even though both are represented in the same genome and nuclease could be used to destroy physically trapped or poorly-paired RNA. Ribosomal RNA, as well as the transfer RNA's, was proved by molecular hybridization techniques to have its bases specified by distinct sequence segments in cellular DNA. Furthermore, molecular hybridization experiments proved that when the two strands of DNA are separated in mRNA formation only one of the two strands of the DNA is transcribed in any particular segment (see chapter 6, p. 78).

RNA-DNA hybridization techniques became one of the most important tools of molecular biology in the past decade. Spiegelman introduced its use to search for evidence of viral genomes in human cancer, and was able to demonstrate that human leukemias, lymphomas, sarcomas, and breast cancer contain RNA molecules with base sequences homologous to the RNAs of tumor viruses causing similar cancers in mice. The relationship of viruses to cancer has moved in other directions in recent years, due to the impact of the elegant research of Dulbecco, Baltimore, and Temin.

Dulbecco has clarified the molecular events in the transformation of oncogenic DNA viruses to cancer. Crucial to quantitative studies was the development of assay techniques. He showed that in certain cultures polyoma virus would grow, or be *permissive,* and in others it would induce a cancer-like state, not grow out as virus, or be *non-permissive.* The induction of a cancer-like state in vitro was called *transformation.* Transforming DNA virus proved to be cyclical or circular in shape. The circle would be broken and the entire DNA chain would be integrated and covalently bonded as a complete unit into the DNA of the cell. *Integration* was essential to virus-induced cell transformation, and explained the subsequent ability of this integrated viral particle to code for transformation as well as for the production of identifiable viral coat proteins, specific viral antigens. The viral DNA of the SV 40 DNA, and other papovaviruses studied, was integrated into the cell as a *provirus,* and is, therefore, genetically transmitted and serves as the template for transcription into mRNA. The integration of the viral DNA takes place in two parts, an early integration which codes for cancer-like transformation (the A gene) and a later integration which codes for other aspects of viral proteins (the B gene).

Working with SV 40 DNA, the search for the viral transforming protein in the A gene was begun by studying the so-called T antigen. T antigen is about 94,000 daltons in molecular weight, is specified for by viral DNA, and is affected by mutations of the A gene. Transforming protein was found to control both the initiation and maintenance of transformation, but the need for transforming protein decreased once transformation took place. This suggests a self-stabilization of the state of gene expression as a general property of animal cells to preserve differentiation, and leads to work on the cellular events in transformation. Is this self-stabilization a matter of functional change in gene activation and repression through operator and repressor genes, or is it an actual mutation? Functional changes could be produced by binding of transforming proteins to DNA; mutations would alter the sequence of bases in DNA. The methodology of molecular hybridization techniques is still not good enough to answer this question, but the emerging methodology of recombinant DNA (discussed in detail later) could explore and hopefully answer this important question. Through recombinant DNA, cellular DNA fragments can be cloned in phages or plasmids and quantitatively used to probe this problem.

The important role of cell mutation in the viral transformation of cells was explored by Dulbecco. With the papovaviruses, viruses frequent chromatid breaks appear early in transformation, but malignant transformation seems to occur in steps. The cells that are transformed immediately may have undergone promutations from other promutagens prior to viral infection. Conversely, cells fully transformed by SV 40 virus can revert to relatively normal phenotypes, although they still contain normal viral DNA and T antigen, the transforming protein. Observations of this type reveal the important role of cellular mutations in cell transformation induced by different carcinogens. The experimental enhancement of transforming activity of viruses by mutagenic agents fits in well with clinical observations that some genetic diseases have an increased frequency of cancer (hereditary polyposis of the colon, for example) and that most carcinogens, either physical or chemical, are promutagens and must be acted upon by cellular metabolism to induce cancer. Nevertheless, the *provirus theory,* the persistence of viral DNA in transformed cells, permits us to test whether a given DNA virus is a possible agent in human cancer.

However, we still need more knowledge of the normal regulation of growth of animal cells and its deregulation by carcinogens and viruses. Growth regulation involves a complex chain of both extracellular and intracellular events. The extracellular regulators of whatever kind must interact with the cell membrane; cell membranes through their chemical and physical properties must permit penetration of extracellular regulators, perhaps even in a modified way; cytoplasmic mediators must carry both extracellular and intracellular regulators to the cell nucleus, where DNA binding proteins and direct mutations influence the physical and chemical activation of DNA through structural, activator, or repressor changes. All of these complex events are coming under investigation. But first, how do RNA viruses as well as DNA viruses code for cancer?

RNA tumor viruses are called retroviruses. The basic needs of any virus are two: (1) a nucleic acid core, a genome, to be transmitted from generation to generation; and (2) a mRNA to direct the synthesis of viral proteins. The critical proteins that the mRNA must encode are the ones that coat the genome and those that help replicate the genome. New viruses require specific RNA or DNA polymerases, chemically unique and identifiable, to synthesize the virus-specific nucleic acids in their core. The retroviruses, the RNA viruses coding for cancer, have a unique style for replication and for the induction of cancer, subjects which yielded to understanding through the imaginative research of Baltimore and Temin (fig. 3). Historically, the picornaviruses, which produce diseases like poliomyelitis and the common cold, were studied first and the retroviruses were later explored to relate the biochemistry of the RNA virus to oncogenicity.

Picornaviruses, like poliomyelitis virus, were early shown to be

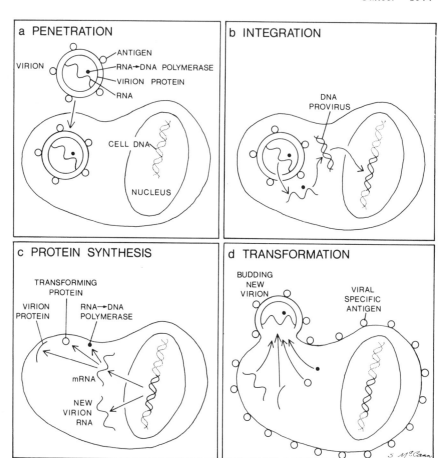

FIGURE 3. *Schematic Outline of Interaction of RNA Virus with Cells to Introduce Carcinogenic Material into DNA: (A) The RNA virion penetrates the cell together with the RNA–DNA polymerase. The virion RNA is transcribed to a provirus. B) The RNA provirus, through RNA–DNA polymerase, is transformed into DNA provirus. The DNA provirus can penetrate the nucleus of the cell and code for cancer. C) Protein synthesis by the cell produces new virion RNA. The altered cell can now produce through its transformation a cancer cell in an appropirate oncogenic environment, as well as new virion RNA proteins. D) Transformation is complete. The altered cell has become a cancer cell, genetically altered by the RNA virion. The cancer cell can also bud off new viral particles, and the cancer cell carries on its surface the viral specific antigens of the original RNA virion.*

capable of shutting off the nuclear synthesis of cellular RNA after infecting the cell, only to initiate new RNA synthesis in the cytoplasm which appeared to represent production of viral RNA. No pure enzyme able to make picornavirus RNA has ever been isolated, so the details of viral RNA synthesis must still be pursued in infected cells. Precise *in vitro* analysis with infected cells disclosed that the poliovirus genome RNA is the messenger RNA for the synthesis of viral proteins. The whole viral genome is first translated into a single continuous polypeptide or polyprotein. This incoming strand of RNA polyprotein serves as a plus strand from which a complementary minus strand is synthesized, which in turn synthesizes a series of plus strands. From the minus strand viral specific proteins emerge which give specificity to the virus and also produce the capsid proteins to form a new virion. Some of the minus strand, however, is converted into a double-stranded RNA. This much was known about poliovirus when work began on vesicular stomatitis virus (VSV), another RNA virus.

Work with multiple RNA's produced by VSV infection in cells showed that the major VSV-induced RNA's in infected cells were complementary in base sequence to the initial virion RNA. The viral mRNA, in other words, was in infected cells complementary to the virion RNA. Since there was no known RNA to RNA transcription, they postulated that a RNA polymerase entered the cell with the virus, or the cell contained a RNA polymerase. A virion RNA polymerase was then confirmed, a RNA dependent RNA polymerase. The demonstration of this enzyme, subsequently called *reverse transcriptase,* soon led to the realization that a huge class of viruses, called negative-strand viruses, all carry the strand of RNA complementary to the messenger RNA as their genome and carry also an RNA polymerase able to copy the genome RNA, converting it into a double-stranded piece of viral DNA, which then serves as the source of multiple messenger RNA's.

After the discovery of reverse transcriptase, the search began for virion polymerases in the retroviruses, in an effort to explain their replication and their oncogenicity. Others, notably Temin, had already postulated, but never proved, that there was a DNA intermediate in the replication of RNA tumor viruses. Baltimore returned to a study of Rous sarcoma virus, now almost 50 years after it had been abandoned by Rous because of its complexity, and demonstrated that RSV contained a ribonuclease-sensitive DNA polymerase. The capability of making a DNA copy of the RNA genome was contained within the virons of the RNA tumor virus itself. Reverse transcriptase converted the viron RNA into viron DNA (fig. 4). A fraction of the DNA can be recovered as closed, circular DNA, and that circular DNA presumably integrates into the cellular DNA of the host, again as a provirus.

The proviral DNA can now be expressed in accordance with the central dogma: DNA is transcribed to mRNA which is translated into protein by the cytoplasm. Two types of products have already been characterized: (1) the new virion RNA; and (2) the mRNA's for the other viral proteins. The virus-specific proteins also have two known functions: (1) the genomal RNA may transform the cell from a normal cell into a cancer cell; and (2) the normal viral proteins supply the coat and other needed proteins for new viral articles. RSV is a defective or incomplete virus in the sense that infection with RSV may convert a normal cell to a cancer cell by remaining as a provirus in the normal cellular DNA rather than killing the cell and emerging as a new complete virion.

The retroviruses attack a cell in two distinct time periods: the first short, lasting only a few hours; and the second long. In the short phase, reverse transcription—formation of a closed circular duplex DNA—and integration of the provirus into the cellular DNA occur. The second phase starts when the integrated genome or provirus begins making viral RNA. Synthesis of viral proteins and progeny virions continues thereafter in concert with the cell cycle. The retrovirus becomes a tumor virus, if one of the viral proteins made by the infected cell is capable of changing the growth properties of the cell. The key possessed by the retrovirus that enables it to initiate this unique life cycle is reverse transcriptase (see fig. 3, p. 300).

Reverse transcriptase, like most DNA polymerases, is primer-dependent and makes DNA in a 5′ to 3′ direction. Primer-dependence means that it can only elongate nucleic acid molecules; it cannot initiate DNA synthesis *de novo*. The viral genome RNA carries with it the primer RNA molecule to initiate the copying of viral RNA by reverse transcriptase. Reverse transcriptase, however, differs from normal DNA polymerase in 3 important ways: (1) it has a unique polypeptide sequence; (2) it can make copies of RNA templates as well as DNA templates; and (3) ribonuclease H activity associated with it is capable of degrading the RNA-DNA strand,

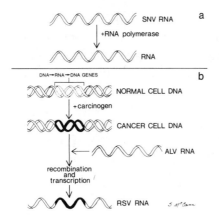

FIGURE 4. *Schematic Concept of the Protovirus Hypothesis on the Possible Origin of Cancer: The Possible Origin of Rousa Sarcoma Virus, as Postulated by Temin: A) The RNA spleen necrosis virus under the influence of RNA–DNA polymerase synthesizes a strand of RNA virion. B) In the genes of many normal cells there is a site where-in a piece of DNA can be converted to a piece of RNA and can be reconverted back to DNA through the reverse transcriptase enzymes (RNA–DNA polymerase). A carcinogen, whatever its nature, produces an oncogene in the normal cell at that site. The oncogene is further altered by a harmless piece of RNA produced by a non-carcinogenic avian leukosis virus. Recombination and transcription take place. The heavy lines indicating DNA involved in information transfer of DNA to RNA to DNA are transformed by the combination of the carcinogen and the harmless RNA virion to produce an oncogenic RNA virus, the Rous sarcoma virus. The protovirus hypothesis predicts the origin of oncogenic RNA viruses by recombinations and transcriptions at normal sites of DNA where RNA to DNA to RNA coding occurs. Normally, according to this Temin postulate, this DNA site codes for cell surface phenomena and intracellular antigenic modulation.*

leaving only the DNA to form a DNA-DNA double strand. This DNA-DNA strand, if it is circular or cyclical, can then be integrated into the host genome as the provirus. Once the provirus has been integrated into the host genome, it need not be expressed or activated but can be replicated indefinitely in the host genome as a silent or repressed gene.

In the retroviruses, DNA provirus is comparable to the "minus strand" in the picornavirus genetic system. DNA provirus is believed to be the clue to cancer induction by RNA viruses. It becomes hereditable genetic material which can be carried as a repressed gene, or can induce cancer ultimately in the cell by: (1) attaching or recombining with other genetic material in the cell nucleus or plasmids of the cell cytoplasm to form a recombinant DNA which codes for cancer; (2) making a specific type of transforming protein which alters normal cellular growth and regulation; (3) being susceptible as a promutagen to cellular or environmental carcinogens; or (4) enabling direct mutations in the cell, transforming the cell to a cancer. The proviral stage in the life cycle of retroviruses enables cells to harbor RNA viruses as genetically silent DNA molecules. This may well account for the findings by molecular hybridization experiments that normal cells and cancer cells have fragments of DNA related to one or more types of retroviruses. The significance of these genes that resemble retroviruses in normal and cancer cells remains a challenge to cancer virology. Temin has addressed himself beautifully to this challenge in his research.

Temin began working with RSV virus in association with Rubin in 1956. He formulated the DNA provirus hypothesis in 1960, discovered the RSV virion DNA polymerase in 1969, and confirmed the DNA provirus hypothesis in the 1970's. He beautifully summarized our knowledge of the mechanism of formation of DNA provirus as follows: "After infection of susceptible cells by RSV, the virion DNA polymerase synthesizes a DNA copy of the viral RNA, probably using a cellular transfer RNA molecule associated with the viral RNA as a primer for the DNA synthesis (see fig. 4, p. 303). After the formation of the RNA-DNA hybrid molecule, there is synthesis of a second strand of DNA, perhaps after degradation of the viral RNA by the ribonuclease H activity of the virion DNA polymerase. Double-stranded closed circular viral DNA appears. Viral DNA becomes integrated with the host DNA. However, neither the mechanism for integration nor whether virion-associated enzymes are involved in integration is known" (Temin, 1975).

Since 1975 Temin has continued his research on the origin of ribodeoxyviruses, and their mutation and recombinations in and out of cells. He has worked with spleen necrosis virus (SNV), avian leukosis virus (AVL), and Rous sarcoma virus (RSV), the last being a retrovirus. Temin, prior to 1970, observed that the recombination between viruses and cells does not appear to be random, but is primarily dependent on endogenous ribodeoxyvirus-related genes which are part of the normal cellular DNA. Indeed, in 1970 he proposed a hypothesis to explain the origin of ribodeoxyviruses— the *protovirus hypothesis*. This new protovirus hypothesis attempted to explain the increasingly-frequent demonstration by molecular hybridization experiments that many cells, both normal and cancerous, contain nucleotide sequences in their DNA complementary to viral RNA. The protovirus hypothesis states that ribodeoxyviruses evolved from normal cellular components. The normal cellular components which give rise to RNA viruses are the normal endogenous genes which have the capability of transferring information from DNA to RNA to DNA, and, therefore, probably also code for reverse transcriptase. These normal genes coding for normal DNA to RNA to DNA information transfer exist not to code for RNA viruses but probably to control through cellular mechanisms cell growth, differentiation, antibody formation, gene recombination and activation. Temin has also proposed that small animal DNA viruses evolve from unintegrated bits of DNA formed by reverse transcriptase in the RNA to DNA step in viral development. The protovirus concept is an interesting one in explaining the origin of RNA viruses and possibly DNA viruses, but also has important implications for the origin of cancer.

The protovirus hypothesis holds that RNA tumor virus replication is not directly related to cancer formation by RNA tumor viruses, the retroviruses. However, strongly transforming RNA tumor viruses, like RSV, introduce genes into the cell which are prime targets for later cancer formation, by mutation or recombination with other oncogenic genes. Rous-associated virus or spleen necrosis virus replicates like RSV, but these viruses do not contain genes for cancer. The protovirus concept further proposes that Rous sarcoma, for example, appeared before Rous sarcoma virus. Events not involving the virus lead to the formation of an oncogene, a gene for chicken sarcoma. This sarcoma was infected by an avian leukosis virus, ubiquitous AVL, and RSV was formed by a rare recombination between the oncogene and AVL, resulting in RSV which codes for both the AVL protein and the contained cancer gene. Relating this concept to human cancer, Temin proposes that the majority of human cancers are not caused by retroviruses, like RSV, but probably by non-viral carcinogens. These non-viral carcinogens probably mutate a special target in the cell DNA and convert this segment of DNA to an oncogene, a gene coding for cancer. The targets for the non-viral carcinogens are the genes involved in information transfer from DNA to RNA to DNA (see fig. 4, p. 303). Reverse transcriptase, or RNA directed DNA synthesis, would be involved in forming genes for cancer, whether the cancer gene originated from a retrovirus or from a carcinogen of non-viral origin. Cellular recombinations of transcripted DNA by reverse transcriptase, as well as direct nuclear mutations in existing DNA, could introduce cancer genes into the cell code or could be the site for targeting of mutations by external carcinogens.

In summary, both DNA viruses and RNA viruses can produce cancer in experimental animals. The RNA viruses that code for cancer are called retroviruses and Rous sarcoma virus is a prime example of a strongly transforming retrovirus. DNA viruses infect a cell, and the viral DNA becomes integrated into the host genome as a provirus capable of producing cancer. RNA viruses that code for cancer carry into the infected cell the viral RNA genome and an enzyme, reverse transcriptase, capable of converting in the first stage of infection the viral RNA into a circular piece of DNA in a very short time. The circular DNA is integrated in the second stage of infection into the genome of the host cell, and thereafter serves as a provirus. DNA viruses and RNA viruses then both become integrated into the host cell DNA to code for cancer as a provirus.

Inherent in this process is a dual mode of transmission of viral information: (1) horizontal, wherein information flows from RNA to DNA to DNA (RNA virus) or from DNA to RNA (DNA virus); and (2) vertical, wherein for both viruses there is DNA to DNA information transfer from generation to offspring. Molecular hybridization experiments show that both DNA and RNA viral sequences of nucleotides are present in many normal and cancerous cells, particularly in experimental animals but also, less often, in humans. The DNA provirons concept has been proved for both DNA and RNA viruses, but the presence of homologues to DNA and RNA genes in human tumors does not mean that infectious virus resides in or has caused the tumor. A protovirus hypothesis has been proposed, but not proved, that RNA viruses first and DNA viruses later, have originated by evolution from a normal cellular system of DNA to RNA to DNA information transfer. Originally the viral particles are nononcogenic; they become oncogenic by recombination with cellular genes that are either suppressed oncogenes, which they activate, or targeted genes which have already undergone mutation to genes for cancer. Finally, the concept is emerging that the normal role for the cellular system of DNA to RNA to DNA information transfer must be related to cell growth, development, differentiation, immune response, and cell surface and membrane function—in short, evolution.

THE CANCER CELL: CELL SURFACE STRUCTURE, CELLULAR
COMMUNICATION, CELL REGULATION AND CELL DYNAMICS

Cancer cells differ from normal cells in their dynamic behavior and in their cellular growth and communication; they proliferate in an uncontrolled fashion, invade and destroy normal tissue, and metastasize to distant sites. Growth is not inhibited by cell-to-cell contact, cellular communication between cells is lost, and the cancer cell has altered responsiveness to serum factors, hormones, immunological defenses, and agents that exert their effects through the cell membrane. To understand these complex and dynamic factors in cellular growth, communication, and regulation, the structure and function of the cell membrane and its modulation has come under intensive investigation in the last 5 years (Edelman, 1976). Advances in biochemical and electron microscopic technology have again made these studies in cell surface organization possible.

Cell membranes are composed of lipids, proteins, oligosaccharides, and polysaccharides (sugars). Communication between cells is mediated by hormones and enzymes and nerve fibers; once penetration of the cell surface has occurred, communication within the cell is through microtubles and microfilaments (fig. 5). All cellular communications, internal and external, are founded on the information incorporated in the molecules of nucleic acid.

The organization of the lipids, proteins, and sugars in the cell membrane is one which probably requires the least energy to hold the components in position. The lipids (such as phospholipids) have asymmetrical ends; one hydrophobic and excluding water (the hydrocarbon tail), and the other ionic and hydrophilic, seeking

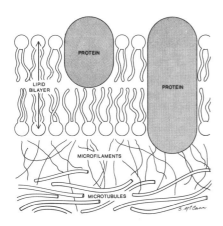

FIGURE 5. *The cell surface consists of a lipid bilayer which contains protein. Through this lipid bilayer and its molecular rearrangements, diverse substances can penetrate the cell membrane. After penetration of the lipid bilayer, the microfilaments and microtubules of the deeper layers carry substances to the cytoplasm and nucleus.*

interactions in the aqueous phase. These interactions favor the lipid being in a continuous bilayer configuration with the hydrocarbon tails avoiding the aqueous phase. The lipids can also segregate into specific domains of average composition, or they can associate with membrane proteins to form lipoproteins. Even though the lipid molecules may be segregated and in specific domains, they tend to remain in a fluid state and be freely diffusable. The membrane proteins are basically of two types: (1) the hydrophobic type interacting with the lipid hydrocarbon tails; and (2) the hydrophilic type. The hydrophobic proteins, which have been termed integral membrane proteins, fold into the membrane to various depths, depending upon their amino acid sequences, and can completely span the membrane from the external surface to the cytoplasmic surface. These integral proteins are essential for membrane stability and are involved in metabolite and ion transport. The hydrophilic proteins are peripheral membrane proteins not involved in membrane stability, and their role is not completely understood. The sugars relate to the proteins as glycoproteins.

The cell membrane, essentially a two-dimensional solution of integral proteins enmeshed in a fluid lipid bilayer, is physically and chemically arranged to permit two unique functional events: (1) the asymmetrical arrangement of the membrane components permits the glycoproteins and the glycolipids to have their carbohydrate residues at the outer surface, where they function as specific receptors for antibodies, hormones, viruses, etc.; and (2) the lipids make the membrane viscous and the components of the membrane can diffuse laterally, but not flip-flop, within the plane of the membrane at diverse rates, permitting variable but reversible changes in membrane topography and chemistry. Cell contact and recognition could depend upon topographic molecular patterns; surface modulation and binding and receptors could be a function of the integral proteins and glycoproteins on the membrane.

Evidence is mounting that the translational mobility of certain classes of integral membrane proteins depends upon their linkage to cytoplasmic microtubules and microfilaments, the cytoplasmic skeletal elements (see fig. 5, p. 307). This concept has been termed trans-membrane cytoskeletal control. The inner cytoplasm then affects, and in part controls, the mobility of integral membrane proteins and the total regulation and function of the cell membrane. The microtubles are large, rigid structures about 25 nn in outside diameter with an inner core of 15 nn diameter. The microfilaments are thin, double helical, 6 to 8 nn in diameter, and have been found to be contractile and related to cell locomotion through actin, myosin, and tropomyosin.

Cell surface receptors can be identified by binding them with multivalent ligands, such as labelled antibodies, hormones, local anesthetics, or lectins (proteins and glycoproteins binding to specific oligosaccharide sequences). These various ligands can either disperse, cluster, coalesce into patches, or form "caps" on the cell surface. For example, it has been shown the binding of immunoglobulin receptors (Ig) on lymphoid cells results in anti-Ig "capping," and the caps are either shed as Ig-receptor-antibody complexes or transported within the cell by endocytosis (fig. 6). Capping of Ig receptors can be reversed by drugs that disrupt microfilaments (fig. 7). Colchicine, for example, dramatically facilitates capping, concanavalin A (Con A) inhibits capping. Some of these drugs alter the microtubules, and others affect the microfilaments. The microtubules and microfilaments are both involved in surface receptor distribution and membrane dynamics.

FIGURE 6. *In the structure of the immunoglobulin molecule, note the light chain and the heavy chain and their sites of fusion and cleavage by papain and pepsin. The antigen binding sites are on the light chain in the Fab fraction. The inner chain bonds are disulfide bonds. There are 5 major classes of immunoglobulins related to the heavy chains and the Fc fragments.*

FIGURE 7. *Changes in the antigens on the cell surface are brought about through the phenomena of patching and capping, producing antigenic modulation.*

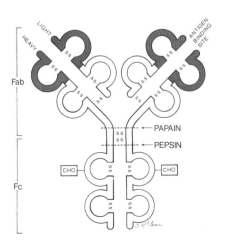

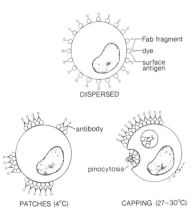

The current model for trans-membrane control mechanisms integrates the physical and chemical structure of the membrane with the cytoplasmic control systems. Microtubule and microfilament arrangements become interconnected into assemblages which are coupled to similar trans-membrane anchorage sites. These anchorage sites serve as regulatory centers for the chemical and physical organization of the membrane into specific domains and receptor sites. The contractile movements of the microfilaments, related to actinomyosin, modulate the anchorage system dictated by the microtubules. The cell surface and its receptors thereby come under the fine regulation of opposing membrane associated cyto-skeletal elements. Cell surface modifications incident to neoplastic transformation can be viewed as an alteration in this normal model. However, despite massive research we are still largely ignorant of the phenotypic changes of tumorigenicity, invasiveness, and metastasis—the stigmata of malignancy.

Experimental controlled studies generally involve tissue culture cells transformed *in vitro* by oncogenic viruses, chemical or physical carcinogens with quantitation of oncogenicity. Cell surface organization is itself affected by cultivation of cells *in vitro*. The complex glycolipids and the glycolipid terminal saccharide residues decrease and the cell becomes more susceptible to antibodies, lectins, and enzymes, but loses contact inhibition. Surface proteins can be labelled with I–125 (iodine 125), and high molecular weight glycoproteins (210,000 to 250,000 daltons) are lost after transformation. This glycoprotein has been called by a variety of names—LETS, galactoprotein a, CSP, component Z, SF 210. The glycopeptides of transformed cells are of higher molecular weight, and resemble the types found after removal of sialic acid from the cell surface by neuroaminadase. Malignant transformation also increases the levels of cell degradative enzymes, such as proteases and glycosidases, and these proteases have been related to loss of growth regulation in malignancy. Transformed cells also show increased transport of sugars and cyclic nucleotides through the cell membrane with increased cellular cyclic nucleotide, cyclic GMP. These cyclic nucleotides may be intracellular messengers altering cytoplasmic enzymes, transport systems, and DNA synthesis, related again to the intracellular RNA to DNA to RNA cycle, which we have discussed previously. The change in the surface receptors is again linked to the cytoplasmic cytoskeletal components, the microfilaments and the microtubules. Alterations in the mobility of surface receptors occurs, the mobility being greater in malignant cells.

The assumption is that important biologic properties of cancer cells depend on the dynamics of the surface receptors and their cytoplasmic controls. This could account for the escape of transformed cells from normal immunologic surveillance, for the shedding of antibodies (antigenic determinants) from the cell surface, for the masking of surface antigens, and for antigenic modulation, making the cell insensitive to the cytotoxic effects of complement. Altered, lost, or coated determinants appear on the cell surface to defy normal immunological surveillance; complement fixation is changed; and shed antigen-antibody complexes can occur, making up the so-called "blocking antibodies" found in some cancers. Both the affector and effector arms of the immune system are involved.

Contact inhibition of cell movement is lost after neoplastic transformation. This could stem from changes in both the surface receptors and the trans-membrane communication, as the cytoskeletal assemblages control cell locomotion through the microfilaments and the microtubules. The tumor cell has a loss of substrate dependency and lack of intercellular communication through the surface adhesive receptors. The redistribution of surface receptors into larger ligands may allow attachment of hormones, serum factors, and mitogens, which then gain access to the microtubules and microfilaments to alter cell growth by transmission to the cell nucleus and its DNA. Information transfer systems within the cell yield to extracellular and transmitted signals. Altered cellular growth, release of substrate dependency, and ultimately invasiveness and metastasis result in the cancer cell. Cell-to-cell recognition, cell adhesiveness, cell positioning within tissues, cell growth independent of substrate, cell invasiveness, and cell metastasis become explicable on cell surface phenomena and intercellular transport systems. Cell proteases probably play a major role in these changes by altering the cell surface and its membrane and changing the linkages of the surface receptors to the cytoskeletal trans-membrane control elements.

Cancer, then, may not involve acquisition of new surface elements and surface receptors, but merely topographic modification and rearrangement of existing surface components with secondary alteration of the trans-membrane linkages to intracellular control mechanisms. Cell proteases probably play a major role in this alteration. The subsequent changes within the cell and its nucleus alter the DNA of the cell, the information transfer system both at the DNA to mRNA to protein level and the RNA to DNA to RNA line, all of which control cell growth and invasiveness. If proteases trigger this change in the cell membrane and its surface receptors, future research may hopefully identify their nature. But of even greater excitement inherent in the possibility that cancer may arise from topographic rearrangement of existing normal components of the cell surface is the dream that cancer is a reversible phenomena. Alterations in topographical patterns of the cell surface are comprehensible and analyzable. Cell surface molecules code for normal cell recognition, growth regulation, and social behavior; alterations in the topographical pattern engender behavioral characteristics of unregulated growth, invasiveness, and metastasis. Cancer, the asocial behavior of cells, is potentially reversible through future research on the dynamics of cell surface organization.

Cell surface organization plays a highly significant role in the immunological reactions of cells; and the basic advances in our knowledge of cellular immunity deserve attention, since immunotherapeutic considerations offer hope in the prevention and treatment of cancer.

CANCER IMMUNOLOGY: 1972–1977

Our previous explorations into cancer immunology prior to 1972 started with the necessity of understanding the difference between histocompatability antigens and cancer-specific antigens. Once inbred strains of animals were developed, it was clearly demonstrated that cancer-specific antigens and antibodies exist and that they are quite distinct from transplantation antigens. A single cell was found to produce a single antibody. From this discovery, the clonal selection theory of Burnett emerged, essentially stating that a single antigen stimulated a single cell to grow out in a clonal fashion and produce single antibodies against it. Acquired immunological tolerance was proved by Medawar, when he showed experimentally that exposure of an embryo to a foreign antigen (not self) prior to immunological maturation permitted that host thereafter, even as a mature adult, to remain tolerant of that foreign antigen and recognize it as self. Balances between antigens and antibodies were important, and immunoparalysis was possible by overwhelming the antibody producing cells with antigen.

The immune system, which had the capacity to respond to thousands of diverse and non-self antigens whether bacterial, viral, or just foreign large molecules, responded in two possible ways: (1) it made special classes of proteins, called antibodies, from the plasma cells, and these antibodies circulated freely as humoral antibodies; and (2) it produced special sensitized cells, the small lymphocytes, which carried cell-bound antibodies on their surface (fig. 8). The binding of either free humoral or cell-bound antibodies on sensitized cells to antigen, like a key fitting a lock, initiated a series of reactions destroying the antigen and eliminating it from the host, thereby sparing the host from death or destruction.

Suppression of the immune responsiveness of the host, by irradiation, cortisone, specific drugs like immuran or anti-lymphocyte globulin, permitted foreign tissue or organs to be transplanted and live in an allogeneic host, yet the incidence of lympho-recticular cancers rose strikingly in the transplanted recipient. The antibody was determined chemically to be an immunoglobulin of diverse

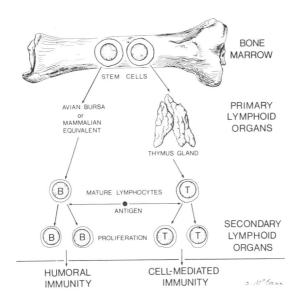

FIGURE 8. *The immune system arises from a primordial stem cell. The stem cell can become either a B cell or a T cell, depending upon its subsequent commitment. The B cells arise from the gut and spleen, homologues of the avian bursa of Fabricius. The T cells receive their commitment from the thymus gland. The B cells are responsible for humoral immunity. The T cells mediate cellular immunity.*

types, but antibodies were divalent, capable of binding two antigenic particles per antibody, and were composed of two long chains
shaped in the form of a Y (see fig. 6, p. 309). The stem of the Y had
no antigen binding site, but each arm of the Y had another short
chain attached to it, and at the end of each arm away from the stem
of the Y was an antigen binding site. It became possible to split the
Y into 3 separate parts with papain, the two arms and the stem.
The two arms, each now claiming one antigen binding site, were
called the Fab fragments, and the free fragment, without a binding
site, was called the Fc fragment. The complete antibody could then
cross-link antigens through the two binding sites; the monovalent
Fab fragments could not.

The general aspects of cancer immunology had several curious
features. Immunosuppression of the host, presumably by abrogating
normal immunologic surveillance, predisposed to cancer formation.
Repeated transplants of the same cancer tissue into allogeneic hosts
often results in the cancer growing out in an enhanced fashion, a
phenomenon called *enhancement*, probably due to coating of the
transplanted cancer cell antigens with just the right amount of
humoral antibody from prior exposure to permit them to grow as
self rather than non-self. Cancers of chemical or physical origin,
such as those arising from dimethylbenzanthracene (cigarette tars),
did not have a common antigen and common antibody in different
hosts, whereas cancers of viral origin had common antigens and
common antibodies identical in all hosts. These antibodies were
coded for by the viral genome itself, whether the virus was DNA or
RNA in type. Small wonder, then, that clinicians began searching
for viral genetic material in human cancers, for common antigens
and antibodies amongst various types of cancer, and for methods of
enhancing the normal immune response of the host by the use of
BCG, and Corynebacterium parva, known immunological enhancing agents.

The virology of cancer has been reviewed already; the finding of
viral genetic material in human cancers by molecular hybridization
techniques has been evaluated; and the use of immunotherapy in
cancer will be discussed under changing concepts in cancer therapy.
We must now focus on the basic understanding of advances in immunology as they relate to cancer generally. The new knowledge
stems from the availability of new techniques to stain and localize
antibodies, to couple cell antibodies with flourescent dyes, to use

fluorescent staining of the cells for the rapid separation of antibody-producing cells, from the molecular analysis of antibody structure, and the ability to study it in fragments by papain cleavage.

Since 1972 it has been possible, through the use of cell surface markers, to separate living cells by means of antibodies, for antibodies bind to cell surface antigens as the initial reaction in cellular communication. Using antibodies as cell markers, the immune system has been shown to arise from a pluripotential cell, the immunoblast, which ultimately becomes a lymphocyte. These stem cells receive different commitments as they mature, but remain responsible for immune reactions. Some stem cells migrate to the thymus, and mature into T (thymic) lymphocytes, spreading into the peripheral lymphoid tissue and blood, but remaining identifiable by the theta antigen on their surface of thymic origin (experimentally). Other stem cells become committed primarily in the bone marrow (also liver and gut), develop into bone marrow lymphocytes, and then migrate to the peripheral tissues and blood as the B lymphocyte. On antigenic stimulation the T cells are activated to clonal selection and produce cell-mediated immune responses; the B cells are activated by antigenic stimulation to produce humoral antibodies as plasma cells. T and B cells and their interaction and effects on cell surface reactors have been intensively studied in recent years (see fig. 8, p. 313).

The B lymphocytes differentiate further into plasma cells, account for humoral immunity, and synthesize specific antibodies that serve as antigen receptors. In many they comprise about 15% to 30% of the peripheral lymphocytes. The B lymphocytes synthesize immunoglobulins on their surface, largely of the IgM, IgG, and IgA types. B lymphocytes also have on their surface receptors for the Fc fragment of antibodies, the stem of the Y of immunoglobulins, and this Fc receptor is quite distinct from the immunoglobulin molecule synthesized by the cell. (Resting T lymphocytes do not have the Fc receptor but may have it on activation). B lymphocytes, in contrast to T lymphocytes, have cell surface receptors that interact specifically with certain components of complement responsible for killing of cells by cytotoxicity. Sheep red blood cells (E) sensitized with appropriate antibodies (immunoglobulins) (A) attach to the Fc receptors of B cells, and in the presence of complement agglutinate into rosettes—the so-called EAC rosettes which enable their identification as human B cells in peripheral blood.

The molecular arrangement of the receptors on B cells shifts with temperature and with antigenic stimulation, and under certain conditions dispersed receptors are cross-linked and cluster as "caps" on the cell surface. This membrane, or antigenic, modulation is reversible and will be discussed later in this chapter.

The T cells receive their commitment from the thymus during maturation and are responsible for cell-mediated immunity. The receptors on their surface are very infrequent in comparison to B cells and are largely of the monomeric IgM type, but this has not been universally proven. They do have cell surface receptors for nonspecific mitogens, and are stimulated to proliferate by compounds like phytohemagglutinin and concanavalin A (ConA). T cells in man form rosettes with unsensitized sheep red blood cells, aiding in their identification.

Macrophages, large mononuclear phagocytic cells, have been shown to have important interreactions with T cells and B cells in both cellular and humoral immunity (fig. 9). The macrophages possess Fc receptors for the C terminal portion of the immunoglobulin molecule, as well as receptors for complement (see fig. 6, p. 309). For the humoral response in immunity, macrophages process antigens for appropriate presentation to lymphocytes. Antigen binding by T cells probably depends on monomeric IgM. For T-dependent antigens in the humoral response, the IgM-antigen complexes are captured by IgM receptors on the macrophage. The macrophage then presents them appropriately to the B lymphocyte, which produces humoral antibodies through plasma cells for their destruction. T cells activation by non-specific stimuli may also result in factors modulating B cell activity. The interaction of macrophages and T cells in delayed hypersensitivity and transplant reactions permits the foreign antigen to react with both macrophages and T cells such that the T cells become effector cells for cell destruction. This occurs through lymphokines and macrophage inhibitor factors, all of which are involved in cellular immunity, or they can become memory cells responsible for the anamnestic response and destruction of foreign tissue more rapidly on repeated exposure to the antigen.

The T cells and the B cells vary in disease. In chronic lymphocytic leukemia the cells are almost all B cells. In multiple myeloma and Waldenstrom's macroglobulinemia the predominant cell is again the B cell. Acute lymphatic leukemia, however, represents a proliferation of T cells.

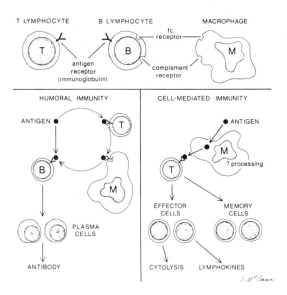

FIGURE 9. *T cells and B cells interact with macrophages to produce humoral immunity or cell-mediated immunity. The ultimate antibody-producing cell of T cell origin is the small lymphocyte. The ultimate producer of B cells are the plasma cells producing humoral antibody. Humoral antibody, cytolysins, and lymphokines result from the interaction of T cells and B cells with macrophages.*

The most interesting recent work has been on the relationship of antigen-antibody reaction on the cell to cell surface modulation and cell surface assembly. Fluorescent labelling of antigen and anti-bodies permits localization of antigen-antibody reactions under the fluorescent microscope. Ferritin labelling of antibody permits local-ization of antigen-antibody reactions on cells by the electron micro-scope. Cells can be studied individually and separated by means of fluorescent antibody labelling.

With these beautiful techniques, antigen-antibody reactions have been shown to take place diffusely on the cell surface membrane, to migrate to segments of the cell membrane, to be temperature de-pendent and to reversibly localize all the immunoglobulin on the cell surface into "caps" (see fig. 7, p. 309). Normal antibody is divalent, but can be split by papain into single or monovalent F ab fragments. The divalent antibody can cross-link multivalent antigen molecules and move the cell surface receptors about in linked groups. The redistribution of surface antigens with divalent anti-body demonstrates readily the clustering of surface antigens into first patches, and then movement of these clusters into one pole of the cell where they form "caps." The actual penetration of the cell membrane of clusters of antigen-antibody by pinocytosis has been clearly visualized, and the movement of proteins within the cell through the actions of the cytoskeletal microfilaments and microtubules has been observed. The bipolar nature of the lipid bilayer of the cell membrane permits the proteins to move through and along the cell membrane, and the cytoskeletal actions of the microfilaments and microtubules facilitate "capping" and non-capping of protein molecule and their reversible distribution within the cell.

Studies of this type in antigenic modulation are now being carried out separately on the T cells and the B cells, and functions and interactions of these immune cells should be elucidated more clearly in the years ahead, along with the interactions between macrophages, T cells, and B cells. Antigen-antibody reactions can now be studied by proteins of known molecular weight and composition, and antigen-antibody anchorage and its modulation can be studied on single cells of the T or B type. This anchorage modulation is known to be mediated by a surface modulating assembly (SMA) consisting of receptors, microfilaments (MF) and microtubules (MT). Local surface modulation can be influenced by proteolytic cleavage enzymes, such as proteases; the interaction between cells is determined by cell-associated molecules (CAM) influenced by proteins, proteolytic enzymes, viruses, and carcinogens.

The sequential expression of enzymes on the cell-associated molecules may be the key to cell growth and differentiation. The redistribution of surface receptors is related to the cross-linking of receptors by divalent antibodies, clustering of similar receptors, and migration of the patches of cross-linked receptors into localized cell caps, where they can be assimilated into the cell by pinocytosis, be shed, or migrate for intracellular functions. The bipolar nature of the cell membrane, combined with the cytoskeletal functions of the microfilaments and microtubules, makes anchorage modulation and capping possible; the microtubules are essential for anchorage modulation but not for capping. The microfilaments provide motion along the membrane; the microtubules permit intracellular transport of assembled molecules.

Immunological studies of this depth are now being conducted on cancer cells, on hybrid cells formed by the fusion of cancer cells with normal cells, and on the interaction of T and B immune cells with cancer cells and viruses. For example, the transplant antigen in animals is the H–2 antigen and in man the HL–A molecules, and is a cell surface antigen or receptor. Recent work has shown that the lysis of tumor cells of viral origin by syngeneic lymphocytes requires the participation of the H–2 antigens on the surface of the tumor cells. The H–2 antigens are the targets in the recognition of the killing event. Capping and patching of the H–2 molecules by appropriately absorbed antiserums that were specific for the H–2 antigen resulted in copatching and cocapping of the viral antigens. The presumption is that the H–2 molecules serve as adaptors that combine with viral antigens in the cell surface to form hybrid antigens containing self (H–2) and non-self (virus). This modulation of the cell surface is recognized by a specific set of antibody receptors on the syngeneic T lymphocytes.

Other experiments have shown that anchorage modulation may be associated with blockade of the commitment of lymphocytes to blast formation and to DNA synthesis. The surface modulating membrane assembly (SMA), particularly its microtubular components, may serve to regulate the biochemical signals inducing cells to mature, undergo mitosis, and divide. The surface modulating assembly controls cell division, movement, and cell-cell interaction. Cell associated molecules (CAM), which may be chemical or viral carcinogens, will interact with the surface modulating assembly and produce the following alterations: cell adhesiveness; immune reactions of cells and their destruction by T and B cells; cell growth and division; contact inhibition and invasiveness.

The investigation of molecular mechanisms of surface modulation in cancer cells in controlled experiments, should clarify cancer immunology. In the meantime, clinicians will continue to work with "cancer-specific antigens," whatever they may be, and with stimulation of normal immune responses by substances like BCG in an effort to enhance immunotherapy in the total treatment of cancer in man.

TUMOR ANGIOGENESIS: 1972–1977

Viruses and antibodies act at the level of the single cell, and their access to the cell is determined by cell surface receptors and cell membrane modulation. Cells in our body are in a continual state of maturation, aging, death and regeneration, but we stay in balance.

Each person regenerates about 10^{20} normal cells every day. A cancer arises from a single deviant cell. It has been calculated that the chance of a single deviant cell becoming a viable growing cancer is in the order of one in 10^{17}. We have explored in detail the molecular basis of quality control in the cell. Folkman has focused his research for a number of years on how a single malignant cell survives and what characteristics it must acquire to become a "successful" tumor (Folkman, 1975).

Folkman has developed simple and beautiful systems for studying tumor growth *in vivo* by transplanting known amounts of tumor into millipore pockets where they can be nourished by diffusion only, and into the cornea and anterior chamber of the rabbit's eye where vascularization can be studied. He also used the chorioallantoic membrane of the chick embryo to study vascularization of tumor implants. Most human cancers arise in the epithelial lining of the bronchus, stomach, colon, uterine cervix, or breast. Normal epithelium is isolated from the vascular system by a basement membrane, and these incipient cancers, termed *in situ* carcinomas, remain harmless and grow very slowly for long periods in an avascular phase.

The critical event that converts a self-contained *in situ* group of malignant cells into a growing cancer comes from vascularization of the tumor. The tumor is no longer nourished by diffusion, but by capillaries and blood vessels richly distributed within it. The vascularization of tumors is triggered by the release of a diffusable chemical into the tumor, a factor not completely isolated and identified as yet, but called tumor angiogenesis factor. This tumor angiogensis factor (TAF) stimulates mitosis in endothelial cells, and rapid formation of new capillaries within the tumor. It is not species specific, has a molecular weight of about 100,000 daltons, and contains 25% RNA, 10% protein, and 5% carbohydrate. It has a lipid coat, is unharmed by trypsin, but is rapidly destroyed by R.N. ase and by heating. Its characteristics permit changes in the surface modulating assembly of the cell membrane and information transfer through R.N.A. No group of malignant cells can reach a size of 33 mm. diameter or greater without producing TAF.

TAF has not been found in normal tissues, in inflamed tissues, nor in tissues stimulated to heal through injury. Some tissues, like cartilage, remains avascular, and cartilage has been shown to have a factor inhibitory to TAF, but this factor has not been accurately identified. Of even greater interest is the relationship of TAF to dormancy in tumors and to tumor progression. The growth of avascular tumor spheroids *in vitro* in nutrient media, with daily changes of fresh media, stops when the spheroid diameter is only 3 to 4 mm., about 10^6 cells. Newly-generated cells at the periphery of the spheroids balance those lost by necrosis in the center. Vascularization of the tumor is impossible and nourishment is only by diffusion. The tumor becomes dormant in the absence of vascularity, and this "dormant diameter" is reached when diffusion of fresh nutrients and elimination of catabolites into the center of the spheroid is reached. The same occurs in man.

The first stage of a tumor is an avascular phase, and the number of growing cells is diffusion-limited. The tumor remains dormant until a humoral factor, TAF, is released and capillary formation is elicited from the host. The tumor is then nourished by capillaries from the host, and the most actively dividing cells are located within 100 microns of the nearest capillary. Typical healthy tumor cells can be adequately supplied with oxygen by diffusion from capillaries for a distance of about 150 microns. The central necrosis of the tumor is then related to the growth of tumor cells in a spheroidal fashion around the capillary until the tumor exceeds 150 microns or 10,000 tumor cells. The cells excessively removed from the capillaries then die from either pressure or lack of oxygen. The vascularized tumor, however, remains malignant, and as growth continues, the cells acquire increasingly harmful properties. Tumor invasion and metastases occur.

Tumors start in an avascular or dormant phase. The penetration of tumors by new capillaries from the host is in response to a humoral stimulus secreted by solid tumors, the tumor angiogenesis factor, TAF. Invasiveness and metastases follow the vascular phase. As the tumor proliferates, variants in the tumor cell arise with increasing malignancy and capabilities for invasiveness and metastases. Malignant growth depends upon TAF, which is an identifiable biochemical product. These concepts point the way to a new approach to cancer therapy, for, in theory, an "antiangiogenesis" factor should limit tumor growth. This substance may be isolated from cartilage, a tissue which remains avascular throughout its normal life. Another possibility is the production of an antibody against TAF, and this now occupies the research efforts of Folkman.

ENVIRONMENTAL CARCINOGENESIS: 1972–1977

We have reviewed in some detail the general problem of carcinogenesis and how cancers of chemical, physical, viral, and other origin ultimately affect the cell membrane and the intracellular apparatus for coding and replication. There is a period of initiation where one of the following ultimately produces cancer: (1) physical agents (X-rays and ultraviolet light, etc.); (2) chemicals, ranging from hydrocarbons to aromatic amines, alkylating agents, nitrosoamines, anesthetic agents, aflatoxins, and plastics; and (3) oncogenic viruses of either the DNA or RNA type, working through an oncogene. But between the initiation and the clinical cancer is a highly variable latent period in which a host of promoting agents, ranging from hormones, mutagens, environmental vectors, dietary habits, and cooking predilections influence the evolution and transmission of the somatic mutation. This whole area might best be called environmental carcinogenesis or co-carcinogenesis. Curiously, it has led to some of the most bitter controversies in our current war on cancer, as administrators, budget analysts, and program planners can envision the prevention of vast numbers of cancers by cleaning up the environment and through targeted research in environmental carcinogenesis. But to scientists it is not an exciting area of basic research, and scientists cannot, with basic knowledge alone, control the economic, emotional, industrial and societal implications of their work. For example, cigarette smoking has long been known to contribute to the growing frequency of lung cancer, but smoking continues undiminished with inconsequential warnings on each pack of cigarettes.

A general list of known environmental carcinogens is listed in Table 1, updated from 1972 (Ryser, 1974). The cyclamate ban continues, but a clear-cut association between cyclamates and cancer has not been proved. It has led many to feel that the laws for newly-introduced, man-made products are far more severe than those applying to natural products and traditional food additives, which might be just as carcinogenic if subjected to the same set of exhaustive tests. The vinyl chloride story, however, has forced controlling government agencies to take a new attitude toward occupational hazards and to react quickly at the first evidence of harm; it also raised the issue of the type and extent of animal research and its significance in the decision-making process. The vinyl chloride risk was widely known even before the first death from liver angiosar-

Table 1: Chemical Carcinogens

Major Classification	Chemical Comopnds	Carcinogenic In Man[18] ($\sqrt{}$)
Polycyclic Aromatic Hydrocarbons	Benzo(a)pyrene Dibenz(a,h)anthracene 7,12-Dimethylbenz(a)anthracene 3-Methylcholanthrene Soots Tars Cigarette smoke	 $\sqrt{}$ $\sqrt{}$ $\sqrt{}$
Aromatic Amines	2-Acetylaminofluorene (AAF) N-Methyl-4-aminoazobenzene (MAB) 2-Naphthylamine N, N-Bis(2-Chloroethyl)-2-naphthylamine Benzidine 4-Aminobiphenyl 3-Hydroxyanthranilic acid 3-Hydroxyxanthine	 $\sqrt{}$ $\sqrt{}$ $\sqrt{}$ $\sqrt{}$
Aklylating Agents	β-Propiolactone Diepoxybutane and other epoxides Ethylene imines Methylmethane-sulfonate and other sulfones Nitrogen mustard and derivatives Mustard gas (bis(2-Chloroethyl)sulfide)	 $\sqrt{}$ $\sqrt{}$
Nitrosamines and Other Nitroso-compounds	Dimenthylnitrosamine Diethylnitrosamine 4-Nitroquinoline-1-oxide N-Methy-N'-nitro-N-nitrosoguanidine 4-Nitrobiphenyl	 $\sqrt{}$
Naturally Occurring Products	Aflatoxin B_1 Cycasin Pyrrolizidine alkaloids Safrole 3-Hydroxyanthranilic acid Griseofulvin Mitomycin C Actinomycin D Betel nut	$\sqrt{}$
Drugs	Nitrogen mustards (Ex. cyclophosphamid, chlorambucil, etc.) Griseofulvin Hycanthone Metronidazole Diethylstilbestrol	$\sqrt{}$
Metals	Nickel compounds Chromium compounds Cadmium compounds Asbestos (calcium-magnesium silicate fibers)	$\sqrt{}$ $\sqrt{}$ $\sqrt{}$ $\sqrt{}$
Industrial Carcinogens	Vinyl chloride Chloromethyl methyl ether	$\sqrt{}$ $\sqrt{}$
Miscellaneous	Ethionine Carbon tetrachloride Ethyl carbamate (Urethane) Thiourea	

coma was reported. It was recognized that vinyl chloride workers suffered more frequently from numb hands and fingertips, a condition called acro-osteolysis, than the normal population, and experimental studies trying to produce acro-osteolysis showed that rats exposed to 250 parts per million vinyl chloride developed liver cancer. The Russians had reported hepatitis-like changes in 1949, abnormal liver function tests were detected in the 1950's, and Dow chemical found that exposure to greater than 50 parts per million could induce changes in liver function. It was not until 1973, however, that information of this type reached the doctors caring for vinyl chloride workers or the U.S. National Institute for Occupational Safety and Health. However, after the first recorded liver deaths from angiosarcoma in man in November of 1973, in a Goodrich plant in Kentucky, Dr. Creech met with the company officials, and by January 1974 Goodrich informed the National Institute of Occupational Safety and Health. The swiftness of response with new research, and a federal investigation focusing on ways to mitigate the vinyl chloride problems and avoid future problems of that type, has been unprecedented. Vinyl chloride gas has virtually been eliminated from both industrial and everyday environment. How different from cigarette smoke!

Environmental and occupational health has become a high-priority item in the prevention of cancer. Refrigeration is credited with a decline in the incidence of stomach cancer by reducing the conversion of nitrate to nitrite in foods. Colon cancer is almost unheard of in Africa, but very common in Western countries, apparently related to the low fibre content of Western food. This low fibre content lengthens intestinal transit time, and increases the anaerobic bacteria in stool. These bacteria degrade bile salts and result in toxic products which are carcinogenic, so current theory goes. Gastric cancer is higher in Japan and Russia, related to carcinogens in their pickles, bracken plant, and seaweed. Rice is often coated with glucose and talc, and the talc contains asbestos-like compounds, known carcinogens. Smoked fish and mutton contain various carcinogenic benzpyrenes, and these same compounds are present in coal soot. One quarter of the drugs prescribed for hypertension in the U.S. have a reserpine base, and concern has been expressed that reserpine and other Rauwolfia synthetics increase two or threefold the likelihood of developing breast cancer. Leukemia seems higher in incidence to those exposed in synthetic rubber plants and also to those working with constant X-ray exposure. Acrylic and plastic plant workers have a higher incidence of cancer generally. Many of the aniline derivatives and chemicals that comprise hair dyes and sprays are polycyclic hydrocarbons that could be carcinogenic. Multivariant statistical analysis indicates that in Louisiana those drinking water from the Mississippi River have a higher incidence of total cancer, cancer of the urinary tract, and gastrointestinal cancer than those who drank water from other sources, linking carcinogens in drinking water to cancer. Materials used in fire-proofing children's clothing, water, food, asbestos, vinyl chloride, and commonly used plastics, all have carcinogenic consequences either in their production or consumption. Evidence is mounting that prolonged exposure to multiple carcinogens has an accelerating effect on the incidence of cancer. Even saccharin is being banned from widespread use as a food sweetener. Nicotine still is permitted widespread use, with just minimal admonitions to the smoker; yet 93,000 new cases of cancer of the lung still appear every year in our statistical analysis of lung cancer.

The relationship of hormones to cancer deserves special analysis from both etiologic and therapeutic implications. The use of female sex hormones, both natural and synthetic, is widespread for a host of common gynecologic problems, ranging from contraception to menopausal complaints. Evidence is mounting to support the belief that female sex hormones are truly environmental carcinogens, and their ubiquitous, protracted use can be related to three cancers: (1) the uncommon vaginal adenosis or clear-cell carcinomas in the vaginal epithelium of young girls; (2) carcinoma of the endometrium or body of the uterus, which has a rising incidence in recent years; and (3) carcinomas of the breast. The relationships are complex, however, and since hormones may also have beneficial effects in the treatment of certain cancers, the entire subject of hormones and cancer will be discussed in a separate section on *Hormones and Hormonal Therapy of Cancer.* (See pages 361–368)

The relationship of fallout irradiation to thyroid cancer has recently been reviewed in followup studies on a group of Marshall Islanders and Japanese fishermen in Rongelap. The fallout on their skin, food, and water has been estimated at 220–450 rads to adults and 700–1400 rads to children, in terms of iodine isotopes going to the thyroid. By 1974, 27 of 86 exposed people on Rongelap had thyroid nodules, the heaviest incidence being in those exposed under

10 years of age. Twenty-four of these nodules have been operated upon with 3 cancers being found, of the papillary type, and cervical metastases were present in two. Thyroxine did not inhibit development of the tumors, but apparently reduced their frequency. The incidence of thyroid tumors per rad is higher in children because the gland is smaller and the radiation dose larger. Radio-iodine treatment of hyperthyroidism is not to be compared to these figures, for the dose is so much greater, and the thyroid cell is destroyed rather than stimulated. (Parker, Belsky, Pamamoto, *et. al.,* 1974).

Tobacco radioactivity and cancer in smokers has also been explored in the past 5 years. Low concentrations of 210 Po (polonium 210), an alpha emitting particle, have been observed in tobacco and cigarette smoke. The cumulative a-radiation dose from inhaled 210 Po to bronchial epithelium may well be a factor in the carcinogenesis of cigarette smoke, as plutonium 210 becomes highly concentrated in insoluble smoke particles and has a half-life of over 20 years. The insoluble particles accumulate in the lung and lymph nodes and add to the carcinogenicity of tobacco tars. Direct mutations of the chromosomes occur in areas surrounding the insoluble plutonium 210 particles, probably from alpha irradiation.

In the last 5 years, cancer has come to be regarded as a social disease, with its causative factors rooted in environment, diet, water, plastics, fertilizers, herbicides, hair sprays, industrial chemicals, hormones, and atmospheric pollutants; in short in our technology and our economy. We are continually being led into new health hazards through unknown chemical compounds brought into our environment for the benefit of comfort, ease of living, science, industry, labor, government, and mankind. But we cannot afford to release many products which in 25 to 30 years will cause, in America alone, over 80,000 deaths per year—the lung cancer death rate at the moment. Prevention of this type of cancer will require the coordinated efforts of government, the scientific community, industry, labor, and epidemiological centers linked to appropriate data-collecting systems. Excluding additional carcinogenic factors from our environment is imperative, but the relentless, yet painfully slow, progression from carcinogen to cancer makes knowledge about each agent hard to come by. The relationship of chemicals to industry, technology, and science, and to the economy of our society, is such that we do not wish to exclude their production and use unless they are an imminent hazard to society. How do we test for carcinogenicity and imminent hazards?

The traditional way to test a chemical for carcinogenicity is to see whether it causes cancer in inbred animals of low cancer strains. It takes controlled experiments over a 2 to 3 year period at a cost of over $100,000 per chemical. Not to be ignored is the fact these test animals live under sex-free, no exercise conditions, with unknown virus contamination. Quick and inexpensive tests are being developed, but their value is controversial. The best one at the moment is the Ames test, based on the premise that carcinogenic agents produce mutations and damage to the DNA of the cell. A bacterial system is employed, based on the fact that Salmonella typhinurium has lost its ability to make the amino acid histidine. In a histidine-free culture medium, any mutation of the bacterium exposed to mutagenic chemicals enables the organism to again make histidine, and thereby grow in a histidine-free culture medium. It is quick, simple, and inexpensive, but man is not a bacterium, and false positives and false negatives can occur. Nevertheless, the test costs only $200, takes 3 days to perform, and is now being used as a screening agent. Chemicals giving a carcinogenic reaction are further tested in experimental animals. But responses in the human population is what we must know; that can only be obtained by recording the cancer history of men exposed to chemicals at work and to drugs in their daily existence. We must, through epidemiological studies in man, discover the existing factors in our environment that account for the 50% of cancers thought to be due to environmental chemicals. Appropriate laboratory facilities, linked to epidemiological data-recording with integration of knowledge, will serve man far better than quick tests in cells and animals.

EARLY DIAGNOSIS OF CANCER: 1972–1977

In the United States there are about 665,000 new cases diagnosed and 360,000 deaths each year from cancer. If detected early enough, half of the cancers could be cured by existing methods of treatment —surgery, irradiation, chemotherapy, hormonal therapy, and immunotherapy, used alone or in combination. Early detection is the key to saving more lives among those succumbing to cancer. Cancer of the breast and cancer of the uterine cervix are the two most common cancers in women. Cancer of the breast remains the leading cause of cancer death in women. There are about 89,000 new cases a year, and the death rate is 33,000 a year; but most distressing is the fact that the age adjusted death rate per 100,000 population has remained the same—22 to 25 per 100,000—since 1940, in spite of publicity about early diagnosis and improvements in total therapy. There are, on the other hand, about 40,000 cases each year of early diagnosis of uterine cancer through the use of the Papanicolau test. At the early (or *in situ*) stage, uterine cancer is curable by very simple surgical techniques. 46,000 cases of true uterine cancer still occur each year; the death rate is about 11,000 yearly; but the age-adjusted death rate per 100,000 population has dropped from 20 to 9, over 50%, attributed to the widening acceptance of the Pap test as part of a regular, yearly physical examination.

The high-risk groups of women in the U.S. apt to get breast cancer are: (1) those over 35 years of age; (2) those who have never had a child; (3) those who bore their first child after 25; (4) those with a family history of breast cancer; and (5) those with early menarche or late menopause.

Early detection of breast cancer became the major focus of clinical interest and effort of both the National Cancer Institute and the American Cancer Society in 1974. Eradication of breast cancer was seen as the major drive in the war against cancer. It was known that if breast cancer were recognized in the early stages, before it was 2 cm. in size and before it had metastasized to any lymph node (while it was small and localized to the breast), it could be cured in 80% of the cases by existing therapy. Yet, in 1973 about 90% of breast lumps were still detected first by women in self-examination of their breasts. Eradication of deaths from breast cancer depended upon detection and treatment before a lump could be palpated clinically, i.e. before the lump was 1 cm. in size. This required screening of large numbers of women in special centers where the latest diagnostic techniques of thermography and xeroradiography could be combined with clinical acumen. All cases could be detected while still curable.

The National Cancer Institute and the American Cancer Society launched a dramatic attack on breast cancer. Twenty-seven breast cancer detection demonstration projects were established, each to screen at least 5000 cases yearly by: (1) a detailed history; (2) careful clinical examination; (3) mammography with low-radiation X-rays; and (4) thermography, analysis of the heat pattern of the breast. Each center was to screen at least 5000 cases on year one and year two; these 10,000 women were to be followed and rescreened regularly for 10 more years. Nearly 300,000 women would be involved in this unprecedented cancer detection and treatment program, hoping to answer such questions as: (1) Who is in the high risk group? (2) What relation does the pill and hormones have to breast cancer? (3) What is the natural history of breast cancer? (4) Can sophisticated techniques of mammography and thermography accurately detect early cancer? and (5) Does localized breast cancer detected in the *in situ* stage, or prior to reaching a size of 1 cm., require a mastectomy or modified radical mastectomy? The model for these centers was the background experience of Dr. Strax, who had been working in breast cancer detection screening with the Hospital Insurance Plan of Greater New York (HIP) since 1968. The HIP study showed that: (1) the death rate had been lowered in the early detection group by 33%; (2) that 33% of these cancers would have been missed by clinical examination alone; and (3) that of the 44 cancers detected by mammography alone, only 1 patient died in the succeeding 5 years. The news media, television, volunteer workers, and the excitement about preventing deaths from breast cancer filled the demonstration clinics with an abundance of patients.

Thermography would be ideal as a screening tool, for it is safe, simple, inexpensive, and harmless. But, since it is dependent upon detection of temperature variations of very slight degree over the entire breast, the indexes of suspicion are so high and the true-positive levels are so low that it can not be used alone to detect stage 1 or earlier carcinomas of the breast. Furthermore, it does not localize abnormalities in a manner which permits operative removal of the lesion unless the growth can be felt clinically. Mammography, on the other hand, has a high index of suspicion with reasonable accuracy, in fact better than clinical judgment in early cancer. The radiological false positive rate is about 50%; the clinical false positive rate is about 75% in very early or occult breast lesions. The diagnosis of occult breast carcinoma is possible with mammography, and mammography permits accurate localization so that surgical removal of the lesion is straightforward and simple.

The diagnosis of cancer is still a histological one, based upon removal of the lesion for microscopic examination. The early diagnosis of breast cancer has become a combined clinical and radiological study—occult carcinomas are best suspected and detected by mammography, the diagnosis of cancer is dependent upon removal of the lesion surgically. All palpable breast tumors are best subjected to microscopic examination. Perforce, occult lesions appearing on mammography will now be operated upon, and many very early cancers will be detected. Yet at least half of these, and probably many more as statistics grow, will prove to be benign. How long the occult cancers have been present prior to detection is still unknown, and what the best treatment is for occult breast cancer remains to be defined.

The yield in xeromammography, now being done more commonly than film mammography but involving the same accuracy, is about 1 case of occult carcinoma per thousand patients screened (1 per 1000). This includes both symptomatic and asymptomatic cases. Axillary node involvement with tumor has been found in 25% of the cases of occult carcinoma, in contrast to the usual 45% incidence of nodal involvement in cases of non-occult carcinoma. A very early new entity is being found, called carcinoma *in situ,* and the treatment for this remains to be defined. Some carcinoma simply escape detection on xeroradiography, and breast biopsy must still be done, if a clinical suspicion of carcinoma exists. The radiological findings include a localized mass, clustered or linearly arranged tiny calcifications, asymmetrical ductal prominence, and any local disturbance of breast architecture. Everyone agrees xeroradiography finds its greatest indication in following the opposite breast in a woman with known breast cancer, and it is extremely useful in screening patients in the high-risk group for mammary cancer. It serves also as a useful baseline for future clinical and radiological evaluations. Diagnostic accuracy is definitely decreased in dense breasts with relatively little fat, unfortunately the situation in women 35 to 45. The radiological false positive rate is 50%, but this seems acceptable when one considers that the danger is high from missing an early cancer and the risk low from biopsy.

Over 270,000 women have now had one or more breast X-rays in the 27 centers throughout the United States, and the value of mammography in finding early and occult breast cancer, presumably curable, has been established. But, like clinical examination, to be of real value it must be repeated on a yearly basis. Concern over the potential risks and hazards of mammography began to appear early in 1976, when a report on the long term followup of 30,000 women in the Health Insurance Plan of New York patients demonstrated that they had discovered and saved over a 20 year period 12 women from breast cancer, but had possibly induced 11 to 12 new breast cancers from the total irradiation exposure over the 15 year period

(Bailar, 1976). With the initial breast mammograms with conventional techniques, the exposure dose per examination was 4 to 6 rads. Low dose mammography, with films of high sensitivity, deliver 1.5 to 2.5 rads per exposure, and the current techniques of xeroradiography impose a dose of 1.5 to 2.5 rads per examination. Mammography is also less productive in women under 50, as the pre-menopausal breast produces a dense radiologic pattern and tends to obscure underlying disease. Yet breast cancer hits its first peak of occurrence in women 40 to 45.

During the past year the happy assessment of mammography has turned into a perplexing controversy. Of the 270,000 women in the NIH study, with some now having had 3 mammograms on a yearly basis, the yield has been 1100 cancers found—300 in women under 50, but only 100 detected by mammography alone; 800 in women over 50, with 280 attributable to mammographic detection. It has been postulated from current knowledge on women exposed to irradiation (Hiroshima, Nagasaki, fluoroscopy for tuberculosis) that 50 to 100 rads of irradiation to the breast would increase the likelihood of getting cancer by 1%, from 0.07 to 0.0707, over a lifetime. The radiation hazards at this rate for women under 50 exceeds the benefits, and most certainly for women under 35. Furthermore, the statistical review of the HIP data, gathered since 1960, on 62,000 women, half of whom had routine yearly mammograms and the other half who merely had routine clinical examination, showed no change in the mortality rate of women under 50 from breast cancer, whether it was discovered early by mammography or merely routinely on examination. The increased incidence of breast cancer in the irradiated group was slight but noticeable.

Statistics are not the last word, and there are hidden benefits in screening programs other than mortality rates. The educational value alone has been of inestimable value. Less radical treatment has been necessary for the cases detected early with increased pleasure in living, and the concept of exploring cancer diagnosis and treatment on controlled clinical trials may improve tremendously all aspects of cancer diagnosis and treatment. Nevertheless, at the moment the National Cancer Institute affirms the value of mammography in the detection of breast cancer, particularly in high-risk women, but prudently suggests that routine mammography in women under 50 on a regular basis should not be urged until the current data from their 27 screening programs can be more fully evaluated. In women over 50, particularly if they fall in a high risk group for breast cancer occurrence, mammography remains the best diagnostic technique for the detection of early and occult breast cancer. The National Academy of Science report states, in effect, that if a million women are each given a single rad at the end of 10 years, an additional 6 cases of cancer will occur among these women; at present it is believed that each additional rad augments the risk at the identical rate, whether it be rad 3 or rad 43. Final decisions on the National Cancer Screening Program will not be reached until all evidence has been evaluated by 3 special committees during 1976.

Screening programs for organs other than the breast have developed during the past 5 years, but most of them employ endoscopic, cytologic, radiologic, xeroradiographic, radio-isotopic or ultrasonic techniques. They are rather expensive, are site-oriented rather than general, and require a rather large critical size for detection—the tumor must already have been in existence for many doubling times (months to years) before the critical size has been reached for detection. Many scientists are working on tests of universal application irrespective of tumor size and site. But none so far has emerged with adequate sensitivity and specificity. The tests being studied with zeal include: (1) immunological approaches with search for common or specific tumor antigens; (2) macrophage electrophoretic mobility tests (MEM) for cell-mediated responses; and (3) search for embryonic or neo-natal antigens, such as the carcino-embryonic antigen and the foetal globulins. At the moment, no simple general test in blood, urine, or other bodily substances exists. The challenge remains, but most workers believe the answer lies in the onco-fetal antigens. Their use as test antigens in a sensitive cell-mediated immune system (MEM) may someday enable us to diagnose and localize primary tumors through assay of body fluids.

MAJOR METHODS OF CANCER TREATMENT: 1972–1977

The major methods for therapy of malignant disease remain: (1) surgical removal of the tumor; (2) radiological treatment; and (3) chemotherapy. These major therapeutic weapons may be used separately, sequentially, or conjointly, depending upon the nature of the tumor, its origin and sites of metastases. The past 5 years, however, have seen a change in therapy related to earlier diagnosis of many cancers while they are still contained and non-invasive, a better understanding of the kinetics of cell growth (cytokinetics), and a realization that disseminated disease might still be controlled and the quality of life improved for variable periods of time by combinations of therapy and alteration of the environment of the host. The new methods of therapy currently under intensive investigation in the clinical setting are: (1) multi-modality therapy; and (2) immunotherapy. Before we dwell upon the newer concepts of tumor therapy, it might be well to review the principles of established therapy in each therapeutic approach in light of current knowledge. The model for discussion will again be the most common cancer in women, that of the breast, for cancer of the breast and malignant melanoma have been the two cancers in which controlled clinical experiments in newest methods of therapy have been vigorously studied.

SURGICAL THERAPY

There are basically two stages in a malignant disease. In the first stage the tumor is still localized and is potentially curable by adequate or radical local surgery. In the second stage the disease becomes disseminated and local therapy alone can not cure the illness. Dissemination can occur through the blood stream, in which event only the defenses of the host or chemotherapy could possibly control it. Dissemination can be halted, if it occurs through the lymphatics, by the regional lymph nodes, which are the first line of defense in the immunological containment of tumor. Once the regional lymphatic barrier is breached, the tumor spreads from the regional lymph nodes into the blood stream. The classical surgical approach to cancer has been to remove the local tumor widely, together with the regional lymph nodes to which it first tends to spread.

In the last 5 years, the role of the regional lymph nodes in the immunological defense of the host against the spread of tumor into the blood stream has led many surgeons to feel that if they are not involved with tumor, there is no need to remove them. Indeed, possible harm may ensue from breaching a normal immunological barrier. If they are involved with tumor, they might harbor the last remaining tumor cells in the host, in which event their removal would be curative; or tumor cells might already have escaped from them into the blood stream, in which event their removal would not be helpful. Clearly, what is needed is a method of detecting tumors at all sites in the body, whether they be primary or secondary. The results obtained with the best present methods are helpful, if positive, but disappointing in the frequency with which they fail to detect small deposits of metastatic tumor. Isotopic techniques are currently the most reliable, and include the bone scintigram, liver scans, gallium scans, and special isotopes for organs like the brain and thyroid. Radiological examinations of the lungs and bones are also desirable, and supplement scintographic studies.

Concerns of this type, about the significance of the lymph nodes in immunological defense against cancer and the inability to detect distant metastases in 15 to 20% of the cases prior to surgical removal of breast cancer, have led surgeons to be more conservative in their approach to surgical eradication of breast cancer. The most common operation done today for operable breast cancer is the modified radical mastectomy. This entirely removes the breast and the axillary lymph nodes, but preserves the pectoral muscles of the chest wall in the hope of preventing complications of the radical classical mastectomy, particularly the problems of post-operative swelling of the arm. Controversy exists, however, and some notable surgeons remove only the breast, and do not touch the axillary lymph nodes unless they seem involved at the time of simple mastectomy. They claim no harm is done by waiting until the lymph nodes become engorged by tumor prior to removing them, and removal of the lymph nodes is done at a second stage, if and when they become clinically enlarged. National protocols with random selection of patients are being conducted in America and in England in an effort to decide which surgical procedure is best for the early stages of breast cancer. Until these controlled studies yield a definitive answer, most surgeons are currently doing the modified radical mastectomy.

Equally important is the question of whether or not adjuvant chemotherapy should be routinely given to control any unknown distant metastases. The use of routine, post-operative X-ray therapy as a surgical adjunctive treatment has led to the conclusion that such routine therapy might reduce the incidence of local recurrence of cancer in the operative area; but it does not prevent silent distant metastases from growing, and, indeed, may weaken normal immunological defenses of the host to the point that these silent metastases may grow out more rapidly. The 5-year survival results are statistically a little less favorable after routine post-operative

X-ray therapy in both the groups with and without positive lymph node metastases. The hope is that adjuvant chemotherapy will kill off distant silent metastases and improve the 5-year survival rates after surgery in all patients, whether or not the regional lymph nodes are involved (Fisher *et al.,* 1975). These national protocols are being conducted at the present time, and the initial results after 2 years of effort will be discussed under the new approach of multimodality therapy.

The emphasis on early diagnosis of breast cancer has led to the recognition of a clinical group of cases called "minimal breast cancer." These include the very early cancers found in the microcalcifications on xeroradiography, and the cases with microscopic cancer in masses no greater than 0.5 cm. in size, or the histological types called lobular carcinoma *in situ,* lobular carcinoma, noninvasive lobular or ductal carcinoma, and the intra-cystic carcinomas or multiple papillomatosis. These are cancers in the preclinical stage both non-infiltrating and infiltrating in type which most phsyicians believe are highly curable. Many feel that even the modified radical mastectomy is unnecessary for cure in this group, and are doing only partial mastectomy or simple mastectomy without gland dissection and, indeed, later breast reconstructions in these minimal breast cancer patients. A whole new spectrum of breast cancer in its formative stages has been disclosed by these ancillary diagnostic techniques of xeroradiography and sensitive-film mammography. It may be that we are merely detecting these breast cancers at an earlier time period in the natural history of the disease, and statistics still do not show any change in the mortality rate of women under 50 from current therapy of breast cancer.

Most breast cancers are of multi-focal origin in the involved breast, leading most surgeons to perform simple mastectomy for even the early minimal cases. Unfortunately, if the patient lives long enough the likelihood of developing a cancer in the opposite breast ranges between 15 to 30%, depending upon the histological type of the tumor. Some surgeons favor doing a mirror biopsy of the opposite breast routinely in all patients of reasonable age, but most surgeons prefer to follow the opposite breast carefully with repeated clinical examinations every few months and xeroradiograms at yearly to longer intervals. If there is a strong family history of breast cancer, or if the patient falls into the high-risk group for developing cancer in the opposite breast prophylactic, simple mastectomy is commonly done. The emotional attitude of the patient towards contralateral biopsy and prophylactic simple mastectomy is of overriding importance in making a definitive decision, and this decision must be a cooperative venture between physician and patient based upon an individual assessment of uncertain risks and emotional consequences, varying from patient to patient.

Surgery is simple and direct. Whatever is removed is 100% destroyed. Inherent in the operation for cancer is the optimistic possibility of removing every last living cancer cell in the patient. If every last living cell is removed, the cancer is cured. The earlier the cancer is operated upon, the more likely it is to be completely removed, as the less likely it is that the cancer has spread to the lymph nodes or to the blood stream, making surgical cure less likely or impossible. At best surgery cures; at worst it decreases the tumor burden proportional to its total reduction of tumor mass or debulking of the tumor burden. Operative reduction of tumor burden improves the success of multimodality therapy of cancer.

RADIATION THERAPY

Just as surgery for cancer is being influenced by the evolving concepts of staging and invasiveness, lymph node functions, adjunctive therapy, and immunological concepts of tumor-host interaction (reducing the tumor-burden or debulking of cancer), so radiation therapy has been responsive to its changing role in the total spectrum of cancer therapy. The radiation therapist has had to broaden his perspective and become a radiation oncologist, sensitive not only to the role of irradiation in the induction of cancer, but to the benefits of combining radiation therapy with surgery, chemotherapy, hormonal therapy, and immunotherapy of cancer in the treatment of cancer.

Radiation therapy, like surgery, is a local, not systemic, type of treatment. It destroys cancer in a local area, focusing and distributing the electromagnetic particles from the therapy machines so that the maximum dose is received by the cancer and minimal damage is done to surrounding tissues. The high-energy machines, the cobalt machines, and the linear accelerators have definitely and completely achieved pride of place in conventional therapy. Their 2 million to 4 million volt high-energy electromagnetic particles can be easily focused, have little side scatter as they penetrate the tissues, and produce minimal damage to skin and surrounding structures.

They are best given in fractionated divided doses, 200 rads a day, 5 days a week, as a general rule. The usual cancers require 5000 to 6000 rads for destruction. The more primitive or embryological the tissue, the more sensitive it is to destruction by irradiation. Hypoxia adds to the radioresistance of irradiated cells. Oxygen comes through the capillaries, and cells more than 120 mu from capillaries receive little or no oxygen and become radioresistant. Oxygen is a requirement for the killing effect of electromagnetic irradiation, a photon type of irradiation rather than particle irradiation. In the absence of oxygen, 3 times as much irradition, regardless of energy source of the electromagnetic particle, is required for killing of the cell. The photons, as they pass through tissue in the presence of oxygen, cause ionization, and the ionization produces active radicles which are combinations of ions and oxygen. These active radicles destroy the DNA of the cell and result in cell death. Tumor angiogenesis factor determines the oxygenation of tissue; irradiation in the presence of oxygen destroys the DNA of the cell.

The relationship of radiosensitivity to oxygen tension of cells led to irradiation treatment in chambers of high-oxygen tension. Hyperbaric oxygen chambers, however, have not proved practical in irradiation therapy, and controlled studies in the clinical setting have never been completed to show improved results from hyperoxygenation. This work has now been abandoned, as the field has moved in other directions exploring new radiation particles, which may not be oxygen dependent—the pi mesons, for example.

Irradiation kills cells in a logarithmic manner. The bigger the tumor, the greater the difficulty in killing every last tumor cell, as large tumors have many areas of low oxygenation and large numbers of live cells regenerating from incomplete destruction. Debulking of the tumor by surgical or chemotherapeutic means is, therefore, an adjunct to irradition therapy; these techniques not only reduce the number of tumor cells to be killed by irradition, but the smaller size of the residual tumor also enhances its oxygenation.

The cell cycle has become increasingly important in radiotherapy, for cells are most susceptible to the damaging effects of irradiation in the beginning of the G1 phase and most resistant at the end of the S phase. The synchronization of cell growth into a uniform cell cycle would also be extremely valuable in chemotherapy. But from the practical clinical standpoint, it has not been achieved for either irradiation therapy or chemotherapy. Debulking of the tumor, combined with irradiation therapy and chemotherapy, has proved most valuable in the management of malignant sarcomas and myosarcomas of the soft parts.

The logarithmic kill of tumor cells by irradiation, and the advantage of starting radiation therapy with the smallest possible number of tumor cells, has led to an increasing use of prophylactic irradiation therapy to regional lymph nodes in selected cancers. This is particularly true in cancers of the head and neck, inner quadrant cancers of the breast which may well spread to mediastinal lymph nodes, and cancers of the cervix and testes. The staging of tumors has been particularly important in the lymphoblastomas and in Hodgkin's disease. For example, it is so important to know the status of the spleen, liver, and retroperitoneal nodes that exploratory lapartotomy is used in addition to scintigraphic and lymphangiographic techniques in staging. All localized tumor which is radiosensitive can then be treated with accuracy, and cases with non-localized tumors can be treated by combinations of radiotherapy and chemotherapy.

The crucial and limiting factor in radiation therapy remains the difference in radiosensitivity between the cancer cell and the normal cell. The new machines enable proper penetration of the radiation beam to the site of the tumor with sharp localization of the maximal effects of ionizing radiation to the cancer. However, normal surrounding tissues are also affected to varying degrees. Modern simulators enable accurate calculation and plotting of isodose curves of radiation as the ionizing particles penetrate the tissue, but one must always stop the irradiation before irreparable damage is done to the normal surrounding tissue. The spinal cord, kidney, heart, lungs, and bowel may also be easily damaged by doses of irradiation required to kill adjoining cancers, and limit the total dose of irradiation which can be administered to neighboring cancers. Skin necrosis is rare now with modern machines, but radionecrosis of bone is still a difficult problem in treating mouth, breast, and extremity cancers.

Current research in radiotherapy envisions the possibility of using non-electromagnetic particles which would escape the oxygen effects discussed above. The oxygen effect is not so apparent in particle irradiation with neutrons, negative pi mesons, and stripped helium ions. Much money and equipment of a very expensive nature is required to develop radiation beams with these particles, yet Negative pi meson generators are now being constructed. A target can be activated by a highly energetic electron beam of about 700 million electron volts generated by a 250 foot linear accelerator. The target emits nuclear particles of many types, and the negative pi mesons can be gathered and focused by electromagnetic fields. These negative pi mesons can then be introduced in the patient through innumerable small ports around the circumference of the patient, and discharge their maximal energy into the delineated area of the cancer. Machines of this type are now being tested with respect to the radiation physics and biological consequences of these new irradiation particles. The future of radiation therapy with new types of non-electromagnetic particles is rich in promise.

CHEMOTHERAPY

Cancer chemotherapy has become increasingly effective in the past 5 years. The indications for treatment of particular malignant diseases have been clarified; new anti-cancer drugs and drug combinations have emerged; new ways of utilizing drugs in association with radiation therapy and surgery have developed; and the relationship between drug-kinetics and tumor-cell kinetics has passed from scientific theory to clinical usefulness. But drugs remain toxic, have harmful side-effects on normal cells, and, with few exceptions, attenuate but do not completely eradicate the cancer. Effective cancer therapy however, almost invariably includes chemotherapy as a further dimension to multi-modality cancer therapy.

Most chemotherapeutic agents affect DNA synthesis of the cell, and the percentage of cells growing and the rapidity of their growth determines in part the effectiveness of the agent. Unfortunately, the normal cells of the bone marrow, gastro-intestinal tract, and the hair follicles also turn over rapidly, and these agents produce toxicity characterized by anemia, leukopenia (infection) thrombocytopenia (bleeding), diarrhea, vomiting, surface ulcerations, and baldness. Fortunately, the toxic symptoms revert on alteration or cessation of drug administration. We need new agents that act specifically against tumor cells rather than normal cells; these specific agents should be active regardless of the state of the cell cycle, that is against resting cells as well as active cells synthesizing DNA. This goal has not been achieved, but in recent years therapy has been modified through this better understanding of the role of cell-cycle in treatment.

The cell undergoes mitosis or divides at the G2 phase. Following the D phase is a variable period of time, the G1 phase, a growth phase during which active RNA synthesis and protein synthesis occur. The duration of G1 phase is the most variable in any cell, is short in very rapidly proliferating cells and in malignant cells, but is long in slow growing cells. From G1 the cell passes into the S phase, or phase of DNA synthesis. This phase requires purine and pyrimidine biosynthesis, and other enzymes necessary for nucleic acid and DNA synthesis. The S phase continues until the DNA content of the cell doubles, and then the cell passes over into the G2 phase. RNA synthesis and protein synthesis occur in the G2 phase, before the cell can construct a mitotic apparatus and begin division (Kaplan, 1964). Replicating cells are most sensitive to attack by the anti-metabolites during the S phase; mitotic inhibitors exert their influence during the G2 phase. In recent years, although the distinction is not absolute, agents have been classified into *cell-cycle specific* or *phase specific* and *cell-cycle non-specific* or *phase non-specific agents,* and chemotherapists try to use combinations of agents which will kill cancer cells during both proliferative and resting phases. Analysis of new drugs requires the most careful clinically-controlled studies wherein adequate numbers of patients can be soundly analyzed with biostatistical support. The problems which controlled clinical trials help solve include: (1) the appropriate timing of administration of the agent in the cell cycle; (2) the advantages of multiple agent therapy, each acting in a different manner at a different stage of the cell cycle; (3) interaction of drugs with normal host defense mechanisms; and (4) methods of detecting and destroying the last remnants of partially-destroyed cancers.

No chemotherapeutic agent is yet available that can kill cancer cells selectively without damaging normal cells to some degree; nor is any anti-neoplastic drug capable of killing all cancer cells at any given exposure. Cancerocidal drugs kill in a log fashion. In advanced malignancy the tumor burden may be 10^{17} cells, approximately 1 Kg. of tumor. The best one can accomplish with a single maximal exposure to a cancer-killing drug is between 2 to 5 logs of cell kill. It is apparent that treatment must be repeated many times in order to achieve even partial control, particularly since not all cells are active and at identical stages of the cell cycle. Indeed, chemotherapeutic agents may never be capable of totally eradicating any given population of tumor cells. Immunological therapy, in theory, does not face this restriction, but it is most effective against small amounts of tumor in the order of 1mg. or less. The possible advantage of combining chemotherapy and immunotherapy is immediately apparent, in theory.

Most of the commonly used anti-cancer drugs suppress both cellular and humoral immunity. We have already emphasized the increased occurrence of lymphoreticular types of cancer in the immunologically-suppressed patient who has lost normal immunological surveillance. Fortunately, the immunosuppressive effects of most drugs do not extend for prolonged periods of time beyond the period of active drug administration. The distribution, route of administration and absorption, biotransformation, excretion, interaction, and resistance to the drug are all of extreme importance. Intermittent, intensive courses of chemotherapy appear to suppress immune competence much less than continuous, low-dose chemotherapy. Response to chemotherapy also correlates with the normal immunological responsiveness of the host. Combination chemotherapy increases the log kill and permits attack at different phases of the cell cycle. The scheduling of chemotherapeutic agents has moved in recent years into short, intensive courses of therapy with combined agents given at intermittent, repeated intervals. Not only is destruction of the cancer cells increased and more normal immunological surveillance preserved, but the susceptibility to unusual fulminating infections has also been reduced by skillful and judicious use of combination chemotherapy, pulsed, and intermittent. Medical oncologists understand all these problems best, for drug scheduling, combination chemotherapy, and multi-modality therapy have become the order of the day.

The treatment of any specific case of cancer requires the skill and judgment of a knowledgeable physician. The diversity of problems in most cancers demands cooperation between surgeon, radiation therapist, chemotherapist, and immunotherapist for optimal total care of the cancer patient. Before proceeding to discuss the concepts of a multi-modality therapy, it might be well to review the classes of chemoterapeutic agents currently available and the current status of clinical cancer chemotherapy shown in the excellent charts taken from Cline and Haskell's recent book, *Cancer Chemotherapy*.

Table 2: Classes of Chemotherapeutic Agents

Class of Compound	Examples	Diseases in Which Useful
Alkylating agents	Nitrogen mustard, chlorambucil, cyclophosphamide, busulfan	Lymphomas, many solid tumors, chronic leukemia, multiple myeloma
Antimetabolites	1. Methotrexate 2. 6-Mercaptopurine 3. Cytosine arabinoside 4. 5-Fluorouracil	1–3. Acute leukemia 1. Choriocarcinoma, head and neck cancer 4. Carcinoma of breast, carcinoma of G.I. tract
Antibiotics	1. Actinomycin-D 2. Adriamycin	1. Wilms' tumor, choriocarcinoma 2. A wide spectrum of tumors
Plant alkaloids	1. Vincristine 2. Vinblastine	1. Acute leukemias, lymphomas 2. Reticuloendothelial malignancy, lymphomas
Adenocorticosteroids	Prednisone	Lymphocytic leukemias, lymphomas, carcinoma of breast
Other steroid hormones	Estrogens Androgens Progestins	Carcinoma of prostrate Carcinoma of breast Carcinoma of endometrium
Enzymes	L-Asparaginase	Acute lymphatic leukemias, lymphomas
Miscellaneous Agents Methylhydrazine	Procarbazine	Lymphomas
Nitrosoureas	BCNU CCNU	Lymphomas Brain tumors, many solid tumors
Hydroxyurea	Hydroxyurea	Chronic leukemia, ? acute leukemia

Table 3: Current Status of Clinical Cancer Chemotherapy

Disease	Agent	Benefit
Malignant Diseases Usually Response (>50%)		
Trophoblastic tumors	Actinomycin-D, methotrexate, vinca alkaloids, alkylating agents	Permanent regression in 90% of cases
Acute lymphoblastic leukemia	Adenocortiscosteroids, vincristine, 6-mercaptopurine, methotrexate, cyclophosphamide, L-asparaginase	Initial remission 80%; prolonged survival
Chronic leukemia: Myelocytic	Busulfan, 6-mercaptopurine, hydroxyurea	Clinical improvement in >70%; occasional prolonged survival
Lymphocytic	Alkylating agents, adrenocorticosteroids	Clinical improvement; occasional prolonged survival
Hodgkin's disease	Alkylating agents, vinca alkaloids, procarbazine, adrenocorticosteroids	Clinical improvement in >70%; prolonged survival
Lymphocytic lymphoma	Alkylating agents, adrenocorticosteroids; vinca alkaloids	Clinical improvement in >50%; prolonged survival
Histiocytic lymphoma	Alkylating agents, vinca alkaloids, adrenocorticosteroids	Clinical improvement in about 50%; occasional prolonged survival
Carcinoma of breast	Estrogens, androgens, 5-fluorouracil, alkylating agents, combination chemotherapy, methotrexate, adriamycin	25–50% response; prolonged survival
Carcinoma of prostate	Estrogens	>80% response; prolonged survival
Wilms' tumor	Actinomycin-D, alkylating agents, vincristine	>60% response; prolonged survival
Ewing's sarcoma	Cyclophosphamide, actinomycin-D, vincristine	>50% response; prolonged survival when combined with radiation therapy

Table 3: Current Status of Clinical Cancer Chemotherapy (*Continued*)

Malignant Diseases After Responsive (20–50%)

Acute myelocytic leukemia	Daunorubicin, 6-mercaptopurine, vincristine, cytosine arabinoside, 6-thioguanine	Clinical improvement in 40–50%; prolonged survival
Multiple myeloma	Alkylating agents; adrenocorticosteroids	Objective response in 40–50%; prolonged survival
Carcinoma of ovary	Alkylating agents	Clinical improvement in 45–60%
Carcinoma of endometrium	Progestins	Clinical improvement in 20–50%
Testicular carcinoma, germinal cell	Actinomycin-D, vincristine, methotrexate, chlorambucil, vinblastine, bleomycin	Clinical improvement in approximately 30–60%
Adrenal carcinoma	o,p'-DDD	Frequent clinical improvement, sometimes prolonged
Differentiated sarcoma in adults	Actinomycin-D, cyclophosphamide, adriamycin	15–50% objective response
Carcinoma of bowel and stomach	5-Fluorouracil	Clinical improvement in 20–25%

Minimal Response (<20%)

Melanoma	Alkylating agents, vinca alkaloids, DIC	5–25% objective response depending on disease site; little prolongation of survival
Head and neck tumors	Bleomycin, adriamycin, methotrexate	10–30% objective response
Bronchogenic carcinoma	Alkylating agents, methotrexate	5–10% objective response
Carcinoma of cervix	Alkylating agents, methotrexate	<20% objective response

Table 4: Pharmaclogic Characteristics of Selected Anti-cancer Drugs

Drug	Cell Cycle Phase Specificity	Plasma T ½	Plasma Protein Binding	Entry Into CNS	Biotransformation Activation	Biotransformation Degradation	Main Route of Excretion
Alkylating Agent							
Cyclophosphamide	NS	6.5 hr.	10%	Moderate		Oxidized by hepatic microsomal enzymes to biologically active and inactive products	Renal
Antimetabolites							
Methotrexate	S	12 hr.	50%	Minimal	None	None	Renal
6-Mercaptopurine	S	90 min.	10–20%	Moderate	To nucleotide	Oxidation to 6-thiouric acid via xanthin oxidase	Renal
Cytosine arabinoside	S	2 hr.	Negligible	Moderate	To nucleotide	Deamination to uracil arabinoside	Renal
5-Fluorouracil	NS	20 min.	? Negligible	Extensive	To nucleotide	Extensive	Lung and renal
Vinca Alkaloids							
Vincristine	S	A few minutes	? Negligible	? Negligible		? Extensive	Bile
Antibiotics							
Dactinomycin	NS	A few minutes	? Negligible	Low	None	None	Bile
Adriamycin	NS	27 hr.	Extensive	? Negligible	Extensive biotransformation to active and inactive metabolites		Bile
Hormones							
Prednisone	NS	24 hr.	90%	Low	—	Conjugation and reduction in liver	Renal

Abbreviations:

S—Phase-specific
NS—Phase-nonspecific
CNS—Central nervous system
T ½—Half-time of plasma clearance
?—Undetermined or estimated from known properties of the drug or a closely related drug

Table 5: Alkylating Agents

Compound	Chemical Characteristics	Clinical Considerations	Route of Administration	Available Preparations
Nitrogen mustard (Mustargen; HN_2)	Bis-(chloroethyl) amine	Rapidly acting; vesicant action	I.V.; intra-cavitary	Powder (untable after hydration), 10 mg vials
Cyclophosphamide (Cytoxan)	Phosphoric acid derivative of HN_2	Effective orally with slow onset; rapid I.V. effect; requires metabolism by liver; produces alopecia and cystitis	Oral; I.V.	50mg ablets; powder, 100, 200, and 500 mg vials
Chlorambucil (Leukeran)	Phenylbutyric acid derivative of HN_2	Slow onset; usually easy to control	Oral	2 mg tablets
Melphalan (Alkeran; PAM)	Phenylalanine derivative of HN_2	May have rapid effect and be difficult to control	Oral	2 mg tablets
Busulfan (Myleran)	Alkyl sulfonate	Appears to be selectively myelosuppressive; effective in chronic myeloproliferative disorders; thrombocytopenia often difficult to manage	Oral	2 mg tablets

Table 6: Antimetabolites

Compound	Chemical Characteristics	Clinical Considerations	Route of Administration	Available Preparations
Methotrexate (MTX)	Folic acid antagonist	Renal excretion; absorbed from meningeal surfaces; toxicity for marrow, G.I. tract, and buccal mucosa; renal toxicity at high dosages; hepatic toxicity with prolonged administration	Oral; I.V.	2.5 mg tablets; powder, 5 and 50 mg vials
6-Mercaptopurine (Purinethol; 6-MP)	Purine analogue	Xanthine oxidase metabolism and renal excretion; marrow and hepatic toxicity	Oral	50 mg tablets
6-Thioguanine (Thioguanine, Tabloid; 6-TG)	Purine analogue	Marrow and hepatic toxicity	Oral	40 mg tablets
5-Fluorouracil (Fluorouracil; 5-FU)	Fluoropyrimidine	Hepatic metabolism; marrow and G.I. toxicity frequent	I.V.	500 mg in 10 ml vials
Cytosine arabinoside (ara-C; Cytosar)	Pyrimidine nucleoside analogue with an altered sugar moiety	Rapidly excreted in urine	I.V.	Powder, 100 and vials 500 mg

Table 7: Antibiotics

Compound	Origin	Clinical Considerations	Route of Administration	Available Preparations
Actinomycin-D (dactinomycin; Cosmegen)	*Streptomyces*	Hematopoietic and G.I. toxicity; locally irritating	I.V.	Powder, 500 μg/vial
Mithramycin (Mithracin)	*Streptomyces*	Hemorrhagic diathesis; hematopoietic and G.I. toxicity	I.V.	Powder, 2500 μg/vial
Bleomycin (Blenoxane)	*Streptomyces*	Pulmonary fibrosis; skin and mucous mebrane toxicity	I.V.	Powder, 15 units/vial
Adriamycin (Doxorubicin)	*Streptomyces*	Hematopoietic and G.I. toxicity; alopecia; cardiac damage; locally irritating	I.V. or I.M.	Powder, 10 mg/vial

Table 8: Vinca Alkaloids

Compound	Origin	Cinical Consideration	Route of Administration	Available Preparations
Vincristine (Oncovin)	Plant alkaloid	Neurotoxicity; severe constipation	I.V.	Powder, 1 and 5 mg/vial
Vinblastine (Velban)	Plant alkaloid	Bone marrow toxicity	I.V.	Powder, 10 mg/vial

Table 9: Antitumor Hormones

Compound	Chemical Characteristics	Clinical Considerations	Route of Administration	Available Preparations
Estrogen				
Diethylstilbestrol	Nonsteroidal estrogen	Potent estrogen; active by mouth; slow degradation; fluid retention and G.I. disturbances; feminization; uterine bleeding	Oral	Tablet, 0.1–25 mg
Steroid Compounds				
Progestins				
Hydroxyprogesterone caproate (Delalutin)	Progestin	Minimal fluid retention; changes in epithelium of female genital tract and acinar cells of breast	I.M.	In oil, 125 and 250 mg/ml
Medroxyprogesterone acetate (Depo-Provera)	Progestin	Fluid retention; changes in epithelial and acinar cells	I.M.	Suspension, 50 mg/ml 10 mg
(Provera)			Oral	Tablets, 2.5 and
Megestrol acetate (Megace)	Progestin		Oral	Tablets, 20 mg
Androgens				
Testosterone propionate (Oreton propionate)	Testosterone ester	Virilization; fluid retention; change in libido	I.M.	In oil, 100 mg/ml
Testosterone enanthate (Delatestryl)	Testosterone ester	Same	I.M.	In oil, 200 mg/ml
Testosterone cypionate (Depo-testosterone)	Testosterone ester	Same	I.M.	In oil, 50, 100, and 200 mg/ml
Fluoxymesterone (Halotestin)	Halogenated derivative	Same, plus oral absorption and hepatic toxicity	Oral	Tablets, 2, 5, and 10 mg
Calusterone (Methosarb)	Dimethyltestosterone derivative	Same, plus oral absorption and hepatic toxicity	Oral	Tablets, 50 mg

Table 9: Antitumor Hormones (*Continued*)

Compound	Chemical Characteristics	Clinical Considerations	Route of Administration	Available Preparations
Corticosteroids				
Prednisone	Sythetic analogue of adrenal cortical steroid	Undesirable side-efiects: potassium loss, sodium and fluid retention, diabetes mellitus, psychosis, gastric bleeding	Oral	Tablets, 1, 2.5, 5, and 20 mg
Dexamethasone (Decadron)	Synthetic analogue of adrenal cortical steroid	Undesirable side-effects: potassium loss, sodium and fluid retention, diabetes mellitus, psychosis, gastric bleeding	Oral	Tablets, 0.25 mg, 0.5 mg, 0.75 mg, 1.5 mg
			I.V.; I.M.	1, 5, and 25 ml vials containing 4 mg/ml

Table 10: Selected Miscellaneous Agents

Compound	Chemical Characteristics	Clinical Considerations	Route of Administration	Available Preparations
Procarbazine (Matulane)	Isopropylmethlhydrazine	Marrow depression; central nervous system toxicity; monoamine oxidase inhibitor; hemolytic anemia	Oral	Capsules, 50 mg
Hydroxyurea (Hydrea)	Urea analogue	Marrow depression; G.I. disturbances	Oral	Capsules, 500 mg
Mitotane (Lysodren)	*o,p'*-DDD, an insecticide	G.I. disturbances; central nervous system toxicity; rashes	Oral	Tablets, 500 mg

NEW METHODS OF CANCER TREATMENT—1972–1977

MULTI-MODALITY CANCER THERAPY

The theory of multi-modality therapy in the treatment of cancer is based on logical principles. Many cancers come under treatment at a time when the local tumor can still be eradicated by either surgery or irradiation, but a few cancerous cells have escaped from the local tumor, either into the lymphatics or into the general circulation, and the balance between the invasiveness of the tumor and the resistence of the host will determine the ultimate fate of the host. Surgery is obviously curative in very early localized tumors, for what is completely removed is permanently eradicated from the host. Similarly, irradiation therapy destroys cancerous tissue in the field of irradiation under proper circumstances. It cannot hope to destroy widespread metastases of even a few cancerous cells that have gained access to the general lymphatic or vascular circulation. Surgery has the advantage of removing cancerous cells 100%; irradiation has the advantage of not mutilating in many important areas of the body, and of being cosmetically more attractive in many situations; but it has the disadvantage that irradiation kills in a log-kill fashion.

The destruction of the tumor cells is sensitive to the oxygen tension of the tumor tissue. Both surgery and irradiation reduce the bulk of the tumor in a safe and simple way, and thereby, the total body burden of cancer cells. Oftentimes, however, neither surgery nor irradiation eradicates every last living cancer cell in a patient. The two major courses for destruction of cancer—surgery and irradiation—are capable of destroying tumor in a localized area and debulking tumor burden; but they do not eliminate cancer cells already spread outside of the field of their local application. The future may permit us to deliver radiation particles selectively to cancer cells in the body wherever these cells might be distributed; but for the moment, the cells remaining outside of the zone of local destruction by either surgery or irradiation must be attacked by chemotherapeutic agents, hormones, or immunological approaches. The concept of multi-modality therapy then relies upon surgery and/or irradiation to reduce the bulk of the tumor, minimize rapidly the total burden; chemotherapy, hormone therapy, or immunotherapy to destroy every last living cell of cancer in the patient. The tumor-host relationship is altered favorably with respect to the host by combinations of cancer therapy.

Chemotherapy, and combinations of chemotherapy, attempts to destroy cancer cells that are spread diffusely throughout the body. Pulsed doses of combinations of chemotherapeutic agents have the advantage of destroying tumor cells in different phases of the cell cycle, and also embarrass to a lesser degree the normal immunological responses of the host against the tumor. The lack of an absolute differential in sensitivity between the responsiveness of a normal cell and the cancer cell to chemotherapeutic agents makes it very difficult to truly cure cancer by killing every last living cancer cell in the patient. It is most effective when the tumor burden is small. It works well against some cancers, but poorly against others. Cure is limited by the toxicity of the agents for normal cells as well as tumor cells, and the inability to put the agent in the exact phase of the cell cycle wherein all tumor cells will be destroyed simultaneously. Multi-modality therapy combining surgery, irradiation, and chemotherapy has tremendously improved the treatment of many tumors in children, particularly tumors of the kidney, adrenal, and malignant tumors of the soft parts, such as myosarcomas and fibrosarcomas of the extremities. Chemotherapy again kills in a log-kill fashion. It never kills 100% of all of the cells at the same time. The log-kill nature of chemotherapeutic action and the relationship of sensitivity of the cells to the phase of the cell cycle limit further the ability of chemotherapy to cure and eradicate every last living cancer cell.

Improved results obtained with multi-modility therapy of childhood rhabdomyosarcomas of the head, neck and extremities, Wilms' tumors, osteogenic sarcomas, Ewing sarcomas and Hodgkin's disease have been gratifying, but still not curative. The ultimate cure of cancer seems to involve some active participation of the host against the tumor so that the host can contain or destroy the final few remaining tumor cells. This concept of host-tumor interaction is best visualized in immunological terms. The significance of the immune system in cancer in the past few years has progressed to clinical usefulness, and immunotherapy has emerged as an additional arm of treatment in the multi-modality approach to cancer.

In theory, immunotherapy is capable of destroying every last living cancer cell. Unlike surgery, radiation therapy, and chemotherapy, which utilized together may reduce the tumor-cell burden from 10^{11} to 10^5 to 10^3 or less, the immune system has the potential for specific destruction of every last living cancer cell. It is not surprising that clinical attempts to employ immunotherapy have become the most recent adjunct to the multi-modality concept of cancer therapy. With minimum tumor burden remaining, that is less than 10^5 cancer cells, immunologic intervention might permit total eradication of neoplastic cells, cure of the cancer without damage to the host. The multi-modality treatment of cancer can only be evaluated in the clinical setting. Time has established the role of surgery, radiation therapy, and single agent chemotherapy in a large variety of cancers.

During the last 5 years, the concepts of debulking of the tumor by surgery and/or irradition, combined with early chemotherapy with multiple agents, has been tested with important clinical trials in cancer of the breast. Breast cancer is an excellent clinical model in which to conduct these studies, for we have accumulated a tremendous amount of data on the results of treatment in cancer of the breast with respect to its size and lymph node mestastses in the areas of surgical treatment and irradiation therapy, either alone or combined. The first of the studies on multi-modality therapy is the L–PAM Study in the United States. The second is the Combination Chemotherapy Study by the National Tumor Institute in Italy, sponsored by our National Institutes of Health. The L–Pam Study has been coordinated by Dr. Fisher (1975); the Combination Chemotherapy Study in Italy has been coordinated by Dr. Bonadonna (1976). Both studies have been running for 28 to 30 months, a time period too short for final conclusions about the effectiveness of early chemotherapy with a single agent (L–PAM), or early chemotherapy (CMF Studies); and both are prospective randomized clinical trials permitting biostatistical evaluation of the information obtained.

The Fisher, or L–PAM, study in the management of primary breast cancer demonstrates in the first 30 months of the study that L–PAM is effective in the treatment of women with primary breast cancer, particularly those who are pre-menopausal. In the pre-menopausal patients, those receiving placebos have the recurrence of the disease in 30% of the patients within a 30 month period, but in those receiving L–PAM the recurrence rate was only 3%. There was a similar trend in the post-menopausal patients, but the difference in the treated and untreated group in the post-menopausal patient was not statistically significant. Thus the overall treatment failure in the untreated group was 22%; the overall treatment failure in the treated group was 9.7%. The L–PAM study with a single agent produced essentially no toxicity, was well tolerated, and was particularly effective in the pre-menopausal patient who already had nodal involvement at the time of surgical removal of the tumor.

The CMF, Combination Chemotherapy Study, or Bonadonna Study, consisted in the prolonged administration of three chemotherapeutic agents—cyclophosphamide, methotrexate, and 5-fluorouracil—as adjuvant treatment to radical mastectomy in primary breast cancer. After 28 months of study, treatment failures occurred in 24% of the control group and in 5.3% of the group receiving combination chemotherapy. Particularly impressive was the effect of this chemotherapy in patients who had four or more positive axillary nodes. In the patients with more than four nodes involved, only 25% remain clinically free of disease after 28 months; in the treatment group 80% remained free of disease after 28 months. There was no difference in this series between women who were pre-menopausal or post-menopausal. However, the toxic manifestations from multiple drug therapy with CMF was between 30% and 50%, and included leucopenia, loss of hair, conjunctivitis, blistering of the oral mucosa, cystitis, and amenorrhea.

It must be pointed out that these studies have only been running for 28 to 30 months, a time interval too short to state whether there is any difference in survival rates ultimately versus immediate rates of recurrence. It is also impossible at this early date to state whether there is any difference in the results between the L–PAM Group and the CMF Group, but certainly the toxicity is much less in the L–PAM Group, a single agent treatment. Finally, the long-term side effects of prolonged chemotherapy remain unknown, particularly the effects on the immune system, which has such an important bearing on the ultimate containment of cancer. Theoretical observations still leave considerable doubt that one can eradicate every last living cancer cell in the patient even by combination chemotherapy. Immunotherapy, however, has within it the theoretical possibility of killing every last cancer cell.

IMMUNOTHERAPY OF CANCER

Hopes have run high in the past 5 years that our burgeoning knowledge of the immune system would soon permit destruction of every last living cancer cell in cancer patients by immunotherapy, either alone or in combination with other methods of treatment.

Tumor cells have been shown to contain specific surface antigens. These antigens make each tumor different and specific, and they induce immune responses in the host. These immune responses are often weak and valueless, but can serve as specific targets for attack by immunotherapy. Cancers of viral origin have a common antigen coded for by the virus; cancers of chemical or physical origin have individual-specific or organ-specific antigens. Inherent in immunological theory is the potential for total destruction of cancer cells in cancer patients with the least possible morbidity, for immunological agents kill a constant number of cells per dose administered (zero-order kinetics), rather than a constant fraction of cells per dose administered (first-order kinetics)—characteristics of both irradiation therapy and chemotherapy. The smaller the number of cells remaining to be killed by immunotherapy the better. Hence, the importance of debulking the tumor burden by surgery, irradiation, and chemotherapy and the combined use of immunotherapy in the multi-modality approach to eradication of every last living cancer cell in the therapy of cancer patients.

Two systems of immunity protect the body from the hazards of cancer: (1) the cell-mediated response, a function of lymphocytes; and (2) the humoral response, a function of free circulating antibodies produced by plasma cells. All immune cells have a common cell of origin, the stem cell, which originates early in embryonic life from the yolk sac, and migrates through the fetal thymus, liver, spleen, and bone marrow to receive different commitments from these organs to make it mature into a T cell or a B cell. The T cells receive a commitment from the thymus and become the cells for cell-mediated immunity, the small lymphocytes; the B cells receive a commitment from the foetal liver and spleen and become the B lymphocytes, which can either interact with T cells and produce lymphokines, or mature into plasma cells which produce humoral immunity with free-circulating immunoglobulins. The complex interactions between the T cells and B cells and the macrophages, and their interrelationship to complement have been reviewed earlier. Knowledge of this type may have a tremendous bearing on the immunological response of any given cancer. We can review clinical progress in immunotherapy of cancer generally, but specific immunotherapy requires detailed information about each specific and disparate cancer. Clinical immunotherapy, however, operates within the general immunological principles we have learned about earlier—acquired immunological tolerance, the clonal selection theory of antibody production, balances between antigens and antibodies in the enhancement of tumor growth, immunoparalysis, the role of immunosuppression in elimination of normal immunological surveillance, and the potential of immunological stimulation for the enhancement of immunological destruction of small foci of dispersed cancer cells.

The various immunotherapeutic approaches to cancer in the past 5 years can be placed into three broad categories: (1) *non-specific immunotherapy,* which involves non-specific stimulation of the immune system of the host by bacteria (BCG—bacillus Calmette, Guerin, Corynebacterium parvum, and MER—the methanol extraction residue of BCG), drugs (Levamisole), and cell products, such as polysaccharides (Lentinan), polynucleotides, and cell-wall products; (2) *active specific immunotherapy,* which includes active stimulation of the immune system by tumor vaccines and immune RNA; and (3) *passive and adoptive immunotherapy,* which transfer antisera, immune lymphoid cells, or subcellular fractions from allogeneic immunized hosts exposed to cancer-specific antigens.

Non-specific immunotherapy. An International Registry of Tumor Immunotherapy has been established in an effort to rapidly gather data of a meaningful nature, and as of June 1975 there were over 200 protocols registered, 74 of which were from the National Institutes of Health, supplying a variety of non-specific adjuvants such as BCG, MER–BCG, and Cornynebacterium parvum.

The most widely used immunotherapeutic agent has been BCG, a microbial material developed early in the 1900's by Calmette and Guerin at the Pasteur Institute for vaccination against tuberculosis. It is safe and millions have received it in the prophylaxis against tuberculosis. It produces a non-specific stimulation of the immune system, and has been found to have anti-tumor activity in both the experimental and clinical setting. BCG has been most widely used in the treatment of malignant melanoma. It has been studied by direct injection into melanotic lesions, as a surgical adjuvant in early disease by repeated intracutaneous inoculations through skin scratches or specially devised grids to permit intracutaneous inoculations, and in the chemotherapy of advanced disease.

The role of BCG in cancer therapy still needs clarification. The best controlled studies with BCG in melanoma suggest that direct injection is effective against the injected nodule in about 50% of the cases, but that it has little effect upon the metastases (less than 10% of cases), and it may even occasionally produce fatal shock (Eilber and Morton, *et al.,* 1976). Distant intracutaneous inoculation retards the appearance of metastases and inhibits their growth for a period of 6 months to a year, but it does not cure the disease.

BCG has also been used in lung cancer and in lymphoma and leukemia patients. In lung cancer intracutaneous or intrapleural injection may well reduce the establishment or growth of distant metastases for several months to a year. In lymphomas fewer patients relapse and the relapse time is lengthened by over a year, but little effect has been substantiated in the treatment of either acute lymphatic or myeloid leukemia. BCG may also be helpful in retarding recurrence in breast cancer, if used in association with multi-modality chemotherapy.

Definitive answers on BCG are hard to come by because of so many variables involved in its use—preparation, dosage, route of delivery, ratio of live to dead bacteria, and duration of treatment— again suggesting that carefully controlled clinical trials must be established, rather than indiscriminate use. These variables must be standardized, if proper evaluation is to take place.

The use of live bacteria in BCG has raised some questions, and in an effort to avoid difficulties from BCG a non-viable methanol extract has been developed, MER–BCG. MER–BCG is being supplied by the National Institutes of Health in nineteen clinical trials. It is uniformly active and standardized in preparation, and is being compared with BCG. The systemic effects of chills, fever, malaise, skin rash, hives, nausea, and myalgia seem less than from BCG. Its use in leukemia seems promising in association with chemotherapy, but it, too, can only kill a small number of remaining cells in a synergistic fashion.

Corynebacterium parvum heat-killed cells are also being used as non-viable material for immunostimulation. They produce an increase in the number of macrophages, a stimulation of macrophage chemotaxis, lymphocyte trapping, and proliferation of antigen-triggered lymphocytes. Dose, timing, and route of administration alter its effects, and improper administration may even be immuno-suppressive.

Levamisol and ettramisole are chemical compounds which are immunopotentiators. Clinical trials are beginning with these compounds. However, it must be emphasized that the mechanism of action of all immunopotentiators of the non-specific types discussed above are complex and are mediated through the interaction of macrophages, B lymphocytes, and T lymphocytes—the last category including subpopulations of cytotoxic, helper, and suppressor cells. Improper dosage, routes of administration, and scheduling may result in immunosuppression rather than immunopotentiation. Misuse and misinterpretation of the effects of these compounds can only be avoided by carefully controlled and conducted clinical trials, with full and unbiased analysis of all evidence of their actions.

Active specific immunotherapy. This second type of immunotherapy has been thwarted by the lack of common antigens among tumors of similar histological type, failure to identify any virus as a causative agent of cancer in man (although it is suspected in several types of tumors), and the inability to isolate tumor-specific antigens from most tumors in sufficient amount to prepare a vaccine. Studies are just beginning with the use of tumor cells inactivated by irradiation, mitomycin C, freezing and thawing, and heat treatments of various types. Unfortunately, these treatments also inactivate tumor-specific antigens. Coupling of tumor cells with highly antigenic carriers, unmasking of antigens with neuraminidase and concanavalin A are being studied, but as yet standardization of vaccines and assessment of administrative techniques has been impossible and ignored for widespread trials.

Passive and adoptive immunotherapy. Passive immunotherapy is currently being explored with the use of either anti-tumor sera or sensitized committed lymphoid cells. There is no solid work which indicates the clinical effectiveness of any anti-tumor serum. The use of sensitized and committed lymphoid cells has been somewhat effective in experimental studies, but this approach carries with it all of the problems of tissue and organ transplantation; for the transferred live lymphocytes are allogeneic cells which are rejected by the recipient host, and they can in large numbers initiate a graft versus host reaction. The problems of tissue typing and cell typing and the immunological problems of transplantation of foreign tissue must be solved before passive transfer of live immunocompetent cells can be realistically employed.

Adoptive immunotherapy is theoretically simpler and may have some advantages over other forms of immunotherapy. This currently involves (1) non-specific stimulation of lymphocytes of the tumor-bearing host with agents like phytohemagglutinin, or specific sensitization of thi esolated host lymphocytes with tumor cells *in vitro* with subsequent reintroduction of the sensitized acceptable cells back into the original host; and (2) administration of extracts from sensitized cells in the form of *transfer factor* or *immune RNA*.

Transfer factor has been studied most widely in bone tumors called osteosarcomas, but it is also being explored in the treatment of malignant melanoma, and breast cancer. Transfer factor is a dialyzable non-cellular extract of sensitized leukocytes from a donor that transfers cellular immunity to a non-sensitive recipient. Its chemical nature is unknown, but it is exceedingly potent, transfers cellular immunity only through systemic action, introduces skin test sensitivity, specific lymphocyte stimulation, and the capacity to produce migratory inhibitor factor, but does not transfer antibody reactivity in the form of blocking antibodies or enhancing factors. Transfer factor confers cellular immunity without further antibody production and enables the patient to recognize the tumor for the foreign body that it is. It acts by replacing or restoring the ability of the patient's T cells to reject foreign antigens. Its specificity is not known. Most of the clinical trials have been predicated upon the theory that a specific antigen stimulates a specific type of transfer factor. Tumor antigen of a given tumor type is used to stimulate donor lymphocytes of autologous source to produce a specific transfer factor, and then the non-cellular dialyzable factor is used to transfer molecular immune factors programmed to kill specific malignant cells. However, some work suggests that transfer immune factor may be a non-specific stimulator of T cells. Non-specificity would make it possible to produce transfer factor through commercial blood banks as another blood product with the potential for immunostimulation of T cells. Studies with transfer factor thus far indicate that it does modify cellular immunity and occasionally produces striking tumor regression, but further knowledge is needed, as well as controlled clinical trials. The areas to be explored include donor and recipient selection, quantitation and dosage, initiation, timing, and length of administration, and above all clearer characterization of the molecular nature of transfer factor.

Immunogenic ribonucleic acid, or immune RNA, is the brightest hope on the immunological horizon (Pilch *et al.*, 1976). Ribonucleic acid (RNA) extracted from the lymphoid tissue of animals previously immunized with tumor cells is called immune RNA. It is capable of inducting tumor-specific immune responses *in vitro* and *in vivo.* Immune RNA is a non-cellular fraction which is effective whether derived from syngeneic, allogeneic, or xenogeneic sources. Most interesting has been the demonstration that normal, non-immune human lymphocytes can be converted into effector cells cytotoxic for human target cells by incubation with xenogeneic immune RNA extracted from the lymphoid tissue of sheep immunized with the same human tumor cell line. The immune reaction is abolished by ribonuclease, not desoxyribonuclease: so it is an RNA, not a DNA fraction. Immune RNA is a cytoplasmic fraction, an RNA-antigen complex, which apparently interacts with the DNA genome of the host to code for the continued production of immuno-specific messenger RNA. It is non-cellular and does not carry histocompatability antigens. It does not transfer blocking or serum factors, does not induce a graft versus host reaction, and is a very weak antigen so that resistance against it is minimal. Allogeneic immune RNA can be derived from patients; xenogeneic immune RNA can be derived from animals specifically immunized with human tumor.

Clinical studies are just being initiated wherein xenogeneic immune RNA derived from sheep is being given to human subjects with renal cell carcinoma. Toxic reactions have been minimal, and sensitization to sheep proteins was not disturbing. There has been a suggestion of clinical improvement with preliminary *in vitro* evidence of enhanced autitumor immunity specific for the given tumor. The initial explorations with immune RNA seem worthy of sustained effort, but clinical data is still insufficient to evaluate its ultimate place in immunotherapy of human cancer.

Immunotherapy of cancer has tremendous future potential, but at present its fundamental premises have not been adequately proved in the clinical setting. The basic premises that must still be proved with respect to man are: (1) tumors have antigens that distinguish them from normal tissue; (2) specific immune responses can be developed against these antigens; (3) immune responses can selectively kill tumor cells in adequate numbers and volume (recognizing only 1 cm. of tumor contains over a billion cells); and (4) modification of the host immune responses can increase host resistance to the cancer. Is immunotherapy tumor specific? Can immunotherapy kill or halt tumor growth wherever it might be disseminated, or are there resistant sanctuaries defying immunological invasion? Can immunologic reactivity in current tests be correlated with successful immunotherapy in man? What are the proper doses and schedules of treatment? Should it be used alone or as a part of multi-modality therapy? A tremendous amount of future work is essential to begin to resolve the potential of immunotherapy in the treatment of cancer in man.

HORMONES AND HORMONAL THERAPY OF CANCER

We alluded earlier to the possibility of hormones serving as environmental carcinogens in certain uncommon cancers of the vaginal epithelium in young girls, and in the rising incidence of cancer of the endometrium in adult women. Hormones also play a very important role in the treatment of cancer, notably cancer of the breast and cancer of the prostate. The alteration of the hormonal environment of the individual may promote cancer or may inhibit it, depending upon specific circumstances which must be defined for each cancer in each individual. Four specific cancers will be discussed to evaluate these complex interrelationships: (1) cancer of the breast; (2) cancer of the prostrate; (3) cancer of the vaginal epithelium in young girls; and (4) cancer of the endometrium in adult women.

Cancer of the Breast. The relationship of hormones to cancer has been studied most extensively in breast cancer as the growth and function of the mammary cells are subject to influence by a variety of hormonal agents. We referred earlier to the initial observation of Bateson in 1895 on the effects of bilateral oopherectomy on the regulation of growth of experimental mouse mammary cancer. Huggins and Bergenstal, in the early 1940's, demonstrated that hormonal deprivation affords striking regression of advanced breast cancer in some humans. They won for this the Nobel Prize, and a new era in understanding the treatment of cancer was heralded by this work. Clinical experience has shown, however, that somewhat less than half of the patients with breast cancer in the pre-menopausal years can expect to benefit from removal of the ovaries, and only 25% of post-menopausal patients with breast cancer respond to endocrine ablative procedures, including oophorectomy, adrenalectomy, and hypophysectomy. During the last 5 years, the estrogen profiles of patients with breast cancer have been intensively investigated. Efforts have been made, by studying the estrogen-binding receptors of the excised breast cancers, to predict which breast cancers might be hormone-dependent, so that endocrine therapy or endocrine ablation could be restricted to the cases in which it has a reasonable chance of success. Three main questions remain to be answered: (1) Do breast cancers arise more frequently in women receiving prolonged doses of estrogens for menopausal or other disorders? (2) Are there patterns of metabolism of the estrogenic hormones which might enable us to predict which women would be predisposed to breast cancer through available analyses of the end products of estrogen metabolism in the urine? (3) Is it possible to predict, on the basis of hormone receptors in breast tissue and in breast cancers, whether or not the cancer will respond to endocrine ablative therapy, that is, oophorectomy, hypophysectomy and/or adrenalectomy?

Breast cancers are lower in parous than in nulliparous women, and the lowest risk is associated with the first pregnancy at an early age. The nature of the protective factor of pregnancy is unknown. The most plausible suggestion is that it may be either progesterone or estriol, both of which are markedly elevated during gestation. The urinary end-products of estrogen in the urine are estrone (E1), estradiol (E2), and estriol (E3). E1 and E2 have been demonstrated to be mammary carcinogens in experimental animals; E3 has not. Asian women, who excrete a much higher proportion of E3, have been found to have a lower risk of breast cancer than North American women, who excrete higher proportions of E1 and E2. A 1976 study of women in Honolulu, age 15 to 39, showed that the Oriental women in Asia have the highest excretion of estriol (E3). The Oriental women of Hawaii have an intermediary excretion of estriol (E3), and the Caucasians of Hawaii have the lowest excretion of estriol, equal to that of the Caucasians on the North American mainland. This study from the National Cancer Institute concluded that there is a correlation between the excretion of urinary estriols and breast cancer risk. The women who excrete large amounts of E3 have the lowest risk; the women who excrete large amounts of E1 and E2 have the highest risk (Dickinson *et. al.,* 1974).

The relationship of menopausal estrogens and breast cancer has similarly been studied in a group of approximately 1900 women given conjugated estrogens for the menopause and watched for the incidence of breast cancer over the ensuing 12 years (Hoover *et. al.,* 1976). In this group of women, 49 cases of breast cancer were observed; the expected incidence was 39.1 on the basis of rates in the general population. This led to a relative risk of breast cancer of

1.3 during the first 12 years after consumption of menopausal estrogen, and this risk rose to 2 after 15 years. There was no clear dose-response relationship to accumulated years of use. The relation of risk of breast cancer to the strength of medication was studied. Women who used 0.30 milligrams and those who used 0.265 milligrams had about the same relative risk, whereas those who used more than 1.25 milligrams of estrogen daily had a considerably higher risk. The risk was also increased by taking higher doses several times a week, rather than on a daily schedule. The relative risk rose as high as 4.7 for women who used the large doses of medication on other than a daily basis. In comparison, women who used 0.30 milligrams or 0.265 milligrams had a relative risk of 2.7.

It must be emphasized that the increased risk of breast cancer was not of epidemic proportions, but was only 30% greater than expected. However, women who took estrogens lost the low-risk factors associated with multiparity and oophorectomy. Similarly, women who developed benign breast disease, such as fibrocystic disease or mammary dysplasia, after the initiation of estrogens had a risk of developing cancer which was 2 to 5 times that of the normal population. The findings of this National Institute of Health Study indicate that menopausal estrogen use does not protect against breast cancer. The Study also raises the possibility that there is a definite risk of increased cancer associated with taking estrogens. The risk appeared some 10 to 15 years following administration of estrogens, particularly in the higher and non-daily dose regimens. Further evaluation of this problem will require studies of the latent period and the total accumulated dosage of estrogen. There is no clear dose-response relation to accumulated years of use, but higher risk occurs in women using higher dose tablets and taking the medication on other than a daily basis. Even harder to understand is the fact that after 10 years of followup, the low risk of breast cancer in multiparous and oophorectomized women seems to be lost. Estrogen use curiously produces an especially high risk of breast cancer among women in whom benign disease develops after they have started the drug.

The answer to the first two questions posed about breast cancer would seem to be: (1) the taking of large doses of estrogen on a non-daily basis increases the risk of breast cancer and eliminates the protective effects of oophorectomy and multiparity; and (2) the presence of high amounts of estriol in the urine is inversely correlated with the development of breast cancer. Hormones, however, are useful in the treatment of many breast cancers. Estrogen-responsive tissue of laboratory animals contains characteristic estrogen-binding receptors. In an effort to predict *a priori* which breast cancers are hormone-dependent, techniques have been developed in the last few years for measuring estrogen-receptor sites, or estrogen-binding sites, in human breast tissue and in human breast cancers. Clinically, some 30% to 40% of patients with primary carcinoma of the breast have a temporary remission when treated by endocrine ablative surgery (oophorectomy, adrenalectomy, hypophysectomy) or by steroid therapy. Using biopsy material from human breast cancers, it has been possible to demonstrate that some, but not all, malignant tumors contain protein receptor molecules in the cytoplasmal and nuclear cellular compartments of the tissue that bind estradiol specifically. The presence of estrogen receptors in human breast cancer, whether they are primary or metastatic, furnish useful information to the clinician in deciding which patient will respond to endocrine manipulation. Unfortunately, the success rate is only about 50% with current methods of discovering estrogen receptors, but those containing estrogen receptors have a much better chance of responding to endocrine ablation or to additive steroid therapy.

Our knowledge in this field is just beginning, and recent studies suggest that measurement of progesterone receptors might be far more valuable than estrogen receptors in furnishing useful information about the endocrine susceptibility of tumors (McGuire, Carbone, Vollmer, 1975). Estrogen receptor is the initial step in the binding of the hormone to the tissue. The elaboration of progresterone is a measurable product of hormone action, rather than the initial binding step. The presence of progesterone receptors in tumors would indicate that the tumor is capable not only of binding the estrogen, but of synthesizing at least one end product under estrogen regulation, and that the tumor is indeed endocrine whether it binds estrogen or not. The clinical correlation between progesterone receptors and estrogen receptors is being studied. Progesterone receptors are found in 56% of tumors with estrogen receptors, but are absent in tumors without estrogen receptors. The clinical correlation shows that only those tumors with progesterone receptors regress after endocrine therapy. The hope is, as our knowledge becomes more complete on the ability of breast tissue and cancerous breast tissue to bind the various steroid receptors, that we will soon be able to predict on a chemical basis which tumors will or will not respond to endocrine alterations of the environment. Estrogen antagonists, progesterone antagonists, and certain types of androgens might then prove equally effective to oophorectomy, adrenalectomy, and hypophysectomy in the treatment of breast cancer.

Cancer of the Prostate. There is very little new material on the relationship of hormones to cancer of the prostate. It is still clear, on the basis of clinical experience, that about 80% of men who have carcinoma of the prostate will have improvement in the disease by the administration of estrogens. Their survival is further prolonged by adding orchiectomy to estrogen administration at appropriate stages in the disease. This again is further proof that alteration of the hormonal environment of the patient has a great bearing on the rate of growth and progression of cancer of the prostate.

Cancer of the Vaginal Epithelium in Young Girls. Diethylstilbesterol, a synthetic version of one of the natural feminizing sex hormones called estrogens, was synthesized in the early 1940's. It has been used extensively for 30 years as a good agent to prevent miscarriages in pregnant mothers (Manber, 1976). Since 1971 young women under 20 have been found in increasing numbers to have a clear-cell adenocarcinoma of the vagina. Adenocarcinoma occurs in glandular tissue of a type not normally found in the vagina. It is postulated that the diethylstilbesterol (DES) led to the formation of this special glandular tissue in the female genital tract in early fetal development, and exposed these young girls to this special type of cancer. Over 250 of these cases have now been found in young girls under 20; until 1970 such cancers had never been found in women under 25. However, 25% of these young girls with these vaginal cancers have had no exposure to DES. This special type of glandular tissue appears in many young women in a precancerous state called adenosis, and can be removed by special surgical techniques to prevent later cancerous change. DES was rarely used in 1976, despite its advantages in preventing miscarriages, treating abnormal vaginal bleeding in early gestation, or maintaining pregnancies in diabetics.

There is no doubt that vaginal adenosis is common in young girls whose mothers took DES, but its significance and treatment is still controversial. Many gynecologists remove the vaginal adenosis by limited surgery or laser destruction; others merely observe it, as evidence does not unequivocally exist at the moment for an increased incidence of squamous cell cancer among DES-exposed females. The more years that these DES patients are followed, the less certain is the risk of squamous cell cancers. Squamous cell cancers are very rare, and the clear-cell adenocarcinomas are now running about 4 to 1000. Recently, animal studies with DES show males to have a high rate of male genital abnormalities and infertility. Unfortunately, also, its use in animals to prevent miscarriages has not been successful. Sons of DES mothers may be aspermic, but here again numbers are so small as to be inconclusive. DES is best banned, although the truth may not emerge for another 40 years, despite intense epidemiological studies under way in many parts of the country.

The precise mechanism by which hormones influence the origin and growth of mammary, vaginal, uterine and other tumors remains obscure. The issue is further clouded by the changing attitudes of women towards pregnancy and lactation. Thousands of years ago the mature female was usually pregnant or lactating. Today oral contraceptives and birth control complicate the problems of female existence. Most of the oral contraceptives are hormones; these may theoretically increase cancer risk because of their hormonal activity or because they are directly carcinogenic. Cancer risks can only be studied meaningfully in humans by epidemiological means, for the female experimental mouse or rat on oral contraceptives overeats, gets obese, and this in itself increases the incidence of tumors in the liver, uterus, and ovaries. Women without children are more prone to mammary cancer than those who have them. Absence from sexual intercourse reduces the risk of cervical cancer, but increases the risk of fibroids and endometrial cancer. The whole issue has been further complicated by the appearance in 1973 of hepatic adenomas in women on oral contraceptives. Since 1973, over 50 cases of benign liver nodules have been reported (Kelso, 1974). The liver tumors are of two types: (1) localized, solitary hepatic adenomas which can rupture and bleed; and (2) focal, nodular hyperplasias which are multi-nodular and small and invariably benign, with a small central area of necrosis probably from thrombosis of estrogen origin. The incidence is sparse for both types, regression occurs if the contraceptives are stopped, and the direct causation by the pill is still open to question.

Until further sound epidemiological data is available in young women, they should be aware of the fact that if their mothers took diethylstilbesterol, (DES), they have a chance of developing clear-cell adenocarcinoma of the vagina at an early age. They should also be warned that if they develop benign adenosis (the presence of glandular epithelium in the vagina or cervix), which occurs in about half the patients who are exposed to DES *in utero,* this is apparently a premalignant lesion. These young women should then have both a Papanicolaou smear and vital dye staining of the entire cervix and vagina at regular intervals between 20 and 30, and the abnormal areas of vaginal epithelium should be eradicated early by surgical excision, cauterization, or cryosurgery. If true malignancy develops, they should be treated vigorously by surgery and high radiation radiotherapy. The cure rate in these patients is high, if treatment is initiated early and the incipient cancer completely eradicated.

In addition, young women taking contraceptive pills regularly should be aware of the problems of hepatic adenomas, as well as the problems of venous thrombosis which now can be correlated with the regular administration of birth control pills.

Adenocarcinoma of the Body of the Uterus. The incidence of adenocarcinoma of the body of the uterus is steadily rising (adeno-carcinoma of the endometrium). It is associated with a high frequency of sterility and an unusual frequency of increased bleeding during the menopause. This particular tumor is not recognized by the Papanicolaou smear, and requires biopsy of the endometrial cavity for diagnosis. It is felt that the increased frequency of adeno-carcinoma of the body of the uterus may be related to the taking of hormones, in particular birth control pills, over an extended period of time (Swerdloff *et. al.,* 1975). The evidence for this is indirect, related to the observation that progestational agents (hydroxy-progesterone, delalutin, methoxyprogesterone-depo-privera) are helpful in the treatment of this disease once it has appeared. These progestational drugs must be continued if they induce remission.

OVERALL SUMMARY OF HORMONES AND CANCER

The last 5 years have demonstrated that the taking of large doses of estrogen on a non-daily basis increases the risk of breast cancer, and eliminates the protective effects of oophorectomy and multi-parity. The presence of high amounts of estriol in the urine is inversely correlated to the appearance of cancer.

The exposure *in utero* of the female fetus to diethylstilbesterol predisposes to the development of adenosis of the vagina and cervix and to the occasional appearance of clear-cell adenocarcinoma of the vagina in young girls.

The incidence of carcinoma of the body of the uterus is increasing. The taking of birth control pills over extended periods of time may be a factor in the rising occurrence of cancer of the endometrium. The progesterones have a protective effect against cancer of the body of the uterus; the birth control pills have a stimulating effect.

The ability to detect estrogen receptors and progesterone receptors in normal breast and other tissues, as well as in cancerous tissue, may give us valuable information concerning the use of hormones in the treatment of certain cancers. The hormonal treatment of cancer has its most useful place in the treatment of cancer of the breast and cancer of the prostrate at the present time.

EMERGING FUTURE RESEARCH: 1975 TO WHEREVER THE SOLUTION MAY EXIST

We have reviewed some of the brilliant advances in cancer research and in the application of this knowledge to the clinical care of cancer patients during the past 5 years. Cancer, however, still remains an unsolved clinical problem. The more we gain in information the less certain seems the immediate solution and understanding of the true nature of cancer. Several bright new future avenues of research have emerged.

The true nature of cancer, the fundamental change in the genetic machinery of the cancer cell, remains unanswered. The subject that now captures the imagination of scientists, and the one that has the greatest bearing on the future of cancer research, is the notion of genetic engineering. The ability to manipulate the genes within certain cells and to change the character, structure, and attributes of a living cell is here. Genetic manipulation has evoked the greatest concern, as well as the liveliest excitement, in the complex relationship between advancement of scientific knowledge to social purposes. The regulation of genetic manipulation is moving from the scientific realm into the public domain, and just as each physician must now deal with his patients through the mechanism of informed consent in the light of existing knowledge, so the public must begin to join with the scientists in making informed judgments about future prospects in scientific research.

The public has the right to be assured that experiments in the manipulation of genes will not endanger social health and welfare. The risks and benefits of acquiring new knowledge in the area of genetic manipulation must be carefully balanced. The freedom of the individual scholar to select and pursue the subject of his research must be preserved to enhance scholarly creativity; yet the public must be aware of both the processes and consequences of research, as the precise outcome of important experiments on public safety cannot be predicted. Nevertheless, preoccupation by society with unknown risks and consequences of accumulating knowledge must not deny scientists the tools and techniques for preventing, curing, or favorably treating diseases of genetic alteration.

RECOMBINANT DNA

The area where the challenges to scientists are the greatest, and where their responsibility for the consequences of research are the most frightening, is that of *recombinant DNA*. Two scientific breakthroughs have occurred within the past 5 years which have made it possible to break, splice, and rejoin pieces of a DNA chain in a variety of different ways. For the first time the species barrier can be broken. New genetic material from one living organism can be introduced into another completely unrelated organism, even of a different species. Dr. Herbert Boyer and his colleagues first isolated an enzyme that can break the DNA from chromosomes into bits in which the pieces contain only 1 to 10 genes in each bit. Mertz and Davis later established the fact that the enzyme breaks the DNA in a special way, leaving sticky ends which can be rejoined in a variety of different ways. Dr. Stanley Cohen and his associates then found that some bacteria contain small extra chromosomes in addition to their major chromosomes; these small extra chromosomes are called *plasmids*. A plasmid is a piece of DNA that exists as a circular molecule. It is possible to cleave the circle of plasmid DNA, introduce into it a piece of foreign genetic material of almost any origin, reestablish the circular integrity of the plasmid, and then have this plasmid carry this totally new genetic information into the DNA chain of the host cell (fig. 10). The bacterium then propogates the new genetic material as if it were a part of its own genetic machinery; and, since bacterial cells divide every 20 minutes, within a day billion of bacteria carrying copies of the foreign DNA propogate and produce pure segments of this new yet foreign genetic material.

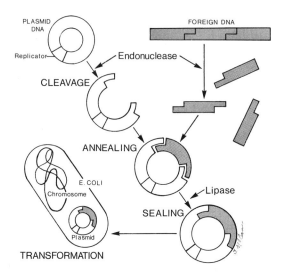

FIGURE 10. *Recombinant DNA: Plasmids are extra-chromosomal frag-ments of DNA which can be cleaved with endonuclease. Foreign DNA can then be introduced into the plasmid and the plasmid again annealed and sealed. The recombined plasmid DNA can next be introduced into the cell of origin to transform it and produce a DNA–Recombinant within the cell consisting of the original plasmid, the foreign DNA fragment, and the original DNA of the cell. The foreign DNA is replicated by virtue of the replication functions of the plasmid.*

E. Coli is a ubiquitous bacteria in man and animals and it is the bacterium used for the introduction of new genetic material by several plasmids that it contains. One can immediately see the pos-sibility of introducing cancerous DNA into this ubiquitous E. Coli organism and having E. Coli DNA coding for cancer spread widely throughout the human and animal population. Inherent in the alter-ation of genetic functions of bacteria, however, is the opportunity of taking plant material, which codes for the production of food supplies unique to the plant kingdom, and having an innocent and harmless bacterium suddenly produce the types of food or hormones which could have immense usefulness to man. Unpredictable, but potentially dangerous, mutations could, thereby, be formed which could escape from the laboratory into the environment of man.

For the first time we have the possibility of mutations bridging the barrier between the eukaryocytes and the prokaryocytes which will produce a radically new class of organisms. In nature mutations occur within a given class of organisms, or a given species; and the mutants survive by being transformed into an organism more compatible with the total environment—the Darwin Concept of Evolution of the Species with Survival of the Fittest. Recombinant DNA, wherein already genetic material from the toad (Xenopos Lavias) and the fruit fly (Drosophila melanogastar) have been introduced into the bacterium E. Coli, permits creation in the laboratory of new forms of life. If these new micro-organisms were to escape into nature, their degree of self-propogation would be entirely unknown, and the host of diseases and cancers which they might introduce into man would be completely uncontrollable. Clearly, guidelines have to be established which would be appropriate safeguards of both a biological and physical nature to contain potentially biohazardous agents arising from recombinations of DNA. Physical containment with the use of special laboratories, isolation techniques and hood would be imperative and, in all probability, not enough to limit the escape of new organisms from experimental situations. Most important would be biological containment which would require that: (1) plasmid or viral DNA into which foreign DNA had been inserted should be permitted only in specified bacterial hosts and under defined conditions; and (2) that the bacterial hosts serving as vectors for the recombinant DNA should not be able to survive outside of the laboratory environment.

Knowledge is the product of human experience, research and creativity, and the well spring is individual freedom to explore novel and imaginative avenues of research, growth, and expansion. Accumulated knowledge acquires a social purpose, the prime purpose to benefit the public. A host of imaginative individual scientists are eager to pursue the studies in recombinant DNA. Inherrent in it are: (1) unknown benefits to mankind from the expanded knowledge and its judicious use; (2) specific means of modifying or controlling harmful genes in man, animals, and plants; (3) modification of microorganisms, plants, and possibly animals to improve their usefulness to man; and (4) the mass production by harmless bacteria of compounds of inestimable value to man, such as hormones, (insulin) antibiotics, antibodies, blood fractions, and, compounds indeed for the prevention and control of cancer.

The initial anxiety in the public domain over recombinant DNA was rapidly quelled by the scientists themselves. Scientists agreed, immediately after the discovery of methods to breach natural barriers among species through genetic manipulation, to institute appropriate biological and physical barriers in their research. The public was soon assured that experiments with recombinant DNA would be carried out safely, under appropriate biological and physical constraints to the spread of new organisms. Microbial pathogenicity and communicalibility in nature are complex and depend upon a balanced acclimated genome. The laboratories and their workers would be exposed to far more hazard than anyone else, and the chances of these novel organisms surviving in nature would be small. Weighing the benefits and the risks, appropriate conferences and guidelines were rapidly established and work on recombinant DNA is progressing in a balanced way through a National Institutes of Health Recombinant DNA Molecule Program Advisory Committee. The guidelines protect the people engaged in the experiments, the general public, and the environment. Five types of experiments have been ruled inappropriate and are not to be initiated according to current guidelines. These are: (1) Cloning of DNA from disease-causing organisms or from tumor viruses; (2) recombinations involving genes for the synthesis of potent toxins; (3) recombinations that might increase the virulence, or range, of genes for plant disease; (4) liberation or release of hosts containing recombinence from controlled laboratory environments; and (5) transference of a drug-resistant trait to an organism that does not acquire it naturally, for the transfer might compromise control of the disease.

Permissible experiments must be conducted with appropriate levels of physical containment ranging from an ordinary laboratory condition to sterile, sealed-off conditions used in dealing with the most dangerous living microorganisms. Biological containment has also been invoked. Only those mutations can be produced which will be unlikely or unable to survive except in the laboratory. The combination of physical containment and permissible biological hosts enables extensive research on recombinant DNA in areas which are most likely to be of use and benefit to man. These guidelines will be reviewed and revised frequently, and the hope is that through improved knowledge and studies on recombinant DNA we may come closer to the understanding of the true nature of cancer, its prevention and its treatment. It is still too early to assess the impact of this important area of research on the cancer problem.

DNA SEQUENCING

We have repeatedly emphasized that the DNA chain or helix of the cell is made up of a sequence of 4 purine or pyrimidine bases, and that this sequence of DNA codes for specific genes and for specific functions of the genes along the DNA helix. The purine and pyrimidine bases are adenine, guanine, thymine and cytosine. Any 3 of these codes for a specific amino acid, and in the DNA chain there are a variety of genes coded for by the sequences of these bases. Some of the genes are active, some are inactive; some code the proteins, and some code for cancer. The ability to sequence the purine and pyrimidine bases in a gene would open a new era of understanding in molecular biology. Particularly important would be the knowledge of sequencing of bases in the structural genes, that is those that code for specific proteins or specific functions. Knowing the sequence would also permit an understanding of the control of genetic regulation and expression through the nonstructural genes located along the DNA chain. The ability to do DNA sequencing would enable us to explain how information is encoded in the DNA helix.

Within the past 2 years, fast and simple ways have been developed to determine DNA sequences. Just 3 years ago it took the leading scientists working in this area over 2 years to determine the sequences of a piece of DNA that is only 20 bases long. One of the greatest obstacles in DNA sequencing was the inability to label the entire length of the chain with isotopic or radioactive precursors of individual bases. However, if one could cleave the chain into smaller fragments, it might be possible to label DNA *in vivo* with a specific activity high enough for subsequent analyses, particularly in the segments that were of interest for sequencing. The solution to DNA sequencing rested on 3 crucial features: (1) radioactive labels had to be applied in sufficient concentration to sequences of known size so that they could be subsequently identified; (2) DNA dissecting enzymes had to be found that would cleave the DNA chain at specific bases; and (3) once the DNA dissecting enzymes cleaved the DNA molecule, it would have to be of sufficiently small yet variable lengths that segments could be separated and analyzed.

Two years ago a method was developed to cleave DNA into varying lengths at a given base sequence, to tag one end of that segment with a radioactive label, and gather all lengths of DNA beginning with that particular base. Scientists were able to identify the terminal nucleotide of each initial segment, and sequencing of segments of DNA was then made possible, beginning with initial lengths of a known base composition and sequencing the order of the terminal nucleotides of the initial segments in order of increasing lengths.

Within the last year, restriction enzymes have been discovered that will splice DNA into bits by cutting the DNA at a particular nucleotide along the chain. About 45 enzymes with different specificities for splicing different lengths of DNA have now been developed, and it is possible to get small segments of DNA of varying lengths for labelling and sequencing. With improved methods of gel electrophorosis, one can separate fragments of DNA into lengths of 20 up to 100 nucleotides in length. It is now possible to obtain small DNA fragments of interest from large DNA molecules, to label these initial segments, and to separate them up to 100 nucleotides by length. The sequencing of these small bits can then be done chemically. The bits can be ordered and put back together in accordance with base sequencing, and the entire length of the DNA sequencing can thereby be accomplished.

During the last year another method has been developed for getting controlled fragments of DNA by using enzyme-catalyzed synthesis. A single-stranded piece of DNA is used for copying, and the copies are made to terminate at specific bases through enzyme-catalyzed synthesis. For example, synthesis of a fragment of DNA will be started with cytosine; cytosine will then be removed from the medium and the chain will grow, of course, until the next need for cytosine arises. This permits analysis of the length of all segments that begin with cytosine, and how long they evolve before another cytosine fragment is needed. The reaction can then be started again, and one can synthesize the chain again up to the next required cytosine, analyze it, and gradually reconstruct the entire DNA chain by spreading the elongation of the chain from cytosine base to cytosine base through the use of enzyme catalyzed synthesis.

In short, it is possible to synthesize the DNA chain from a single strand and stop the synthesis at specific bases. It is also possible to break the chain or thymine, depending upon whether a purine cleavage enzyme (adenine and guanine) or pyrimidine cleave enzyme (cytosine and thymine) is used. By combining radioactive labelling of bases with cleavage and synthesis analysis, one can gradually begin to do DNA sequencing over a large length of the DNA chain. At the present time DNA segments of up to 100 nucleotides can be fairly rapidly sequenced. It is hoped within the next year to be able to sequence fragments of 100 nucleotides long by improving the separation of fragments with gel-electrophoresis. The new DNA sequencing methods enable study of a wide variety of DNA segments. It is hoped within the next year that the genes controlling different regions of the bacterium E. Coli will be known.

The methods of chemical cleavage work with both single and double-stranded DNA molecules. Single-stranded DNA molecules can be copied from an RNA molecule with a reverse transcriptase. Hopefully, one will be able to sequence the DNA in both the DNA viruses and the RNA viruses that code for cancer. Within the next few years the rapid sequencing of both DNA molecules and RNA molecules will be possible. Between the manipulation of genes and the sequencing of DNA in genes, a clearer understanding of the genetic basis and chemical coding of cancer should emerge.

JUMPING GENES

Traditionally cancer is regarded as a mutation of DNA within a cell, but its frequency and diversity have puzzled scientists. Genetic structures have an unusual stability. Spontaneous mutations in bacteria occur only at frequencies of one per 10^6 divisions. However, it has recently been demonstrated in bacteria that genes and segments of DNA move onto and off of chromosomes, or jump from place to place on chromosomes with frequencies as great as 10^2 divisions. This new phenomenon of "jumping genes" may be extremely important in mutations of cells and their carcinogenic change.

Jumping genes have thus far been studied most intensively in the bacteria, viruses, and plasmids (small pieces of extra-chromosonal DNA that replicate independently and can be directly transmitted from bacterium to bacterium). Two types of jumping genes have been clearly identified: (1) insertion elements, or specific DNA sequences ranging in size from about 700 to 1400 base pairs that can readily be inserted into bacteria. These specific sequences are IS–1, IS–2, IS–3, and IS–4; and (2) larger segments of jumping genes which confer antibotic resistance.

The jumping genes which carry antibody resistance are generally transferred to the bacterium by plasmids, and we have already recounted the role of plasmids in the production of recombinant DNA. Indeed it would appear that in the bacteria there are special plasmids—termed fertility plasmids, or F plasmids—that have a unique capability of integrating into the donor bacterium's chromosome.

Many molecular biologists now propose that these jumping

genes, which carry insertion sequences for antibiotic resistance, attach to plasmid DNA and serve as bridges for the modular construction of chromosomes. The antibiotic resistance genes are transferred from bacterium to bacterium by both plasmid and viruses. These jumping genes, whether they be insertion elements or antibiotic-resistant elements, turn off the expression of blocks of genes, integrate with the DNA of the host, and transform the organism and its characterisics.

The phenomenon of jumping genes seems to occur in higher organisms as well. There are 2 types of evidence for this: (1) structural; and (2) genetic. The structural evidence consists in similarities between the orientations and the sequences of eukaryotic DNA and the orientation of sequences on either end of the antibiotic-resistant jumping genes. The genetic evidence is very recent and comes from studies on the Drosophila genes, wherein certain genes cease to be expressed but can spontaneously regain their function, as if a jumping DNA segment had been inserted. Molecular biologists are beginning to propose that jumping genes are responsible for changes in the development of cells, and their transformation by viruses. These jumping genes could provide the means to shut off gene activity in differentiated cells, and permit them to become undifferentiated or cancerous. The attachment of jumping genes in cells to viruses might permit transformation into a cancerous cell by the integration of the virus into the cell DNA at a site of genetic homology. The mechanism for frequent mutations in the cell resides through insertion, deletion, and alteration of genetic structure by the intervention of jumping genes, plasmids, and viruses. This, of course, is still highly theoretical, but these questions of cellular mutation in eukaryotic cells can now be more readily studied through probing of cell genetics with jumping genes, plasmids, and viruses.

CELL FUSION, GENETIC CARTOGRAPHY, AND CANCER

The importance of molecular hybridization techniques in studying cancer cells has been reviewed in the work of Spiegelman in the section on "Viruses and Cancer." Ten years ago Professor Henry Harris at Oxford discovered that cells from different animal species could be fused to form viable hybrids under the guidance of harmless viruses (Harris, 1967). At first these hybrid cells are binucleate, but simultaneous division of the cells into daughter cells results in a hybrid which contains complete sets of chromosomes from both parent nuclei. Thereafter, chromosomes are progressively lost as the cells replicate. Harris used this technique to demonstrate that the genes for normalcy are dominant over the genes for malignancy. If a normal cell and a malignant cell are fused, the hybrid cell is initially nonmalignant. As chromosomes are progressively lost from the hybrid cell, which is characteristic of the replication of all of these hybrid cells, the cell reverts to a malignant state. By laboriously painful studies on chromosome deletion, and by carefully relating associations between the loss of particular chromosomes to the change in cell function, it is possible to assign genes determining overt phenotypic functions to particular chromosomes. X-ray or ionizing radiation can be used to induce breaks in the cell chromosome. The gene determining a specific measurable function is a marked gene. The analysis of the frequency of chromosomal breaks with function enables determination of the order of the marked genes on the chromosome and the distance between them, so-called chromosomal mapping or genetic cartography. Studies of this type over the past 10 years have been used to map human chromosomes, for it is possible to make human mouse cell hybrids, and in this hybrid the human chromosomes tend to be lost preferentially. Human genetic cartography is now in progress.

The ability of a hybrid cell to multiply and kill its genetic host is a genetic marker of malignancy. With hybrid cells it has been possible to show that malignancy is a recessive trait. Fusion of a malignant cell with a nonmalignant one results in suppression of the malignant phenotype. As long as the resulting hybrid cell contains the full chromosomal compliment of the 2 parent cells, it is possible to suppress the immunity of syngeneic hosts and by using "nude" mice as hosts to show that malignancy is similarly lost when human cancer cells are fused with normal human cells. Unfortunately, as these hybrid cells replicate, malignancy almost invariably appears, after they have lost about ¼ of the total chromosomes. This may well be because chromosomes which neutralize malignancy are lost from the hybrid cells. Tedious and painstaking research is now going on to discover which particular chromosomes control malignancy and which control the dominant gene for normalcy. In the mouse, it has already been shown that chromosome 4 carries some determinant important in controlling cell growth. However, the loss of both chromosomes 4 does not confer malignancy. So malignant transformation and alteration of cell growth are not genetically identical. It has also been shown that malignancy associated with the presence of an oncogenic virus can be suppressed by fusion with a normal cell, in spite of continued replication of the virus in the hybrid cell. This clearly reveals the importance of genetic cartography and the mapping "activator" and "repressor" genes in the chromosomes. Repression of the contained viral genetic information suppresses malignancy, whereas activation of the contained viral information produces a malignant phenotype.

A curious feature of transplanted animal tumor cells is the non-expression of histo-incompatability surface antigens. The recipient host of the transplanted tumor cell apparently does not reject the transplantable tumor cell line because it lacks expression of its surface antigens. Cell fusion studies have shown that such non-expression is not necessarily associated with the loss from hybrids of the chromosomes bearing the relative genes. The suppression of surface antigen production in malignant cells exists even though the genetic information for such production is present. Fusions with cells showing normal expressions of H–2 antigens may restore the antigenicity of the immunoresistant cell lines with reduced expression of the H–2 antigens. This, of course, has tremendous implications for the whole field of immunotherapy, as it may well be that the development of successful immunotherapeutic procedures will depend upon the understanding of how to overcome the immuno-resistance of the growing cancer cells. Genetic cartography and cell fusion techniques will be extremely valuable tools in understanding the nature and immunological characteristics of cancer in the years ahead.

FUTURE IMPLICATIONS OF BASIC MOLECULAR RESEARCH
IN CANCER

With these incipient studies on recombinant DNA, DNA sequencing, jumping genes, and cell fusion cartography, the heart of basic research in cancer is shifting to the molecular level. Support for this basic research stems largely from the federal government, but this research has tremendous implications not only in understanding cancer, but in the changing work orientation and accomplishments of our industrial economy. Recently, Dr. Robert Sinsheimer, Chairman of the Biology Division at Cal Tech, stated before a Senate Investigating Health Subcommittee "what this technology does is to make available to us the complete gene pool of evolution. We can take the genes of one organism and recombine them with those of others in any manner we wish. To my mind, this is an accomplishment as significant as the splitting of the atom" (1976). And his answer to the question, "Are you saying that with all that has gone before, we now have the power to change in some way the evolutionary process?" was "Yes."

Most scientists believe that work of this type should be permitted to proceed under appropriate safeguards. We have reviewed the initial guidelines for research issued by the National Institutes of Health in June of 1976. Public safety with respect to our environment and public health is at stake. For the first time the scientists' absolute right to free inquiry is being questioned, and limits may have to be placed on scientific investigation in the interests of society. In these manipulations of DNA we are approaching the alteration of the core of life itself. It is a way to escape the undesirable impositions of heredity, the molecular determinants of illness and disease, and the harsh impositions of the interactions of man with his environment. Through it man's intellect could be improved and his evolutionary adjustments controlled, but inherent in its injudicious use is the tyrannical shackling of man by man, and man by his environment. We must not rob ourselves of the potential benefits of this future research, but with Sinsheimer we must "begin to see that the truth is not enough, that the truth is necessary, but not sufficient, that scientific inquiry, the revealer of truth, needs to be coupled with wisdom, if our object is to advance the human condition."

To this end we leave the understanding of cancer in 1976. The solution of the cancer problem through individual scientific inquiry may force us as a society to assume the responsibility for life on this earth, and leave us with the dreadful burden of controlling our own future evolution.

REFERENCES TO CANCER—1977

Bailer, J. C. 1976. "Mammography: A Contrary View." *Annals of Internal Medicine,* 84:77–84.

Baltimore, D. 1976. "Viruses, Polymerases, and Cancer." *Science,* 192:632–636.

Bittner, J. J. 1936. "Some Possible Effects of Nursing on the Mammary Gland Tumor Incidence in Mice." *Science,* 84:162

Bonadonna, G., et. al. 1976. "Combination Chemotherapy as an Adjuvant Treatment in Operable Breast Cancer." New England Journal of Medicine, 294:405–410.

Cline, M. J., and Haskell, C. M. 1975. Cancer Chemotherapy. Philadelphia: Saunders, pp. 6, 10.

Conrad, R. A., Dobyns, B. M., and Sutow, W. W. 1970. "Thyroid Neoplasia as Late Effect of Exposure to Radioactive Iodine in Fallout." Journal of the American Medical Association, 214:316–324.

Cooper, M. D., and Lawton, A. E. 1974. "The Development of the Immune System." Scientific American, 23:59–72.

Dickinson, L. E., et. al. 1974. "Estrogen Profiles of Oriental and Caucasian Women in Hawaii." New England Journal of Medicine, 291:1211–1213.

Dulbecco, R. 1976. "From the Molecular Biology of Oncogenic DNA Virus to Cancer." Science, 192:437–458.

Edelman, G. M. 1976. "Surface Modulation in Cell Recognition and Cell Growth." Science, 192:218–226.

Eilber, F. R., Morton, D. L., et. al. 1976. "Adjuvant Immunotherapy With BCG in Treatment of Regional Lymph Node Metastases From Malignant Melanoma." New England Journal of Medicine, 294:237–240.

Ellermann, V., and Bang, O. 1908. "Experimentelle Leukämie bei Hühnern Zentralbl." Bakteriol, 46:595–609.

Fisher, B., et. al. 1975. "1–Phenylalanine Mustard (L–PAM) in the Management of Primary Breast Cancer: A Report of Early Findings." New England Journal of Medicine, 292:117–122.

Folkman, J. 1975. "Tumor Angiogenesis: A Possible Control Point in Tumor Growth." Annals of Internal Medicine, 82:96–100.

Gross, Ludwik. 1974. "The Role of Viruses in the Etiology of Cancer and Leukemia." Journal of the American Medical Association, 230:1029–1032.

Harris, H. 1967. Cell Fusion. Mass.: Harvard University Press.

Hoover, R., et. al. 1976. "Menopausal Estrogens in Breast Cancer." New England Journal of Medicine, 122:20–48.

Kelso, D. R. 1974. "Benign Hepatomas and Oral Contraceptives." Lancet, 2:315–317.

McGuire, W. L., Carbone, P. P., Vollmer, E. P., eds. 1975. Estrogen Receptors in Human Breast Cancer. New York: Raven Press.

Manber, M. M. 1976. Medical World News. August 23, pp. 44–56.

Parker, L. N., Belsky, J. L., Pamamoto, T., et. al. 1974. "Thyroid Carcinoma After Exposure to Atomic Radiation." Annals of Internal Medicine, 80: 600–604.

Pilch, Y. H., et. al. 1976. "Immunotherapy of Cancer With 'Immune' RNA." American Journal of Surgery, 132:631–637.

Rous, P. 1911. "A Sarcoma of the Fowl Transmissible by an Agent Separable From the Tumor Cells." Journal of Experimental Medicine, 13:397–411.

Rubin, H. 1964. "A Defective Cancer Virus." Scientific American, 210:46–52.

Ryser, Hughes J. P. 1974. "Chemical Carcinogenesis: Special Report." A Cancer Journal for Clinicians, 24:351–362.

Sinsheimer, R. L. 1976. "Recombinant DNA: A Critic Questions the Right of Free Inquiry." Science, 194:303.

Spiegelman, S. 1974. "Ribonucleic Acid." Journal of the American Medical Association, 230:1036–1042.

Swerdloff, R. S., *et. al.* 1975. "Complications of Oral Contraceptive Agents." *Western Journal of Medicine,* 122:20–48.

Temin, H. 1976. "The DNA Provirus Hypothesis." *Science,* 192:1075–1080.

Watson, J. D. 1965. *The Molecular Biology of the Gene.* New York: W. A. Benjamin.

GLOSSARY

Ablation. Removal of a part.

Actinic rays. Rays of light beyond the violet end of the spectrum.

Adenine. One of the four bases of DNA (deoxyribonucleic acid). See also *Guanine, Cytosine,* and *Thymine.* One of the four bases of RNA (ribonucleic acid). See also *Guanine, Cytosine,* and *Uracil.*

ADP (Adenosine diphosphate). A product, along with organic phosphates, of the hydrolysis of adenosine triphosphate (ATP).

Adrenal glands. Two small glands located just above the kidney that produce hormones essential for life.

Adrenalectomy. Removal of the adrenal glands.

Aerobic system. An oxygen-dependent respiratory system. Cells in the animal kingdom operate on an aerobic system; they are utterly dependent on oxygen for their life.

Agglutination. Collection into clumps of the cells distributed in a fluid.

ALG (Anti-lymphocyte globulin). Powerful immuno-suppressive agent made against the lymphocytes or the lymphocyte globulins.

Alkaptonuria. Excretion in urine of alkapton bodies, causing the urine to turn dark.

Alkylating agents. Chemical carcinogens. Other cancer-producing chemicals are: the *Nitroso compounds,* the *Lactones,* the *Azo dyes* and the *Polycyclic hydrocarbons.*

Alleles. Dominant or recessive forms of the same genetic trait on the chromosomes.

Allogenic grafting. Transplantation of tissues between genetically nonidentical animals belonging to the same species.

Alpha helix. Name given to the helical configuration of proteins by Linus Pauling.

Alpha particles. High-energy particles dispensing their energy in a very limited range within the tissues but highly destructive of the tissues they encounter.

Amino acids. Organic compounds, building blocks of proteins; about 20 amino acids are essential for life.

Anaerobic system. The chlorophyll system of plants. Cells in the plant kingdom do not depend upon oxygen for life but absorb carbon dioxide and
   return oxygen to the atmosphere. Aerobic and anaerobic systems are inter-
   dependent.
Anaphase. The stage in mitosis following metaphase in which the halves of
   the divided chromosomes move apart to the poles of the spindle.
Anaploid cells. Cells containing an abnormal number of chromosomes. They
   are cancerous cells. See also *Hypoploid, Heteroploid, Tetraploid* cells.
Androgens. Male sex hormones.
Anorexia. Lack of the appetite for food.
Antibody. Substance manufactured by cells to fight invading antigens.
Antigen. Foreign substance (such as the antigen of a virus) invading a cell and
   eliciting the formation of antibodies.
Atom. Smallest element of matter having distinct chemical properties. Atoms
   group together into molecules constituting all substances found in nature.
   An atom is made in the form of a miniature solar system: at its center is
   the nucleus around which electrons orbit at enormous speeds.
ATP (Adenosine triphosphate). A nucleotide compound occurring in all cells
   which represents an energy source for cellular function.
Axilla. A small hollow beneath the arm where it joins the shoulder (also called
   the armpit).
Axillary lymph nodes. Lymph nodes in the axilla.
Azo dyes. Chemical carcinogens. See *Alkylating agents.*

Bacteria. Single-celled organisms. Many are infectious.
Bacteriophage. A virus that multiplies in bacteria.
BCG (Bacillus Calmette-Guérin). A vaccine against tuberculosis, consisting of
   attenuated living cultures of bovine tubercle bacilli.
Biochemistry. The chemistry of living organisms or living processes.
Biological predeterminism. Concept expressing the fact that each individual
   organism's response to cancer and other diseases is unique and, to an
   extent, "predetermined."
Biopsy. The removal of a small portion of tissue from the body for examination under the microscope.
Burkitt's lymphoma. A hereditary human cancer of lymphoid tissues, present
   in South Africa in endemic form.

Carcinogen. An agent (viral, chemical, irradiating) capable of inducing cancer.
Carcinogenesis. Development of cancerous cells.
Carcinoma. Cancer.
Catalase. An enzyme which specifically hastens the decomposition of hydro-
   gen peroxide which is found in practically all cells.
Catalyst. A substance that does not initiate but facilitates a chemical reaction.
Cell. Unit of living tissue, both in plants and animals.
Cell-free system. A system which reproduces artificially the composition of
   a cell. All the elements of a cell are present but they are not structured into
   a cell.
Cell fusion. Coherence of adjacent cells.

Cellular antibodies. Or cell-bound antibodies. May circulate throughout the organism but are bound to the cell, generally the lymphocyte.

Centromere. Clear region where the arms of a chromosome meet.

Centrosomes (or *centrioles*). Two small bodies in the cell cytoplasm which travel to either side of the cytoplasm at the time of cell division.

Chalones. Substances produced in an organ which diminish or inhibit function in the organ.

Chemotherapy. Treatment by drugs.

Chlorophyll. Green pigment of plants.

Chromatin strands. The readily stainable portion of the cell nucleus forming a network of fibrils of DNA and serving as the carrier of the genes in inheritance.

Chromatography. Chemical analysis of compounds through examination of the rate of migration on an absorbent column.

Chromosomes. Minute structures in the cell nucleus made up of genes; the carriers of heredity.

Chronic cystic mastitis. Breast disease characterized by nodular cysts; the breast is tender and painful.

Classical radical mastectomy. Operation of Halsted for breast cancer. Removal of the breast with its tumor, together with the pectoral muscles and the lymph nodes of the axilla.

Clone. A strain of cells descended in culture from a single cell.

Compton effect. A change in the wavelength of scattered rays and emission of recoil electrons in deep radiation.

Contact inhibition. A mechanism of growth control in cells, whereby cells cease to grow when they touch each other. Cancer cells have lost the capacity for contact inhibition.

Control genes. Genes that stimulate or inhibit the action of structural genes. (Jacob and Monod). See *Structural genes.*

Crossing-over. Exchange of genes between homologous chromosomes of a hybrid.

Cryogenic. Pertaining to the production of very low temperatures.

Cyclic accelerator (or *cyclotron*). One of the machines producing high-energy radiations.

Cytoplasm. Protoplasm of the cell, its living matter. Makes up the bulk of a cell, excluding the nucleus and membrane.

Cytosine. One of the four bases of DNA—see *Adenine.* One of the four bases of RNA—see *Guanine.*

Defective virus. A virus which does not destroy the cell and replicate itself but which inserts its genome into the cell it attacks.

Dicarboxylic acid. An organic acid having a carboxyl (COOH) group at each end of the organic carbon chain.

Differentiation. The development of form and function in a cell or tissue.

Dimerization. Fusion or joining of two similar purine or pyrimidne bases by cross-linkage of carbon rings.

Diploid cell. A normal cell containing the normal number of chromosomes, in a human being 46 chromosomes.

DNA (deoxyribonucleic acid). The informational macromolecules of the cell nucleus, wound together in the form of a double helix.

Dominant trait. A strong genetic trait.

Double helix. The coil-like configuration of the nucleic acid molecule as demonstrated by Watson and Crick, forming the backbone of DNA.

Dysplasia. Faulty or abnormal development or growth.

Edema. The presence of large amounts of fluid in the intercellular spaces of the body.

Effusion. The escape of fluid into a part or tissue.

Electron. The unit of negative electricity which revolves about the nucleus of an atom or which flows in a conductor to produce an electric current.

Electron microscopy. A technique for visualizing material through the microscope that uses beams of electrons instead of light beams, and thereby permits clearer magnification than is possible with the ordinary microscope.

Electron therapy. Direct cancer therapy by electrons.

Endocrine glands. Glands secreting internally into the blood or lymph.

Endometrium. The mucous coat or lining of the uterus.

Endoplasmic reticulum. System of connected channels in the cell cytoplasm. It is involved in protein synthesis and also has a role in the action of drugs on cells.

Energy metabolism. Cellular processes directly related to the production of energy.

Enzymes. Proteins stimulating cell functions or acting as catalysts.

Epidemiology. The scientific study of factors determining the frequency and distribution of disease.

Epithelium. The external covering of a tissue or organ.

Escape mechanisms (from *immunological surveillance*). Mechanisms through which the body favors tumor growth.

Estrogen. Female sex hormone.

Etiocholanolone. A reduced form of testosterone (hormone produced by testes) excreted in the urine.

F_1 *generation.* First generation cross as demonstrated by Mendel when crossing pea seeds different in a single trait: the first generation shows the characteristics of *one* parent.

$F_2, F_3, F_4, \ldots$ *generation.* Second, third, fourth . . . filial generations in the Mendelian experiments when traits from *both* parents appear.

Femoral. Pertaining to the femur (thigh bone) or to the thigh.

Filial. Pertaining to offspring.

Fractionation. The dividing into fractions.

Gamete. One of two cells, male and female, whose union is necessary to initiate the development of a new individual (in sexual reproduction).

Gamma rays. Electromagnetic radiations of short wavelength emitted by the nucleus of an atom during a nuclear reaction.

Genes. Units of hereditary material grouped into chromosomes and constituted of DNA.

Genetic code. A sequence of purine and pyrimidine bases in DNA which carries the hereditary message for protein synthesis.

Genome. The complete set of hereditary factors contained in the haploid chromosome.

Gonadectomy. Excision of an ovary or testis.

Guanine. One of the four bases of DNA; see also *Adenine.* One of the four bases of RNA; the other three bases of RNA are: *Adenine, Cytosine, Uracil.*

Haploid cell. A germ cell, in human beings, containing 23 chromosomes. In fertilization, when male and female germ cells unit, the total number of chromosomes is again 46.

Heme. The nonprotein, insoluble iron protoporphyrin constituent of hemoglobin (oxygen-carrying pigment of the blood).

Heteroploid cell. A cell containing more than the normal number of chromosomes.

Hodgkin's disease. Disease of the lymphoid tissues.

Homeostasis. The essential stability of an organism.

Homografts (or allografts). Grafts of tissue between genetically different animals of the same species.

Horizontal transmission (of tumors). Transmission from individual to individual. See *Vertical transmission.*

Hormones. Substances secreted by the endocrine glands and discharged through the blood and lymph streams. They stimulate organs (the so-called "target organs") to specific action.

Huggins' tumor. An experimental breast cancer in inbred rats produced by 7, 12 DMBA (7, 12 dimethylbenz (a) anthracene).

Humoral antibodies. Free-circulating antibodies.

Hydroxy acids. Acids containing the hydroxyl (OH) group.

Hydroxy corticoids. Hormones of the adrenal cortex.

Hyperplasia. The abnormal multiplication of cells in a tissue.

Hypophysis. See *Pituitary body.*

Immunity. Rejection of an antigen by the organism.

Immunological surveillance. Body mechanisms for the rejection of foreign cells.

Immunological tolerance. A state of body reaction to antigens varying from total tolerance to total immunity.

Immunology. The science of immunity, or the study of the mechanisms whereby the host reacts to foreign substances in its environment to resist desease, poison, or infection.

Immuno-suppression. Suppression of the body's immune responses. Certain chemicals initiate immuno-suppression.

Initiation (of cancer process). The silent beginning of the cancer process.

In situ. Confined to a small site of origin (cancer *in situ*).

Internal mammary chain. Chain of lymph nodes within the chest.

Interphase. "Resting" period of cell, when it is not dividing.

In vitro. In the test tube.

In vivo. Within the living body.

Ion. Electrically charged atom.

Ionic bond. Organic molecules commonly contain one or more units of net positive or negative charge in a group known as an ionic group or an ionic bond.

Ionizing radiation. X-ray or gamma ray radiation which produces ion pairs in matter.

Isogenic. Of identical genetic composition.

Isotopes. Variants of a given chemical element. Their constitutions are about identical to that of the original element but their nuclei weigh more or less, therefore their atomic weights are different.

Karyotype. Constant grouping of chromosomes in a normal cell; also arrangement in pairs according to length and shape.

Lactones. Chemical carcinogens. See also *Alkylating agents.*

Leucosis (or *leukosis*). Proliferation of leukocyte-forming tissue—the basis of leukemia.

Leukemia. Cancer of the blood cells.

Leukemogenic. Causing leukemia.

Ligation. The application of a ligature.

Linear accelerator. A machine producing high-energy radiations.

Lipid. An organic fatty substance which is insoluble in water but soluble in alcohol, ether, chloroform, and other fat solvents.

Lymph. The watery fluid between the body cells.

Lymph nodes. Glands that produce lymphocytes and act as the sites of defense against infection, or against invasions by foreign agents.

Lymphangiography. Radiography of the lymph nodes after the introduction of an opaque iodinated oil into the lymph channels.

Lymphoblastoma. Tumor of the lymph glands.

Lymphocytes. White blood corpuscles arising in lymph glands and nodes, instrumental in the immunological processes of the body.

Lymphosarcoma. Cancer of lymphoid tissue.

Lysosomes. Bodies situated in the cell cytoplasm, containing enzymes active in the digestion of foodstuff.

Lysozyme. An enzyme within cells which is capable of destroying the cell or certain of its functions.

Male gamete (and *female gamete*). See *Gamete.*

Malignant tumor. An abnormal tissue growth which tends to destroy the host by direct spread or metastasis.

Mammography. Breast X-rays.

Mass spectrometry. Analysis of substances by breaking them down into their basic atoms and measuring the weight, or mass, of the atoms by the rate of their migration in a strong electric field.

Mastectomy. Removal of the breast.

Meiosis. Division of sex (or germ) cells.

Messenger RNA. The messenger between nuclear DNA and the ribosomes of the cell cytoplasm, site of protein synthesis.

Metabolism. All the physical and chemical processes in living organisms necessary for maintaining life.

Metaphase. The middle phase of mitosis during which the lengthwise separation of the chromosomes in the equatorial plate occurs.

Metastasis. Secondary tumor centers at a distance from the original tumor, and resulting from the transportation of tumor cells by blood or lymph streams.

Mitochondria. Fine structure in the cell cytoplasm, "power house" of the cell; center of photosynthesis in plants, and of oxidation of foodstuffs in animals.

Mitosis. Cell division.

Molecule. Small mass of matter, made up of atoms.

Mongolism. Mental retardation associated with flat skull, flat nose, short fingers, wide fingerwebs, and a chromosomal abnormality.

Mutagenesis. The process of genetic changes within the cell.

Mutant. The result of a mutation.

Mutation. Change in a cell which is permanent and transmissible to offspring.

Myelocytic. Related to myelocytes, or marrow cells.

Neoplasia. The process of new growth; commonly cancer formation.

Neoplasm. Cancerous growth.

Neoplastic transformation. The change from normal growth to abnormal growth such as a tumor.

Neurofibromatosis. Familial changes in the nervous system, muscles, bones, and skin, with appearance of soft tumors over the whole body of nerve tissue and fibrous tissue origin.

Nitroso compounds. Compounds containing nitrogen and oxygen in a univalent linkage.

Nuclear sap. Amorphous protein matrix which bathes all the nuclear structures of the cell.

Nucleic acids. DNA (deoxyribonucleic acid) and RNA (ribonucleic acid); chemical constituents of genes, simplest forms of "life" (capable of reproducing themselves).

Nucleolus. A round granular structure found in the nucleus of the cell, which is involved in ribosomal RNA synthesis.

Nucleotide. Purine or pyrimidine base bound to a 5-carbon sugar and a phosphate group.

Nucleus (of cell). A steroid body within the cell which is circumscribed by a thin nuclear membrane and contains nucleoli, granules of chromatin, and the main core of DNA in the cell.

Obstructive edema. Swelling of the limbs due to choking of the lymphatic channels by cancer cells.

Oncogenesis. The development of a tumor or growth.

Oncogenic. Leading to the development of a tumor or growth.

Oophorectomy. Removal of an ovary or the ovaries.

Operator gene. The gene responsible for synthesis of a specific enzyme or protein.

Operon. A genetic unit of functions at the subcellular level under the control of a so-called operator and a repressor.

Oxidation. The act of combining with oxygen, generally consisting in either an increase in the positive charges on the atom or the loss of negative charges.

Oxygen effect. Enhancement of radiosensitivity of cells because of the presence of oxygen.

Ozone. A more active form of oxygen resulting from exposure of oxygen to the silent discharge of electricity.

Palpation. The application of the fingers to the body for the purpose of diagnosis.

Parametrium. Soft tissues adjoining the uterus.

Pituitary body (or *hypophysis*). An endocrine gland situated at the base of the brain; the master gland.

Philadelphia chromosome. An abbreviated chromosome, found in certain leukemias, such as chronic granulocytic leukemias.

Photons. "Quanta" of energy delivered by X-rays and the other rays of the electromagnetic spectrum (Planck).

Photosynthesis. Metabolism of plants. The sunlight energy is captured by the plants' chlorophyll and transformed into chemical energy.

Polycyclic hydrocarbons. Chemical carcinogens. See *Alkylating agents.*

Polyoma virus. A DNA virus inducing a variety of cancers in mammals.

Polymer. Variation of a given chemical compound. In polymerization the molecules of the compound join other molecules of the same compound; in consequence, the polymer has a heavier molecular weight than that of the compound.

Polynucleotide. A linear sequence of nucleotides in which the 3 prime position of the sugar of one nucleotide is linked through a phosphate group to the 5 prime position on the sugar of the adjacent nucleotide.

Polypeptide. A polymer of amino acids linked together by peptide bonds.

Polyposis. The development of multiple polyps in an organ or structure.

Polyvalent vaccine. A vaccine prepared from cultures of more than one strain of virus or bacterium.

Prognosis. The prospect of a disease, its outcome or future.

Progression (of cancer process). The appearance of cancer in clinical form.

Promotion (of cancer process). The intermediate stages of cancer growth wherein the cell is altered by extraneous factors either within the patient or from the environment.

Prophase. Followed by *Metaphase, Anaphase, Telophase;* the four main phases of cell division.

Proteins. Combinations (polymers) of amino acids, constituting animal tissues.

Proton. The unit of positive electricity equivalent in charge to an electron and equal to the hydrogen ion in mass.

Provirus. A latent stage of a virus.

Purine base, pyrimidine base. Organic compounds of carbon, hydrogen, and nitrogen; in cyclic form these are the primary components of DNA.

Rad. A measure of the amount of any ionizing radiation which is *absorbed* by tissues.

Radiation sickness. Illness sometimes caused by radiation therapy; characterized by nausea, lack of appetite, vomiting, and diarrhea.

Radioactive isotopes. Isotopes having radioactive properties.

Radiopaque. Not permitting the passage of X-rays or other radiant energy.

RBE. Relative biological effectiveness of a radiation: the effect of a given radiation on a given tissue is dependent upon the energy absorbed and the wavelength used.

Recessive trait. A weak genetic trait.

Regression. The subsidence of a disease, or symptom.

Replication. Transcription and *translation:* biological processes of the cell. Replication is the self-copying process; transcription, the passage of a message from DNA to RNA; translation, the actual carrying out of the message by messenger RNA.

Repressor gene. The gene suppressing the active, or operator, gene.

Retinoblastoma. A malignant tumor of the retina.

Ribonucleotide. A compound that consists of a purine or pyrimidine base bonded to a ribose sugar which in turn is connected to a phosphate group.

Ribosome. Substance of the cell cytoplasm, site of protein synthesis.

RNA (Ribonucleic acid). Polymer of ribonucleotides.

Roentgen. Unit of radiation (after the name of the German physicist who discovered X-rays).

Roentgen rays. X-rays.

Rous sarcoma virus. An RNA virus, producing cancer in chickens.

Sex-linked. Invariably related to male or female sex.

Structural genes (Jacob and Monod). Genes which determine the complexity and differentiation of a cell. See *Control genes.*

Supraclavicular nodes. Lymph nodes above the clavicle.

Syngenic grafting. Transplantation of tissues between genetically identical animals.

Telecobalt unit. A machine producing high-energy radiations.

Telophase. The last of the four stages of mitosis.

Template surface. Copying surface of the DNA strands; in replication, when the DNA helix unwinds into two separate strands, each of these strands serves as the template on which the second half is paired off.

Thymine. One of the four bases of DNA.

Tolerance. State of acceptance of an antigen by the cell.

Transcription. The formation of messenger RNA from the template DNA.

Transduction. The transfer of a genetic fragment from one cell to another.

Transfer RNA. The adaptor molecule between messenger RNA (bringing DNA's message to the ribosomes) and the ribosomes themselves. It is a free RNA molecule in the cell cytoplasm, which "searches" each required amino acid and brings it to each exact spot on messenger RNA for protein synthesis.

Translation. The formation of protein coded by the messenger RNA.

Triplet. Assemblage of any three of the four bases of DNA (A, G, T, C) codifying the formation of a particular amino acid.

Tumor. An abnormal growth of tissue.

Tumoricidal. Destroying cancer cells.

Univalent vaccine. A vaccine prepared from the culture of one strain of virus or bacterium.

Uracil. One of the four bases of RNA. See also *Adenine.*

Vertical transmission (of tumors). Transmission from generation to generation, from mother to offspring.

Virus. Minute living organism composed of an inner nucleic acid core and an outer protein coat. Parasitic, needs to live in a cell to reproduce itself.

Wilms' tumor. An embryonal tumor of the kidney.

Yttrium. A very rare metal producing isotopes that emit X-rays.

Zenogenic grafting. Transplantation of tissues between animals of different species.

BIBLIOGRAPHY

Alvarez, W. C. 1952. "Care of the Dying." *Journal of the American Medical Association,* 150:89–91.

Ambrose, E. J., and Roe, F. J. C. 1966. *The Biology of Cancer.* New York: Van Nostrand.

American Cancer Society. 1961. *Tobacco.* New York: Published jointly with other organizations.

———. 1966. *Unproven Methods of Cancer Treatment.* New York: American Cancer Society.

———. 1970a. *Index of the American Cancer Society File Material on Unproven Methods of Treatment of Cancer.* New York: American Cancer Society.

———. 1970b. *Cancer Facts and Figures.* New York: American Cancer Society.

Anon. 1961. "Euthanasia." *Lancet,* 1 (12 Aug.): 351–354.

Bard, Morton, 1966. "Clues to the Psychological Management of Patients with Cancer." *Annals of the New York Academy of Sciences,* 125: 995–997.

Bell, Thomas. 1961. *In the Midst of Life.* New York: Atheneum.

Billingham, R. E., Brent, L., and Medawar, P. B. 1953. " 'Actively acquired tolerance' of foreign cells." *Nature,* 172: 603–606.

Bricker, E. M. 1970. "Pelvic Exenteration." In *Advances in Surgery,* vol. 4, pp. 13–72.

Brookes, Peter. 1966. "Quantitative Aspects of the Reaction of Some Carcinogens with Nucleic Acids and the Possible Significance of Such Reactions in the Process of Carcinogenesis." *Cancer Research,* 26: 1994–2003.

Bullough, W. S. 1967. *The Evolution of Differentiation.* New York: Academic Press.

Burnet, Sir Macfarlane. 1961. "The Mechanism of Immunity." *Scientific American,* 204(1): 58–67.

Butcher, H. R., Jr. 1963. Radical Mastectomy for Mammary Carcinoma. *Annals of Surgery,* 157: 165–166.

Butcher, H. R., Jr., Seaman, W. B., Eckert, C. *et al.* 1964. "An Assessment of Radical Mastectomy and Postoperative Irradiation Therapy in the Treatment of Mammary Cancer." *Cancer,* 17: 480–485.

Calvin, Melvin. 1965. "Chemical Evoluation." *Proceedings of the Royal Society (London),* Series B, 288: 441–446.

Calvin, Melvin, and Calvin, G. J. 1964. "Atom to Adam." *American Scientist,* 52 (2): 163–186.

Crile, George, Jr. 1965. Rationale of Simple Mastectomy without Radiation for Chemical Stage 1 Cancer of the Breast." *Surgery, Gynecology, and Obstetrics,* 120: 975–982.

Darwin, Charles. 1959. "Unpublished Letters," ed. Sir Gavin De Beer. *Notes and Records of the Royal Society (London),* 14:12–66.

Ehrlich, P. 1957. *Collected Papers,* ed. F. Himmelweit. 2 vols. New York: Pergamon Press.

Emmelot, P., and Mühlbock, O. (editors). 1964. *Cellular Control Mechanisms and Cancer.* New York: Elsevier Pub. Co.

Everson, T. C., and Cole, W. H. 1966. *Spontaneous Regression of Cancer.* Philadelphia: Saunders.

Ewing, James. 1941. *Neoplastic Diseases.* 4th ed. Philadelphia: Saunders.

Exton-Smith, A. N. 1961. "Terminal Illness in the Aged." *Lancet* 2(5 Aug.): 305–308.

Fedor, S. L. 1966. Panel Discussion: "Retrospects and Prospects." *Annals of the New York Academy of Sciences,* 125: 1032.

Fisher, Bernard *et al.* 1968. "Surgical Adjuvant Chemotherapy in Cancer of the Breast." *Annals of Surgery,* 161: 339–356.

Fitts, W. T., Jr., and Ravdin, I. S. 1953. "What Philadelphia Physicians Tell Patients with Cancer." *Journal of the American Medical Association,* 153: 901–904.

Furth, J., Clifton, K. H., Gadsden, E. L., and Buffet, R. F. 1956. "Dependent and Autonomous Mammotropic Pituitary Tumors in Rats: Their Somatotropic Features." *Cancer Research,* 16: 600–607.

Furth, J., Seibold, H. R., and Rathbone, R. R. 1933. "Experimental Studies on Lymphomatosis of Mice." *American Journal of Cancer,* 19: 521–604.

Gardner, W. H. 1966. "Adjustment Problems of Laryngectomized Women." *Archives of Otolaryngology,* 83: 31–42.

Getzen, L. G., Lobpreis, I., and Holloway, C. K., Jr. 1969. "The Treatment of Breast Cancer: Analysis of Various Therapeutic Modalities." *Archives of Surgery,* 98: 131–137.

Gorer, P. A. *et al.* "Passive Immunity in Mice Against C57BL Leukosis E.L.4 by Means of Iso-immune Serum." *Cancer Research,* 16: 338–342.

Grant, R. N., and Bartlett, Irene. 1966. "Unproven Cancer Remedies: A Primer." In *Unproven Methods of Cancer Treatment.* New York: American Cancer Society. p. 14.

Greene, W. A. 1966. "The Psychological Setting of the Development of Leukemia and Lymphoma." *Annals of the New York Academy of Sciences,* 125: 794–801.

Grinker, Roy, 1966. Discussion of Papers Presented. *Annals of the New York Academy of Sciences,* 125: 874–875.

————. 1966. "Psychosomatic Aspects of the Cancer Problem." *Annals of the New York Academy of Sciences,* 125: 876–881.

Gross, L. 1961. "Induction of Leukemia in Rats with Mouse Leukemia (Passage A) Virus." *Proceedings of the Society for Experimental Biology and Medicine,* 106: 890–893.

Guttman, Ruth. 1967. "Radiotherapy in Locally Advanced Cancer of the Breast." *Cancer,* 20: 1046–1050.

Haagensen, C. D., and Cooley, E. 1963. "Radical Mastectomy for Mammary Carcinoma." *Annals of Surgery,* 157: 166–169.

Hammet, V. B., and Graff, Harold. 1966. "Therapy of Smoking." *Current Psychiatric Therapies,* 6: 70–75.

Handley, R. S., and Thackray, A. E. 1963. "Conservative Radical Mastectomy (Patey's Operation). *Annals of Surgery,* 157: 162–164.

Hillman, James. 1965. *Suicide and the Soul.* New York: Harper and Row.

Hinton, John. 1967. *Dying.* London: Penguin Books.

Holland, J. F. 1967. "The Krebiozen Story. Is Cancer Quackery Dead?" *Journal of the American Medical Association,* 200: 213-218.

Huggins, C. B. 1965. "Propositions in Hormonal Treatment of Advanced Cancers." *Journal of the American Medical Association,* 192: 1141–1145.

Huggins, C. B., and Bergenstal, D. M. 1952. "Inhibition of Human Mammary and Prostatic Cancers by Adrenalectomy." *Cancer Research,* 12: 134–141.

Huggins, C. B., and Dao, T. L. Y. 1953. "Adrenalectomy and Oophorectomy in Treatment of Advanced Carcinoma of the Breast." *Journal of the American Medical Association,* 151: 1388-1394.

Huggins, C. B., Grand, L. C., and Brillantes, F. P. 1961. "Mammary Cancer Induced by a Single Feeding of Polynuclear Hydrocarbons, and Its Suppression." *Nature,* 189:204.

Hutchinson, G. B., and Shapiro, S. 1968. "Lead Time Gained by Diagnostic Screening for Breast Cancer." *Journal of the National Cancer Institute,* 41: 665–673.

Jacob, F., and Monod, J. 1961. "Genetic Regulatory Mechanisms in the Synthesis of Proteins." *Journal of Molecular Biology,* 3: 318–356.

Jacobs, M. A., Knapp, P. H., Anderson, L. S. *et al.* 1965. "Relationship of Oral Frustration Factors with Heavy Cigarette Smoking in Males." *Journal of Nervous and Mental Disease,* 141: 161–171.

Jensen, E. 1967. "Estrogen Receptors in Hormone-responsive Tissues and Tumors." In *Endogenous Factors Influencing Host-tumor Balance,* ed. R. W. Winssler, T. L. Dao, and S. Wood, Jr. Chicago: Univ. Chicago Press.

Kaae, S., and Johansen, H. 1962. "Breast Cancer—Five Year Results: Two Random Series of Simple Mastectomy with Postoperative Irradiation Versus Extended Radical Mastectomy." *American Journal of Roentgenology,* 87: 82–88.

Kaplan, H. S. 1964. "Some Possible Mechanisms of Carcinogenesis." In *Cellular Control Mechanisms and Cancer,* ed. P. Emmelot and O. Mühlbock.

————. 1967. "The Natural History of Murine Leukemia." *Cancer Research,* 27: 1325–1338.

Kinsolving, Lester. 1967. "Some Thoughts on Mercy Killing." *San Francisco Chronicle,* Aug. 26.

Kissen, D. M. 1966. "The Significance of Personality in Lung Cancer in Men." *Annals of the New York Academy of Sciences,* 125: 820–826.

Kornberg, Arthur. 1968. "The Synthesis of DNA." *Scientific American,* 219(4): 64–78.

Lacassagne, A. M. 1932. "Apparition de cancers de la mamelle chez la souris mâle, soumise à des injections de folliculine. *Comptes Rendus, Academie des Sciences (Paris),* 195: 630–632.

Laqueur, G. L., Mickelsen, O., and Whiting, M. G. 1963. "Carcinogenic Properties of Nuts from *Cycas circinalis* L. Indigenous to Guam." *Journal of the National Cancer Institute,* 31: 919–951.

LeShan, Lawrence. 1966. "An Emotional Life-history Pattern Associated with Neoplastic Disease." *Annals of the New York Academy of Sciences,* 125: 780–792.

————. 1966. Panel Discussion: "Retrospects and Prospects." *Annals of the New York Academy of Sciences,* 125: 1050.

Little, J. B. 1966. "Environmental Hazards: Ionizing Radiation." *New England Journal of Medicine,* 275: 929–937.

Lowenstein, W. R., and Kanno, Y. 1966. "Intercellular Communication and the Control of Tissue Growth: Lack of Communication between Cancer Cells." *Nature,* 209: 1248–1249.

Lowenstein, W. R. *et al.* 1967. "Intercellular Communication and Tissue Growth." *Journal of Cellular Biology,* 33: 225–234.

Lukes, R. J., and Butler, J. L. 1966. "The Pathology and Classification of Hodgkin's Disease." *Cancer Research,* 26: 1063–1083.

Lwoff, André. 1965. *Biological Order.* Cambridge, Mass.: M.I.T. Press.

McClennan, C. E., McClennan, M. T., and Bagshaw, M. C. 1967. "Linear Acceleration in the Treatment of Cervical Cancer." *American Journal of Obstetrics and Gynecology,* 98: 675–687.

McWhirter, Robert. 1955. "Simple Mastectomy and Radiotherapy in the Treatment of Breast Cancer." *British Journal of Radiology,* 28: 128–139.

Magee, P. N., and Barnes, J. M. 1956. "The Production of Malignant Primary Hepatic Tumors in Rat by Feeding Dimethylnitrosamine." *British Journal of Cancer,* 10: 114–122.

Marx, R. 1961. *The Health of the Presidents.* New York: Putnam.

Mastrovito, R. C. 1966. "Acute Psychological Problems and the Use of Psychotropic Medicine in the Treatment of the Cancer Patient." *Annals of the New York Academy of Sciences,* 125: 1006–1010.

Maussner, Bernard. 1966. "Report on Smoking Clinic." *American Psychologist,* 21: 251–255.

Mitchison, N. A. 1955. "Studies on the Immunological Response to Foreign Tumor Transplants in the Mouse. I. The Role of Lymph Node Cells in Conferring Immunity by Adoptive Transfer." *Journal of Experimental Medicine,* 102: 157–177.

Moses, Rafael, and Cividali, Nizza. 1966. "Different Levels of Awareness of Illness: Their Relation to Some Salient Features in Cancer Patients." *Annals of the New York Academy of Sciences,* 125: 984–993.

Muslin, H. L., Gyarfas, K., and Pieper, W. J. 1966. "Separation Experience and Cancer of the Breast." *Annals of the New York Academy of Sciences,* 125: 802–806.

Northrup, Eric. 1957. *Science Looks at Smoking.* New York: Coward McCann.

Nowell, P. C., and Hungerford, D. A. 1960. "A Minute Chromosome in Human Chronic Granulocytic Leukemia." *Science,* 132: 1497.

Ochsner, Alton. 1959. *Smoking and Health.* New York: Messner.

Oken, D. 1961. "What to Tell Cancer Patients: A Story of Medical Attitudes." *Journal of the American Medical Association,* 175: 1120–1128.

Paterson, R., and Russell, M. H. 1959. "Clinical Trials in Malignant Disease, Part III, Breast Cancer: Evaluation of Postoperative Radiotherapy. *Journal of the Faculty of Radiologists,* 10: 175.

Peeters, R. G. 1966. *Le Cancer.* Verviers, Belgium: Gerard & Co.

Reid, J. W. 1964. "On the Road to the River." *Canadian Medical Association Journal,* 91: 911–913.

Rhoads, Paul S. 1965. "Management of the Patient with Terminal Illness." *Journal of the American Medical Association,* 192: 661–665.

Rosenblatt, M. B., and Lisa, J. R. 1967. "Bronchogenic Carcinoma." *Medical Science,* 18(8): 37–41.

Ross, W. S. 1965. *The Climate is Hope.* New York: Prentice-Hall.

Rous, Peyton. 1967. "The Challenge to Man of the Neoplastic Cell." *Science,* 157: 24–28.

Rubin, Harry. 1964. "A Defective Cancer Virus." *Scientific American,* 210(6): 46–52.

Russell, Bertrand. 1903. *A Free Man's Worship.* (Reprinted in *Why I Am Not a Christian,* New York: Simon and Shuster, 1957.)

Sacerdote, Paul. 1966. "The Uses of Hypnosis in Cancer Patients." *Annals of the New York Academy of Sciences,* 125: 1011–1019.

Sakshaug, J., Sögnen, E., Hansen, M. A., and Koppang, N. 1965. "Dimethylnitrosamine: Its Hepatoxic Effect in Sheep and Its Occurence in Toxic Batches of Herring Meal." *Nature,* 206: 1261–1262.

Sandberg, Avery A. 1966. "The Chromosomes and Causation of Human Cancer and Leukemia." *Cancer Research,* 26: 2064–2081.

Saunders, Cicely. 1961. "Letter to the Editor." *Lancet,* 2(2 Sept.): 548–549.

Schmale, Arthur, and Iker, Howard. "The Psychological Setting of Uterine Cervical Cancer." *Annals of the New York Academy of Sciences,* 125: 807–813.

Shimkin, M. B. 1967. "End Results in Cancer of the Breast." *Cancer,* 20: 1039–1043.

Smith, R. L. 1968. "New Traffic in Cures for Cancer." *Saturday Evening Post,* 241 (10 Feb.): 62–64.

Snell, G. D. 1952. "The Immunogenetics of Tumor Transplantation." *Cancer Research,* 12: 543–546.

Stewart, Louis, and Livson, Norman. 1966. "Smoking and Rebelliousness." *Journal of Consulting Psychology,* 30: 225–229.

U.S. National Cancer Institute. 1961– . *End Results and Mortality Trends in Cancer.* Washington, D. C.: National Cancer Institute.

Urban, J., and Farrow, H. 1963. "Long Term Results of Internal Mammary Lymph Node Excision for Breast Cancer." *Acta: Unio Internationalis Contra Cancrum,* 19: 1551.

Wald, George. 1964. "The Origins of Life." *Proceedings of the National Academy of Sciences,* 52: 595-611.

Wangensteen, O. H. 1957. "Another Look at the Super-radical Operation for Breast Cancer." *Surgery,* 41: 857–861.

Watson, J. D. 1965. *The Molecular Biology of the Gene.* New York: Benjamin.

————. 1968. *The Double Helix.* New York: Atheneum.

Weisman, A. D., and Hackett, T. P. 1961. "Predilection to Death. Death and Dying as a Psychiatric Problem." *Psychosomatic Medicine,* 23: 232–256.

Wynder, E. L., and Hoffman, D. 1966. "Current Concepts of Environmental Cancer Research." *Medical Clinics of North America,* 50: 631-650.

INDEX

Abbe, Robert, 89
Active specific immunotherapy, 358
Adenine, 14, 290–291
Adenosine diphosphate (ADP), 11
Adenosine triphosphate (ATP), 11, 48
Adrenalectomy, 108, 112; in breast cancer, 176–178; and Bulbrook-Hayword discriminant, 177; and etiocholanolone, 177; and hypophysectomy, 110–114
Aerobic system, 5
Agglutination, 21
Alkaptonuria, 36
Alkylating agents, 100, 209–210, 346; busulfan (myleran), 210, 346; carcinogenesis and, 100; chlorambucil (leukeran), 210, 346; cyclophosphamide (cytoxan), 210, 346; melphalen (alkeran), 210, 346; nitrogen mustard, 209, 346; thiotepa, 210
Allele, 34
Alpha helix, 16
American Cancer Society: and danger signals of cancer, 90, 137–138; and screening programs for early detection of cancer, 287, 328
Ames test, 327
Amino acids, 290
Anaerobic system, 5
Anaphase in cell division, 31
Aniline dyes and bladder cancer, 124
Antibiotics as chemotherapeutic agents, 348
Antibodies. See Cancer immunology
Antibody synthesis: cellular, 61; humoral, 61
Anti-cancer drugs. See Chemotherapeutic agents

Antigen-antibody reactions, 317–319; and capping, 317–318; and cell-associated molecules (CAM), 318–319; and surface modulating assembly (SMA), 318–319
Antigenic determinants, 62
Antigens, 24; action of, 62–64; cancer specific, 229–233, 312, 319; and chemical tumors, 229–233; and clonal selection theory, 62, 312; and enhancement, 314; and viral tumors, 229–233
Antimetabolites as chemotherapeutic agents, 210–211, 347; 5 fluorouracil (5 FU), 211, 347; 6 mercaptopurine, 211, 347; methotrexate, 210, 347; 6 thioguanine, 211, 347
Antitumor hormones as chemotherapeutic agents, 349–350; androgens, 349; corticosteroids, 350; estrogen, 349; steroid compounds, 349
Asepsis, 86
Astbury, W. T., 43
Atomic blasts and cancer: at Hiroshima and Nagasaki, 106; leukemia and, 106; at Rongelap, 325–326
Atomic structure: and electrons, 46; and isotopes, 46; and molecules, 46; and neutrons, 46; and protons, 46
Avenzoar, 84
Averrhoës, 84
Avery, O. T., 45
Azo dyes: carcinogenesis and, 101–102

Bacteriophage, 57
Bacterium, 5
Baetson, G. L., 106–107